Cultural Diversity
in Health and Illness

CULTURALCARE

There is something that transcends all of this
I am I ... You are you
Yet. I and you
Do connect
Somehow, sometime.

To understand the "cultural" needs
Samenesses and differences of people
Needs an open being
See—Hear—Feel
With no judgment or interpretation
Reach out
Maybe with that physical touch
Or eyes, or aura
You exhibit your openness and willingness to
Listen and learn
And, you tell and share
In so doing—you share humanness
It is acknowledged and shared
Something happens—
Mutual understanding

—Rachel E. Spector

Cultural Diversity in Health and Illness

EIGHTH EDITION

Rachel E. Spector, PhD, RN, CTN-A, FAAN

Needham, MA 02494

PEARSON

Boston Columbus Indianapolis New York San Francisco Upper Saddle River
Amsterdam Cape Town Dubai London Madrid Milan Munich Paris Montréal Toronto
Delhi Mexico City São Paulo Sydney Hong Kong Seoul Singapore Taipei Tokyo

Editor-in-Chief: Julie Levin Alexander
Executive Acquisitions Editor: Kim Norbuta
Senior Marketing Manager: Phoenix Harvey
Managing Editor, Production: Central
    Publishing
Production Editor: Saraswathi Muralidhar,
    PreMediaGlobal

Production Manager: Tom Benfatti
Creative Director: Jayne Conte
Cover Designer: Bruce Kenselaar
Composition: PreMediaGlobal
Printer/Binder: RR Donnelley & Sons
Cover Printer: RR Donnelley & Sons

Notice: Care has been taken to confirm the accuracy of information presented in this book. The author, editors, and the publisher, however, cannot accept any responsibility for errors or omissions or for consequences from application of the information in this book and make no warranty, express or implied, with respect to its contents.

The authors and publisher have exerted every effort to ensure that drug selections and dosages set forth in this text are in accord with current recommendations and practice at time of publication. However, in view of ongoing research, changes in government regulations, and the constant flow of information relating to drug therapy and drug reactions, the reader is urged to check the package inserts of all drugs for any change in indications of dosage and for added warnings and precautions. This is particularly important when the recommended agent is a new and/or infrequently employed drug.

Pearson Prentice Hall™ is a trademark of Pearson Education, Inc.
Pearson® is a registered trademark of Pearson plc
Prentice Hall® is a registered trademark of Pearson Education, Inc.

Pearson Education Ltd., London
Pearson Education Singapore, Pte. Ltd.
Pearson Education Canada, Inc., Toronto
Pearson Education—Japan
Pearson Education Australia PTY, Limited

Pearson Education North Asia Ltd., Hong Kong
Pearson Educación de Mexico, S.A. de C.V.
Pearson Education Malaysia, Pte. Ltd.
Pearson Education, Upper Saddle River,
    New Jersey

Library of Congress Cataloging-in-Publication Data
Spector, Rachel E.
   Cultural diversity in health and illness/Rachel E. Spector.—8th ed.
      p. cm.
   Includes bibliographical references and index.
   ISBN-13: 978-0-13-284006-4
   ISBN-10: 0-13-284006-5
   1. Transcultural medical care—United States. 2. Health attitudes—United States.
   3. Transcultural nursing—United States. I. Title.
   RA418.5.T73S64 2013
   610—dc23   2012012708

10 9 8 7 6 5 4 3 2 1

PEARSON

ISBN-13: 978-0-13-284006-4
ISBN-10:   0-13-284006-5

I would like to dedicate this text to

My husband, Manny;
Sam, Hilary, Julia, and Emma;
Becky, Perry, Naomi, Rose, and Miriam;
the memory of my parents, Joseph J. and Freda F. Needleman,
and my in-laws, Sam and Margaret Spector;
and the memory of my beloved mentor, Irving Kenneth Zola.

Contents

PREFACE   xi

ABOUT THE AUTHOR   xvii

ACKNOWLEDGMENTS   xviii

UNIT I   **CULTURAL FOUNDATIONS**   1

Chapter 1   **Building Cultural and Linguistic Competence**   3
National Standards for Culturally and Linguistically
    Appropriate Services in Health Care   8
Cultural Competence   11
Linguistic Competence   11
Institutional Mandates   12
CULTURALCARE   13

Chapter 2   **Cultural Heritage and History**   19
Heritage Consistency   20
Acculturation Themes   29
Ethnocultural Life Trajectories   32
Commingling Variables   34
Cultural Conflict   36
Cultural Phenomena Affecting Health   37

Chapter 3   **Diversity**   43
Census 2010   45
Immigration   48
Poverty   54

Chapter 4   **Health and Illness**   62
Health   63
Illness   74

UNIT II   **HEALTH DOMAINS**   85

Chapter 5   **HEALTH Traditions**   89
HEALTH and ILLNESS   91
HEALTH Traditions Model   92
HEALTH Protection   95
Health/HEALTH Care Choices   102

Folk Medicine 104
Health/HEALTH Care Philosophies 108

Chapter 6 **HEALING Traditions** **120**
HEALING 121
Ancient Forms of HEALING 123
Religion and HEALING 124
HEALING and Today's Beliefs 136
Ancient Rituals Related to the Life Cycle 138

Chapter 7 **Familial HEALTH Traditions** **158**
Familial Health/HEALTH Traditions 160
Consciousness Raising 171

Chapter 8 **Health and Illness in Modern Health Care** **178**
The Health Care Provider's Culture 179
Health Care Costs 182
Trends in Development of the Health Care System 187
Common Problems in Health Care Delivery 191
Pathways to Health Services 195
Barriers to Health Care 197
Medicine as an Institution of Social Control 199

UNIT III **HEALTH AND ILLNESS PANORAMAS** **207**

Chapter 9 **HEALTH and ILLNESS in the American Indian and Alaska Native Population** **210**
Background 211
Traditional Definitions of *HEALTH* and *ILLNESS* 213
Traditional Methods of HEALING 215
Current Health Care Problems 222
The Indian Health Service 228

Chapter 10 **HEALTH and ILLNESS in the Asian Populations** **238**
Background 239
Traditional Definitions of *HEALTH* and *ILLNESS* 241
Traditional Methods of HEALTH Maintenance
and Protection 246
Traditional Methods of HEALTH Restoration 247
Current Health Problems 257

Chapter 11 **HEALTH and ILLNESS in the Black Population** **265**
Background 266
Traditional Definitions of *HEALTH* and *ILLNESS* 270
Traditional Methods of HEALTH Maintenance
and Protection 271

	Traditional Methods of HEALTH Restoration	272
	Current Health Problems	279
Chapter 12	**HEALTH and ILLNESS in the Hispanic Populations**	**291**
	Background	292
	Mexicans	294
	Puerto Ricans	308
Chapter 13	**HEALTH and ILLNESS in the White Populations**	**323**
	Background	324
	German Americans	326
	Italian Americans	330
	Polish Americans	334
	Health Status of the White Population	339
Chapter 14	**CULTURALCOMPETENCE**	**345**
	CULTURALCOMPETENCY	351
Appendix A	**Selected Key Terms Related to Cultural Diversity in Health and Illness**	**354**
Appendix B	**Calendar: Cultural and Religious Holidays That Change Dates**	**364**
Appendix C	**Suggested Course Outline**	**367**
Appendix D	**Suggested Course Activity—Urban Hiking**	**373**
Appendix E	**Heritage Assessment Tool**	**376**
Appendix F	**Quick Guide for CULTURALCARE**	**379**
Appendix G	**Data Resources**	**381**
	BIBLIOGRAPHY	**383**
	INDEX	**403**

Preface

Every book, every volume you see here, has a soul. The soul of the person who wrote it and of those who read it and lived and dreamed with it.

—Carlos Ruiz Zafon,
The Shadow of the Wind, *2001*

In 1977—more than 35 years ago—I prepared the first edition of *Cultural Diversity in Health and Illness*. Now, as I begin the eighth edition of this book—the sixth revision—I realize that this is an opportunity to reflect on an endeavor that has filled a good deal of my life for the past 30 years. I believe this book has a soul and it, in turn, has become an integral part of my soul. I have lived—through practice, teaching, and research—this material since 1974 and have developed many ways of presenting this content. In addition, I have tracked for 40 years:

1. the United States Census;
2. immigration—numbers and policies;
3. poverty—figures and policies;
4. health care—costs and policies;
5. morbidity and mortality rates;
6. nursing and other health care manpower issues; and
7. the emergence and growth of the concepts of health disparities and cultural and linguistic competence.

My metaphors are *HEALTH*, defined as "the balance of the person, both within one's being—physical, mental, and spiritual—and in the outside world—natural, communal, and metaphysical"; *ILLNESS*, "the imbalance of the person, both within one's being—physical, mental, and spiritual—and in the outside world—natural, communal, and metaphysical"; and *HEALING*, "the restoration of balance, both within one's being—physical, mental, and spiritual—and in the outside world—natural, communal, and metaphysical." I have learned over these years that within many traditional heritages (defined as "old," not contemporary or modern) people tend to define HEALTH, ILLNESS, and HEALING in this manner. Imagine a kaleidoscope—the tube can represent HEALTH. The objects reflected within the kaleidoscope reflect the traditional tools used to care for a given person's HEALTH. If you love kaleidoscopes, you know what I am describing and that the patterns that emerge are infinite.

In addition, I have had the unique opportunity to travel to countless places in the United States and abroad. I make it a practice to visit the traditional markets, pharmacies, and shrines and dialogue with the people who work in or patronize the settings, and I have gathered invaluable knowledge and unique items and images. My tourist dollars are invested in amulets and remedies and my collection is large. Digital photography has changed my eyes; I may be a "digital immigrant," rather than a "digital native," but the camera has proven to be my most treasured companion. I have been able to use the images of sacred objects and sacred places to create HEALTH Traditions Imagery. The opening images for each chapter and countless images within the chapters are the results of these explorations. Given that there are times when we do not completely understand a concept or an image, several images are slightly blurred or dark to represent this wonderment.

The first edition of this book was the outcome of a *promesa*—a promise— I once made. The promise was made to a group of Asian, Black, and Hispanic students I taught in a medical sociology course in 1973. In this course, the students wound up being the teachers, and they taught me to see the world of health care delivery through the eyes of the health care consumer rather than through my own well-intentioned eyes. What I came to see I did not always like. I did not realize how much I did not know; I believed I knew a lot. I promised the students that I would take that which they taught me regarding HEALTH and teach it to students and colleagues. I have held on to the *promesa*, and my experiences over the years have been incredible. I have met people and traveled. At all times I have held on to the idea and goal of attempting to help nurses and other health care providers be aware of and sensitive to the HEALTH, ILLNESS, and HEALING beliefs and needs of their patients.

I know that looking inside closed doors carries with it a risk. I know that people prefer to think that our society is a melting pot and that the traditional beliefs and practices have vanished with the expected acculturation and assimilation into mainstream North American modern life. Many people, however, have continued to carry on the traditional customs and culture from their native lands and heritage, and HEALTH, ILLNESS, and HEALING beliefs are deeply entwined within the cultural and social beliefs that people have. To understand HEALTH and ILLNESS beliefs and practices, it is necessary to see each person in his or her unique sociocultural world. The theoretical knowledge that has evolved for the development of this text is cumulative and much of the "old" material is relevant *today* as many HEALTH, ILLNESS, and HEALING beliefs do not change. However, many beliefs and practices do go underground.

The purpose of each edition has been to increase awareness of the dimensions and complexities involved in caring for people from diverse cultural backgrounds. I wished to share my personal experiences and thoughts concerning the introduction of cultural concepts into the education of health care professionals. The books represented my answers to the questions:

- "How does one effectively expose a student to cultural diversity?"
- "How does one examine health care issues and perceptions from a broad social viewpoint?"

As I have done in the classroom over the years, I attempt to bring you, the reader, into direct contact with the interaction between providers of care within the North American health care system and the consumers of health care. The staggering issues of health care delivery are explored and contrasted with the choices that people may make in attempting to deal with health care issues.

When I began this journey in nursing, there were limited resources available to answer my questions and to support me in my passion for knowledge. The situation has dramatically changed and today there is nearly more information than one can absorb! Not only is this information being sought by nurses, all stakeholders in the health care industry are struggling with this concept. The demographics of America, and the world, have changed and perhaps this challenge of building bridges between cultural groups can be seen as a way to open opportunities to do this in many disciplines. Indeed, the content is readily available:

■ Countless books and articles have been published in nursing, medicine, public health, and the popular media over the past 40 years that contain invaluable information relevant to CULTURALCOMPETENCY.

■ Innumerable workshops and meetings have been available where the content is presented and discussed.

■ "Self-study" programs on the Internet have been developed that provide continuing education credits to nurses, physicians, and other providers.

However, **the process of becoming CULTURALLYCOMPETENT** is not generally provided for. Issues persist, such as:

■ Demographic disparity exists in the profile of health care providers and in health status.

■ Patient needs, such as modesty, space, and gender-specific care, are not universally met.

■ Religious-specific needs are not met in terms of meal planning, procedural planning, conference planning, and so forth.

■ Communication and language barriers exist.

As this knowledge is built, you are on the way to CULTURALCOMPETENCY. As it matures and grows, you become an advocate of CULTURALCARE, as it will be described in Chapter 1.

■ Overview

Unit I focuses on the background knowledge one must recognize as the foundation for developing CULTURALCOMPETENCY.

■ Chapter 1 presents an overview of the significant content related to the on-going development of the concepts of cultural and linguistic competency as it is described by several different organizations.

■ Chapter 2 explores the concept of cultural heritage and history and the roles they play in one's perception of health and illness. This exploration is first outlined in general terms: What is culture? How is it transmitted? What is ethnicity? What is religion? How do they affect a person's health? What major sociocultural events occurred during the life trajectory of a person that may influence his or her personal health beliefs and practices?

■ Chapter 3 presents a discussion of the diversity—demographic, immigration, and poverty—that impacts on the delivery of and access to health care. The backgrounds of each of the U.S. Census Bureau's categories of the population, an overview of immigration, and an overview of issues relevant to poverty are presented.

■ Chapter 4 reviews the provider's knowledge of his or her own perceptions, needs, and understanding of health and illness.

Unit II explores the domains of HEALTH, blends them with one's personal heritage, and contrasts them with the Allopathic Philosophy.

■ Chapter 5 introduces the concept of HEALTH and develops the concept in broad and general terms. The HEALTH Traditions Model is presented, as are natural methods of HEALTH maintenance and protection.

■ Chapter 6 explores the concept of HEALTH restoration or HEALING and the role that faith plays in the context of HEALING, or magico-religious, traditions. This is an increasingly important issue, which is evolving to a point where the health care provider must have some understanding of this phenomenon.

■ Chapter 7 discusses family heritage and explores personal and familial HEALTH traditions. It includes an array of familial health/HEALTH beliefs and practices shared by people from many different heritages.

■ Chapter 8 focuses on the health care provider culture and the allopathic health care delivery system.

Once the study of each of these components has been completed, Unit III (Chapters 9 to 13) moves on to explore selected population groups in more detail, to portray a panorama of traditional HEALTH and ILLNESS beliefs and practices, and to present relevant health care issues.

Chapter 14 is devoted to an overall analysis of the book's contents and how best to apply this knowledge in health care delivery, health planning, and health education, for both the patient and the health care professional.

Each chapter in the text opens with images relevant to the chapter's topic. They may be viewed in the CULTURALCARE Museum on the accompanying web page.

These pages cannot do full justice to the richness of any one culture or any one health/HEALTH belief system. By presenting some of the beliefs and practices and suggesting background reading, however, the book can begin to inform and sensitize the reader to the needs of a given group of people. It can also serve as a model for developing cultural knowledge of populations that are not included in this text.

There is so much to be learned. Countless books and articles have now appeared that address these problems and issues. It is not easy to alter attitudes and beliefs or stereotypes and prejudices, to change a person's philosophy. Some social psychologists state that it is almost impossible to lose all of one's prejudices, yet alterations can be made. I believe the health care provider *must* develop the ability to deliver CULTURALCARE and knowledge regarding personal fundamental values regarding health/HEALTH and illness/ILLNESS. With acceptance of one's own values come the framework and courage to accept the existence of differing values. This process of realization and acceptance can enable the health care provider to be instrumental in meeting the needs of the consumer in a collaborative, safe, and professional manner.

This book is written primarily for the student in basic allied health professional programs, nursing, medical, social work, and other health care provider disciplines. I believe it will be helpful also for providers in all areas of practice, especially community health, long-term oncology, chronic care settings, and geriatric and hospice centers. I am attempting to write in a direct manner and to use language that is understandable by all. The material is sensitive, yet I believe that it is presented in a sensitive manner. At no point is my intent to create a vehicle for stereotyping. I know that one person will read this book and nod, "Yes, this is how I see it," and someone else of the same background will say, "No, this is not correct." This is the way it is meant to be. It is incomplete by intent. It is written in the spirit of open inquiry, so that an issue may be raised and so that clarification of any given point will be sought from the patient as health care is provided. The deeper I travel into this world of cultural diversity, the more I wonder at the variety. It is wonderfully exciting. By gaining insight into the traditional attitudes that people have toward health and health care, I found my own nursing practice was enhanced, and I was better able to understand the needs of patients and their families. It is thrilling to be able to meet, to know, and to provide care to people from all over the world and every walk of life. It is the excitement of nursing. As we go forward in time, I hope that these words will help you, the reader, develop CULTURALCARE skills and help you provide the best care to all.

You don't need a masterpiece to get the idea.

—Pablo Picasso

■ Features

- ■ **Research on Culture and Health.** As evidence-based practice grows in importance, its application is expected in all aspects of health care. This special feature spotlights how current research informs and impacts cultural awareness and competence.
- ■ **Unit and Chapter Objectives.** Each unit and chapter opens with objectives to direct the reader when studying.
- ■ **Unit Exercises and Activities.** The beginning of each unit provides exercises and activities related to the topic. Questions stimulate reflective

consideration of the reader's own family and cultural history as well as to develop an awareness of one's own biases.

■ **Figures, Tables, and Boxes.** Throughout the book are photographs, illustrations, tables, and boxes that exemplify and expand on information referenced in the chapter.

■ **Health Traditions Imagery.** These symbolic images are used to link the chapters. The images were selected to awaken you to the richness of a given heritage and the practices inherent within both modern and traditional cultures, as well as the beliefs surrounding health and HEALTH. (HEALTH, when written this way, is defined as the balance of the person, both within one's being—physical, mental, spiritual—and in the outside world—natural, familial and communal, metaphysical.)

■ **Keeping Up.** Selected resources that present information that is frequently published in a timely manner to keep you abreast of data, on such topics as poverty, income, immigration, and so forth, as the facts and figures change. This is a new feature for this edition.

■ Supplemental Resources

■ **CulturalCare Guide.** Previously available as a separate booklet, the contents of this helpful guide are now available for downloading on the Companion Website. The guide includes the Heritage Assessment Tool, Cultural Phenomena Affecting Health Care, CulturalCare Etiquette, and other assessment tools and guides.

■ **Companion Website.** www.prenhall.com/spector. The Companion Website includes a wealth of supplemental material to accompany each chapter. In addition to the complete contents of the **CulturalCare Guide**, the site presents chapter-related review questions, case studies, exercises, and MediaLinks to provide additional information. Panorama of Health and Illness videos accompany many chapters, and a glossary of terms appears for each chapter. Also included is a collection of the author's photographs and culturally significant images in the CULTURAL-CARE Museum.

■ **Instructor's Resource Center.** Available to instructors adopting the book are PowerPoint Lecture Slides and a complete testbank available for downloading from the Instructor's Resource Center, which can be accessed through the online catalog.

■ **Online Course Management.** Built to accompany *Cultural Diversity in Health and Illness* are online course management systems available for Blackboard, WebCT, Moodle, Angel, and other platforms. For more information, contact your Pearson Education sales representative.

About the Author

Dr. Rachel E. Spector has been a student of culturally diverse HEALTH and ILLNESS beliefs and practices for 40 years and has researched and taught courses on culture and HEALTH care for the same time span. Dr. Spector has had the opportunity to work in many different communities, including the American Indian and Hispanic communities in Boston, Massachusetts. Her studies have taken her to many places: most of the United States, Canada, and Mexico; several European countries, including Denmark, England, Greece, Finland, Iceland, Italy, France, Russia, Spain, and Switzerland; Israel and Pakistan; and Australia and New Zealand. She was fortunate enough to collect traditional amulets and remedies from many of these diverse communities, visit shrines, and meet practitioners of traditional HEALTH care in several places. She was instrumental in the creation and presentation of the exhibit "Immigrant HEALTH Traditions" at the Ellis Island Immigration Museum, May 1994 through January 1995. She has exhibited HEALTH-related objects in several other settings. Recently, she served as a *Colaboradora Honorifica* (Honorary Collaborator) in the University of Alicante in Alicante, Spain, and Tamaulipas, Mexico. In 2006, she was a Lady Davis Fellow in the Henrietta Zold-Hadassah Hebrew University School of Nursing in Jerusalem, Israel. This text was translated into Spanish by Maria Munoz and published in Madrid by Prentice Hall as *Las Culturas de la SALUD* in 2003 and into Chinese in 2010. She is a Fellow in the American Academy of Nursing and a Scholar in Transcultural Nursing Society. The Massachusetts Association of Registered Nurses, the state organization of the American Nurses' Association, honored her as a "Living Legend" in 2007. In 2008 she received the Honorary Human Rights Award from the American Nurses Association. This award recognized her contributions and accomplishments that have been of national significance to human rights and have influenced health care and nursing practice.

Acknowledgments

I have had a 35-year adventure of studying the forces of culture, ethnicity, and religion and their profound influence on HEALTH, ILLNESS, and HEALING beliefs and practices. Many, many people have contributed generously to the knowledge I have acquired over this time as I have tried to serve as a voice for traditional people and the HEALTH, ILLNESS, and HEALING beliefs and practices derived from their given heritage. It has been a continuous struggle to insure that this information be included not only in nursing education but in the educational content of all helping professions—including medicine, the allied health professions, and social work.

I particularly wish to thank the following people for their guidance, professional support, and encouragement over the 32 years that this book, now in its eighth edition, has been an integral part of my life. They are people from many walks of life and have touched me in many ways. The people from Appleton-Century-Crofts, which became Appleton & Lang, then became Prentice Hall, and now Pearson. They include Kim Mortimer, Patrick Walsh, and countless people involved in the production of the text. My first encounter with publishing was with Leslie Boyer, an acquisition editor from Appleton-Century-Crofts, who simply said "write a book" in 1976. The experience of preparing this eighth edition has been a formidable one. Most of the new content has been gathered via the World Wide Web. However, the most exciting aspect of this project has been working with people in India throughout the copyediting phase. I was living in Honolulu, Hawaii; the Senior Project Manager, Saraswathi Muralidhar, was in India. We were thousands of miles apart, there was a fifteen and one half-hour difference in time; yet, we have completed this challenge in a most timely manner. Yes, the World Wide Web is an amazing asset. In 1976, when the first edition of this book was conceived, I never dreamt that this is where it would be in 2012. In addition, for this edition I have worked closely with Yagnesh Jani, the development editor in the United States. Without their help, this book would not be here today.

The many people who helped with advice and guidance to resources over the years include Elsi Basque, Billye Brown, Louise Buchanan, Julian Castillo, Leonel J. Castillo, Jenny Chan, Dr. P. K. Chan, Joe Colorado, Miriam Cook, Elizabeth Cucchiaro, Norine Dresser, Marjory Gordon, Orlando Isaza, Henry and Pandora Law, S. Dale McLemore, Anita Noble, Carl Rutberg, Sister Mary Nicholas Vincelli, David Warner, and the late Hawk Littlejohn, Father Richard McCabe, and Irving K. Zola.

I wish to thank my friends and family, who have tolerated my absence at countless social functions, and the many people who have provided the numerous support services necessary for the completion of an undertaking such as this. My husband, Manny, has been the rock who has sustained and supported me through all these years–most of all, I can never thank him enough.

A lot has happened in my life since the first edition of this book was published in 1979. My family has shrunk with the deaths of all four parents, and it has greatly expanded with a new daughter, Hilary, and a new son, Perry, and five granddaughters—Julia, Emma, Naomi, Rose, and Miriam. The generations have gone, and come.

■ Reviewers

Michelle Gagnon, BS, RUT, RDCS
Bunker Hill Community College
Boston, MA

Marie Gates, PhD
WMU Bronson School of Nursing
Kalamazoo, MI

Janette McCrory, MSN
Delta State University
Cleveland, MS

Anita Noble, DNSc
Hebrew University School of Nursing,
Henrietta Zold-Hadassah School of Nursing
Jerusalem, Israel

Unit

I

Cultural Foundations

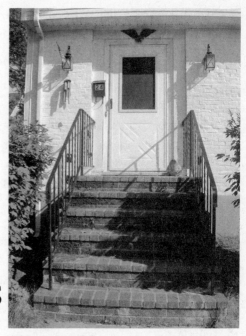

___

Unit I creates the foundation for this book and enables you to become aware of the importance of developing knowledge in the topics of (1) cultural and linguistic competency; (2) *cultural* heritage and history—both your own and those of other people; (3) *diversity*—demographic, immigration, and economic; and (4) the standard concepts of *health* and *illness*.

The chapters in Unit I will present an overview of relevant historical and contemporary theoretical content that will help you climb the first three steps to CULTURALCOMPETENCY. You will:

1. Understand the compelling need for the development of cultural and linguistic competency.

2. Identify and discuss the factors that contribute to heritage consistency—culture, ethnicity, religion, acculturation, and socialization.

3. Identify and discuss sociocultural events that may influence the life trajectory of a given person.

4. Understand diversity in the population of the United States by observing
   - Census 2010 and the demographic changes in the population of the United States over several decades;
   - immigration patterns and issues; and
   - economic issues relevant to poverty.

5. Understand health and illness and the sociocultural and historical phenomena that affect them.

6. Reexamine and redefine the concepts of health and illness.
7. Understand the multiple relationships between health and illness.

Before you read Unit I, please answer the following questions:

1. Do you speak a language other than English?
2. What is your sociocultural heritage?
3. What major sociocultural events have occurred in your lifetime?
4. What is the demographic profile of the community you grew up in? Has it changed; if so, how has it changed?
5. How would you acquire economic help if necessary?
6. How do you define *health*?
7. How do you define *illness*?
8. What do you do to maintain and protect your health?
9. What do you do when you experience a noticeable change in your health?
10. Do you diagnose your own health problems? If yes, how do you do so? If no, why not?
11. From whom do you seek health care?
12. What do you do to restore your health? Give examples.

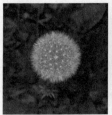 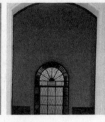 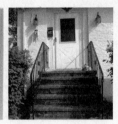

Figure 1–1   **Figure 1–2**   **Figure 1–3**   **Figure 1–4**

Chapter

1

Building Cultural and Linguistic Competence

When there is a very dense cultural barrier, you do the best you can, and if something happens despite that, you have to be satisfied with little success instead of total successes. You have to give up total control. . . .

—*Anne Fadiman (2001)*

■ Objectives

1. Discuss the underpinnings of the need for cultural and linguistic competence.
2. Describe the National Standards for Culturally and Linguistically Appropriate Services in Health Care.
3. Describe institutional mandates regarding cultural and linguistic competence.
4. Articulate the attributes of CULTURALCOMPETENCY and CULTURALCARE.

The opening images for this chapter depict the foundations for the building of CULTURALCOMPETENCE. The first image is that of a dandelion that has gone to seed (Figure 1–1). All of the seeds are united, yet each is a discrete entity—they represent the numerous facets necessary for cultural competence. Figure 1–2 is that of a "fake door" in Vejer de la Frontera, Spain. It is a reminder of personal beliefs that shut out all other arguments and ways of understanding people. Figure 1–3 is a translucent door in Avila, Spain, where it is possible to look into a different reality and because it is not locked—one can open it and recognize the view of others. Figure 1–4 represents the steps to cultural competency. A more detailed discussion of each image follows in the forthcoming text.

In May 1988, Anne Fadiman, editor of *The American Scholar*, met the Lee family of Merced, California. Her subsequent book, *The Spirit Catches You and You Fall Down*, published in 1997, tells the compelling story of the Lees and their daughter, Lia, and their tragic encounter with the American health care delivery system. This book has now become a classic and is used by many health care educators and providers in situations where there is an effort to demonstrate the need for developing cultural competence.

When Lia was 3 months old, she was taken to the emergency room of the county hospital with epileptic seizures. The family was unable to communicate in English; the hospital staff did not include competent Hmong interpreters. From the parents' point of view, Lia was experiencing "the fleeing of her soul from her body and the soul had become lost." They knew these symptoms to be *quag dab peg*—"the spirit catches you and you fall down." The Hmong regarded this experience with ambivalence, yet they knew that it was serious and potentially dangerous, as it was epilepsy. It was also an illness that evokes a sense of both concern and pride.

The parents and the health care providers both wanted the best for Lia, yet a complex and dense trajectory of misunderstanding and misinterpreting was set in motion. The tragic cultural conflict lasted for several years and caused considerable pain to each party (Fadiman, 2001). This moving incident exemplifies the extreme events that can occur when two antithetical cultural belief systems collide within the overall environment of the health care delivery system. Each party comes to a health care event with a set notion of what ought to happen—and, unless each is able to understand the view of the other, complex difficulties can arise.

The catastrophic events of September 11, 2001; the wars in Iraq, Afghanistan, and Libya; the countless natural disasters such as Hurricane Katrina and the earthquakes in Haiti and Japan; and our preoccupation with terrorist threats have pierced the consciousness of all Americans in general and health care providers in particular. Now, more than ever, providers *must* become informed about and sensitive to the culturally diverse subjective meanings of **health/HEALTH**,[1] **illness/ILLNESS**, caring, and **curing/HEALING** practices. Cultural diversity and pluralism are a core part of the social and economic engines that drive the country, and their impact at this time has significant implications for health care delivery and policymaking throughout the United States (Office of Minority Health, 2001, p. 25).

---

[1]This style of combining terms, such as **health/HEALTH**, will be used throughout the text to convey that there is a blending of modern and traditional connotations for the terms. The terms are defined within the text and in the glossary. Furthermore, when terms such as CULTURALCOMPETENCY and CULTURALCARE and others are written in all capital letters, it is done so to imply that they are referring to a holistic philosophy, rather than a dualistic philosophy.

In all clinical practice areas—from institutional settings, such as acute and long-term care settings, to community-based settings, such as nurse practitioners' and doctors' offices and clinics, schools and universities, public health, and occupational settings—one observes diversity every day. The undeniable need for culturally and linguistically competent health care services for diverse populations has attracted increased attention from health care providers and those who judge their quality and efficiency for many years. The mainstream health care provider is treating a more diverse patient population as a result of demographic changes and participation in insurance programs, and the interest in designing culturally and linguistically appropriate services that lead to improved health care outcomes, efficiency, and patient satisfaction has increased.

One's personal cultural background, heritage, and language have a considerable impact on both how patients access and respond to health care services and how the providers practice within the system. Cultural and linguistic competence suggests an ability of health care providers and health care organizations to understand and respond effectively to the cultural and linguistic needs brought to the health care experience. This is a phenomenon that recognizes the diversity that exists among the patients, physicians, nurses, and caregivers. This phenomenon is not limited to the changes in the patient population in that it also embraces the members of the workforce—including providers from other countries. Many of the people in the workforce are new immigrants and/or are from ethnocultural backgrounds that are different from that of the dominant culture.

In addition, health and illness can be interpreted and explained in terms of personal experience and expectations. We can define our own health or illness and determine what these states mean to us in our daily lives. We learn from our own cultural and ethnic backgrounds how to be healthy, how to recognize illness, and how to be ill. Furthermore, the meanings we attach to the notions of health and illness are related to the basic, culture-bound values by which we define a given experience and perception.

It is now *imperative,* according to the most recent policies of the Joint Commission of Hospital Accreditation and the Centers for Medicare & Medicaid Services, that *all* health care providers be "culturally competent." In this context, cultural competency implies that within the delivery of care the health care provider understands and attends to the total context of the patient's situation; it is a complex combination of knowledge, attitudes, and skills, yet

- How do you *really* inspire people to hear the content?
- How do you *motivate* providers to see the worldview and lived experience of the patient?
- How do you assist providers to *really* bear witness to the living conditions and lifeways of patients?
- How do you liberate providers from the burdens of prejudice, xenophobia, the "isms"—racism, ethnocentrism—and the "antis" such as anti-Semitism, anti-Catholicism, anti-Islamism, anti-immigrant, and so forth?

■ How do you inspire philosophical changes from dualistic thinking to holistic thinking?

It can be argued that the development of CULTURALCOMPETENCY does not occur in a short encounter with programs on cultural diversity but that it takes time to develop the skills, knowledge, and attitudes to safely and satisfactorily become "CULTURALLYCOMPETENT" and to deliver CULTURALCARE. Indeed, the reality of becoming "CULTURALLYCOMPETENT" is a complex process—it is time consuming, difficult, frustrating, and extremely interesting. It is a philosophical change wherein the CULTURALLYCOMPETENT person is able to hear, understand, and respect the nonverbal and/or non-articulated needs and perspectives of a given patient.

CULTURALCOMPETENCY embraces the premise that all things are connected. Look again at the dandelion that has gone to seed. Each seed is a discrete entity, yet each is linked to the other (Figure 1–1). Each facet discussed in this text—heritage, culture, ethnicity, religion, socialization, and identity—is connected to diversity, demographic change, population, immigration, and poverty. These facets are connected to health/HEALTH, illness/ILLNESS, curing/HEALING, and beliefs and practices, modern and traditional. All of these facets are connected to the health care delivery system—the culture, costs, and politics of health care, the internal and external political issues, public health issues, and housing and other infrastructure issues. In order to fully understand a person's health/HEALTH beliefs and practices, each of these topics must be in the background of a provider's mind.

I have had the opportunity to live and teach in Spain and to explore many areas, including Cadiz and the surrounding small villages. There was a fake door within the walls of a small village, Vejer de la Frontera (Figure 1–2), that appeared to be bolted shut. The door was placed there during the early 14th century to fool the Barbary pirates. The people were able to vanquish them while they tried to pry the door open. It reminded me of the attempt to keep other ideas and people away and not open up to new and different ideas. Another door (Figure 1–3), found in Avila, Spain, was made of translucent glass. Here, the person has a choice—peer through the door and view the garden behind it or open it and actually go into the garden for a finite walk. This reminded me of people who are able to understand the needs of others and return to their own life and heritage when work is completed. This polarity represents the challenges of "CULTURALCOMPETENCY."

The way to CULTURALCOMPETENCY is complex, but I have learned over the years that there are five steps (Figure 1–4) to climb to begin to achieve this goal:

1. Personal heritage—Who are *you*? What is *your* heritage? What are your health/HEALTH beliefs?
2. Heritage of others—demographics—Who is the other? Family? Community?
3. Health and HEALTH beliefs and practices—competing philosophies
4. Health care culture and system—all the issues and problems

5. Traditional HEALTH care systems—the way HEALTH was for most and the way HEALTH still is for many

Once you have reached the sixth step, CULTURALCOMPETENCY, you are ready to open the door to CULTURALCARE.

Each step represents a discrete unit of study, each building upon the one below it. The steps have been constructed with "bricks," and they represent the fundamental terms, or language, of the content. Table 1–1 lists many examples

Table 1–1 Bricks: Selected CULTURALCARE Terms

Access	Acupuncture	Ageism	Alien
Allopathic philosophy	Amulet	Apparel	Assimilation
Bankes	Borders	Calendar	Care
Census	Citizen	CLAS	Community
Costs	Cultural conflict	CULTURALCARE	CULTURALCOMPETENCY
Culturally appropriate	Culturally competent	Culturally sensitive	Culture
Curandera/o	Customs	Cycle of poverty	Demographic disparity
Demographic parity	Demography	Diagnosis	Diversity
Documentation	Education	*Empacho*	*Envidia*
Ethics	Ethnicity	Ethnicity	Ethnocentrism
Evil eye	Family	Financing	Food
Garments	Gender specific care	Green Card	Gris-gris
Habits	Halal	HEALING	Health
HEALTH	Health care system	Health disparities	HEALTH Traditions
Healthy People 2020	Herbalist	Heritage	Heritage consistency
Heritage inconsistency	Heterosexism	Hex	Homeland security
Homeopathic philosophy	Homophobia	Iatrogenic	Illness
ILLNESS	Immigration	Kosher	Language
Law	Legal Permanent Resident (LPR)	Life trajectory	*Limpia*
Linguistic competence	Literacy	Mal ojo	Manpower
Meridians	Migrant labor	*Milagros*	Modern
Modesty	Morbidity	Mortality	Naturalization
Office of Minority Health	*Orisha*	Osteopathy	*Partera*
Pasmo	Politics	Poverty	Poverty guidelines
Powwow	Procedures	*Promesa*	*Quag dab peg*
Racism	Reflexology	Refugee	Religion
Remedies	Sacred objects	Sacred places	Sacred practices
Sacred spaces	Sacred times	*Santera/o*	*Senoria*
Sexism	Silence	Silence	Singer
Socialization	Spell	Spirits	Spiritual
Spirituality	Title VI	Traditional	Undocumented person
Visitors	Voodoo	Vulnerability	Welfare
Worldview	Xenophobia	*Yin &Yang*	*Yoruba*

of the bricks and the terms are used in the following chapters as appropriate and most are defined in the Key Terms list in Appendix A. These selected terms and many more are the evolving language or jargon of CULTURALCARE.

The railings represent "responsibility and resiliency"—for it is the responsibility of health care providers to be CULTURALLYCOMPETENT and, if this is not met, the consequences will be dire. The resiliency of providers and patients will be further compromised and we will all become more vulnerable. Contrary to popular belief and practice, CULTURALCOMPETENCY is not a "condition" that is rapidly achieved. Rather, it is an ongoing process of growth and the development of knowledge that takes a considerable amount of time to ingest, digest, assimilate, circulate, and master. It is, for many, a philosophical change in that they develop the skills to understand where a person from a different cultural background than theirs is coming from.

This discussion now presents an overview of the significant content related to the ongoing development of the concepts of cultural and linguistic competency as they are described by several different organizations. Presently, there has been a proliferation of resources related to this content and a discussion of selected items is included here. Box 1–2, at the conclusion of the chapter, lists numerous resources.

■ National Standards for Culturally and Linguistically Appropriate Services in Health Care

In 1997, the Office of Minority Health undertook the development of national standards to provide a much needed alternative to the patchwork that has been undertaken in the field of cultural diversity. It developed the National Standards for Culturally and Linguistically Appropriate Services (CLAS) in Health Care. These 14 standards (Box 1–1) must be met by most health care-related agencies. The standards are based on an analytical review of key laws, regulations, contracts, and standards currently in use by federal and state agencies and other national organizations. Published in 2001, the standards were developed with input from a national advisory committee of policymakers, health care providers, and researchers. The CLAS standards are primarily directed at health care organizations. The principles and activities of culturally and linguistically appropriate services must be integrated throughout an organization and implemented in partnership with the communities being served. Enhanced standards are currently being developed but are not yet available. The new standards, *National Standards for Culturally and Linguistically Appropriate Services in Health and Health Care: A Blueprint for Advancing and Sustaining CLAS Policy and Practice* will be available at https://www.thinkculturalhealth.hhs.gov/.

Accreditation and credentialing agencies can assess and compare providers who say they provide culturally competent services and assure quality care for diverse populations. This includes the Joint Commission on Accreditation of Healthcare Organizations (JCAHO); the National Committee on Quality

Box 1–1

Office of Minority Health's Recommended* National Standards for Culturally and Linguistically Appropriate Services in Health Care

The Fundamentals of Culturally Competent Care

1. Health care organizations should ensure that patients/consumers receive from all staff members effective, understandable, and respectful care that is provided in a manner compatible with their cultural health beliefs and practices and preferred language.
2. Health care organizations should implement strategies to recruit, retain, and promote at all levels of the organization a diverse staff and leadership that are representative of the demographic characteristics of the service area.
3. Health care organizations should ensure that staff at all levels and across all disciplines receive ongoing education and training in culturally and linguistically appropriate service delivery.

Speaking of Culturally Competent Care

4. Health care organizations must offer and provide language assistance services, including bilingual staff and interpreter services, at no cost to each patient/consumer with limited English proficiency at all points of contact, in a timely manner during all hours of operation.
5. Health care organizations must provide to patients/consumers in their preferred language both verbal offers and written notices informing them of their right to receive language assistance services.
6. Health care organizations must assure the competence of language assistance provided to limited English-proficient patients/consumers by interpreters and bilingual staff. Family and friends should not be used to provide interpretation services (except on request by the patient/consumer).
7. Health care organizations must make available easily understood patient-related materials and post signage in the languages of the commonly encountered groups and/or groups represented in the service area.
8. Health care organizations should develop, implement, and promote a written strategic plan that outlines clear goals, policies, operational plans, and management accountability/oversight mechanisms to provide culturally and linguistically appropriate services.

Structuring Culturally Competent Care

9. Health care organizations should conduct initial and ongoing organizational self-assessments of CLAS-related activities and are encouraged to integrate cultural and linguistic competence–related measures into their internal audits, performance improvement programs, patient satisfaction assessments, and outcomes-based evaluations.

(continued)

Box 1–1   *Continued*

10. Health care organizations should ensure that data on the individual patient's/ consumer's race, ethnicity, and spoken and written language are collected in health records, integrated into the organization's management information systems, and periodically updated.

11. Health care organizations should maintain a current demographic, cultural, and epidemiological profile of the community as well as a needs assessment to accurately plan for and implement services that respond to the cultural and linguistic characteristics of the service area.

12. Health care organizations should develop participatory, collaborative partnerships with communities and utilize a variety of formal and informal mechanisms to facilitate community and patient/consumer involvement in designing and implementing CLAS-related activities.

13. Health care organizations should ensure that conflict and grievance resolution processes are culturally and linguistically sensitive and capable of identifying, preventing, and resolving cross-cultural conflicts or complaints by patients/consumers.

14. Health care organizations are encouraged to regularly make available to the public information about their progress and successful innovations in implementing the CLAS standards and to provide public notice in their communities about the availability of this information.

---

*CLAS standards are non-regulatory and therefore do not have the force and effect of law. The standards are not mandatory but they greatly assist health care providers and organizations in responding effectively to their patients' cultural and linguistic needs. Compliance with Title VI of the Civil Rights Act of 1964 is mandatory and requires health care providers and organizations that receive federal financial assistance to take reasonable steps to ensure Limited English Proficiency (LEP) persons have meaningful access to services.

CLAS standards use the term patients/consumers to refer to "individuals, including accompanying family members, guardians, or companions, seeking physical or mental health care services, or other health-related services" (p. 5 of the comprehensive final report; see http://minorityhealth.hhs.gov/templates/browse.aspx?lvl=2&lvlID=15).

Source: National Standards for Culturally and Linguistically Appropriate Services in Health Care. Final Report. Washington, DC, March 2001. http://minorityhealth.hhs.gov/templates/browse.aspx?lvl=2&lvlID=15, accessed April 6, 2011.

Assurance; professional organizations, such as the American Medical Association and the American Nurses Association; the Transcultural Nursing Society; and quality review organizations, such as peer review organizations.

In order to ensure both equal access to quality health care by diverse populations and a secure work environment, all health care providers must "promote and support the attitudes, behaviors, knowledge, and skills necessary for staff to work respectfully and effectively with patients and each other in a culturally diverse work environment" (Office of Minority Health, 2001, p. 7). This is the first and fundamental standard of the 14 standards that have been recommended as national standards for CLAS in health care.

■ Cultural Competence

Cultural competence implies that professional health care must be developed to be culturally sensitive, culturally appropriate, and culturally competent. Culturally competent care is critical to meet the complex culture-bound health care needs of a given person, family, and community. It is the provision of health care across cultural boundaries and takes into account the context in which the patient lives, as well as the situations in which the patient's health problems arise.

- **Culturally competent**—within the delivered care, the provider understands and attends to the total context of the patient's situation and this is a complex combination of knowledge, attitudes, and skills.
- **Culturally appropriate**—the provider applies the underlying background knowledge that must be possessed to provide a patient with the best possible health/HEALTH care.
- **Culturally sensitive**—the provider possesses some basic knowledge of and constructive attitudes toward the health/HEALTH traditions observed among the diverse cultural groups found in the setting in which he or she is practicing.

■ Linguistic Competence

Title VI of the Civil Rights Act of 1964 states, "No person in the United States shall, on ground of race, color, or national origin, be excluded from participation in, be denied the benefits of, or be subjected to discrimination under any program or activity receiving Federal financial assistance" (Dirksen Congressional Center, 2011).

To avoid discrimination based on national origin, Title VI and its implementing regulations require recipients of federal financial assistance to take reasonable steps to provide meaningful access to Limited English Proficiency (LEP) persons. Therefore, under the provisions of Title VI of the Civil Rights Act of 1964, when people with LEP seek health care in health care settings such as hospitals, nursing homes, clinics, day care centers, and mental health centers, services cannot be denied to them. It is said that "language barriers have a deleterious effect on health care and patients are less likely to have a usual source of health care, and have an increased risk if non-adherence to medication regimens" (Flores, 2006, p. 230).

The United States is home to millions of people from many national origins. Currently, because there are growing concerns about racial, ethnic, and language disparities in health and health care and the need for health care systems to accommodate increasingly diverse patient populations, language access services (LAS) have become more and more a matter of national importance. This need has become increasingly pertinent given the continued growth in language diversity within the United States. English is the predominant language of the United States and according to the 2010 American Community Survey estimates it is spoken at home by 79.4% of its residents over 5 years of age (U.S. Census Bureau, 2012a). In the total of over 13 million Spanish-speaking households, there are 3.2 million households where no one over 14 speaks English only or speaks English "very well." There are over 5.2 million Indo-European and over 3.7 million Asian and Pacific Island households where no one over 14 speaks English only or speaks English "very well." (U.S. Census Bureau, 2012b). The most common, non-English languages spoken by people over 5 at home are Spanish, Chinese, French, German, and Tagalog. Vietnamese, Italian, Korean, and Russian and Polish are next among the top 10 languages (U.S. Census Bureau, 2012c).

People who are limited in their ability to speak, read, write, and understand the English language experience countless language barriers that can result in limiting their access to critical public health, hospital, and other medical and social services to which they are legally entitled. Many health and social service programs provide information about their services in English only. When LEP persons seek health care at hospitals or medical clinics, they are frequently faced with receptionists, nurses, and doctors who speak English only. The language barrier faced by LEP persons in need of medical care and/or social services severely limits the ability to gain access to these services and to participate in these programs. In addition, the language barrier often results in the denial of medical care or social services, delays in the receipt of such care and services, or the provision of care and services based on inaccurate or incomplete information. Services denied, delayed, or provided under such circumstances could have serious consequences for an LEP patient as well as for a provider of medical care. Some states, for example California, Massachusetts, and New York, recognize the seriousness of the problem and require providers to offer language assistance to patients in health care settings. Language access services are especially relevant to racial and ethnic disparities in health care. A report by the Institute of Medicine (IOM) on racial and ethnic disparities in health care documented through substantial research that minorities, as compared to their White American counterparts, receive lower quality of care across a wide range of medical conditions, resulting in poorer health outcomes and lower health statuses. The research conducted by the IOM showed that language barriers can cause poor, abbreviated, or erroneous communication and poor decision making on the part of both providers and patients (Smedley, B. D., A. Y. Stith, and A. R. Nelson, 2004, p. 3). Each patient must be carefully assessed to determine his or her language needs, and information must be delivered in a manner that is understandable by the patient. When a patient does not understand English, competent interpreters or language resources must be available.

■ Institutional Mandates

Since 2003, the Joint Commission has been actively pursuing a course that ensures that cultural and linguistic competency standards become a part of their accreditation requirements. Since this time, they have published several documents relevant to this topic and in 2010 they published a monograph, *Advancing Effective Communication, Cultural Competence, and Patient and Family*

Centered Care: A Roadmap for Hospitals. The monograph provides checklists to improve effective communication during the admission, assessment, treatment, end-of-life, and discharge and transfer stages of a given patient's hospitalization trajectory. They strongly state that:

> Every patient that enters the hospital has a unique set of needs—clinical symptoms that require medical attention and issues specific to the individual that can affect his or her care. (The Joint Commission, 2010, p. 1)

They implicitly recognize that when a given person moves through the hospitalization continuum, he or she not only requires medical and nursing intervention, but they also require care that addresses the spectrum of each person's demographic and personal characteristics. The Joint Commission has made many efforts to understand personal needs and then provide guidance to organizations to address those needs. They initially focused on studying language, culture, and health literacy needs and presently (as of 2011), they are focusing on effective communication, cultural competence, and patient- and family-centered care.

The Joint Commission defines cultural competency as:

> the ability of health care providers and health care organizations to understand and respond effectively to the cultural and language needs brought by the patient to the health care encounter. (2010, p. 91)

They further recognize that:

> cultural competence requires organizations and their personnel to: (1) value diversity; (2) assess themselves; (3) manage the dynamics of difference; (4) acquire and institutionalize cultural knowledge; and (5) adapt to diversity and the cultural contexts of individuals and communities served. (The Joint Commission, 2010, p. 91)

These principles apply to each segment of the institutional experience from admission to discharge or end of life, and for each facet there are specific actions that must be undertaken. These actions include informing patients of their rights, assessing communication needs, and involving the patient and family in care plans. Each segment is accompanied by a checklist for activities; for example, there is a checklist to Improve Effective Communication, Cultural Competence, and Patient- and Family-Centered Care during admission (The Joint Commission, p. 9).

■ CULTURALCARE

The term CULTURALCARE expresses all that is inherent in the development of health care delivery to meet the mandates of the CLAS standards and other cultural competency mandates. CULTURALCARE is holistic care. There are countless conflicts in the health care delivery arenas that are predicated on cultural misunderstandings. Although many of these misunderstandings are related to universal situations—such as verbal and nonverbal language misunderstandings, the conventions of courtesy, the sequencing of interactions, the phasing of interactions, and objectivity—many cultural misunderstandings are unique to the delivery of health care. The need to provide CULTURALCARE is essential, and providers must be able to assess and interpret a patient's health beliefs and practices and cultural and linguistic needs. CULTURALCARE alters the perspective of health care delivery as it enables the provider to understand, from a cultural perspective, the manifestations of the patient's cultural heritage and life trajectory. The provider must serve as a bridge in the health care setting between the given institution, the patient, and people who are from different cultural backgrounds.

In conclusion, cultural and linguistic competency must be understood to be the foundations of a new health care *philosophy*. It is comprised of countless facets—each of which is a topic for study. CULTURALCOMPETENCY is a philosophy that appreciates and values holistic perspectives rather than, or in addition to, dualistic—modern and technological—viewpoints. CULTURALCOMPETENCY is more than a "willingness"—it is a philosophy that ***must*** be part of an institution's and a professional's mission and goal statement. Within the philosophy of cultural competency, **HEALTH, ILLNESS,** and **HEALING** are understood holistically.

There are countless interrelated facets that include but are not limited to:

1. Language and the regulations of Title VI
2. Demography
3. Gender issues such as gender specific care and modesty
4. Faith and the roles religions play in HEALTH
5. Dietary practices
6. Income—both low and high
7. Heritage
8. Education
9. Social status
10. Spatial factors
11. Immigration—legal and illegal
12. Environmental issues
13. Unnatural causes of diseases
14. Health disparities
15. Manners
16. Socialization—both into the dominant society and into the professional practice disciplines
17. Traditional HEALTH beliefs and practices
18. Use of traditional healers and medicines
19. The human right of a given person/family/community to choose and select the type of health/HEALTH care (modern, traditional, or both) he or she prefers.
20. **Dissonance**—when a practitioner provides culturally and linguistically competent care and this care is not in harmony with his or her allopathic and/or institutional care beliefs and practices.

Each of these topics will be further discussed in various chapters in the remainder of this text.

Indeed, the development of CULTURALCOMPETENCE is an ongoing, lifelong endeavor. This is a topic that requires deep study, reflection, and time. The days when a "bagged lunch" with an hour's lecture or discussion have passed and hours—even a lifetime—must be dedicated to the topics, and countless others, this book presents. A critical question must be asked: "Are health care providers institutional advocates? Modern health care advocates? Or, patient advocates?"

Explore MediaLink

Go to the Student Resource Site at nursing.pearsonhighered.com for chapter-related review questions, case studies, and activities. Contents of the CULTURALCARE Guide and CULTURALCARE Museum can also be found on the Student Resource Site. Click on Chapter 1 to select the activities for this chapter.

Box 1–2: Keeping Up

There are countless references that are published weekly, monthly, annually, and periodically, which may be accessed to maintain currency in the domains of cultural and linguistic competency and with professional organizations concerned with this specialty area of practice. The following are selected suggestions:

American Association of Colleges of Nursing (AACN)

http://www.aacn.nche.edu/Education/pdf/toolkit.pdf

The AACN's Toolkit for Cultural Competent Education provides extensive resources including content and teaching-learning activities.

Health and Human Services (HHS) Data Council

http://aspe.hhs.gov/datacncl/

The HHS Data Council coordinates all health and human services data collection and analysis activities of the Department of Health and Human Services, including integrated data collection strategy, coordination of health data standards and health and human services, and privacy policy activities.

Kaiser FamilyFund

http://facts.kff.org/

Kaiser Fast Facts provides direct access to facts, data, and slides about the nation's health care system and programs, in an easy-to-use format.

(continued)

Box 1–2 *Continued*

http://www.statehealthfacts.kff.org/

The Kaiser Family Foundation has launched a new Internet resource, State Health Facts Online, that offers comprehensive and current health information for all 50 states, the District of Columbia, and U.S. territories. State Health Facts Online offers health policy information on a broad range of issues such as managed care, health insurance coverage and the uninsured, Medicaid, Medicare, women's health, minority health, and data and slides about the nation's health care system and programs, in an easy-to-use format.

National Breast and Cervical Cancer Early Detection Program (NBCCEDP)

http://www.cdc.gov/cancer/NBCCEDP/CDC

NBCCEDP provides access to critical breast and cervical cancer screening services for underserved women in the United States, the District of Columbia, 4 U.S. territories, and 13 American Indian/Alaska Native organizations.

Office of Minority Health (OMH)

http://minorityhealth.hhs.gov/

The OMH was created in 1986 and is one of the most significant outcomes of the 1985 *Secretary's Task Force Report on Black and Minority Health.* The Office is dedicated to improving the health of racial and ethnic minority populations through the development of health policies and programs that will help eliminate health disparities. The OMH was reauthorized by the Patient Protection and Affordable Care Act of 2010 (P.L. 111-148). In addition the new standards, *National Standards for Culturally and Linguistically Appropriate Services in Health and Health Care: A Blueprint for Advancing and Sustaining CLAS Policy and Practice* will be available at https://www.thinkculturalhealth.hhs.gov/.

Robert Wood Johnson

http://www.countyhealthrankings.org/

The Robert Wood Johnson Foundation has launched an online tool that ranks state counties by health status, taking into account clinical care, socioeconomic and environmental factors.

The National Center for Health Statistics (NCHS)

http://www.cdc.gov/nchs/

The NCHS provides quick and easy access to the wide range of information and data available, including HHS surveys and data collection systems.

The Joint Commission

http://www.jointcommission.org/facts_advancing_effective_communication/
Since 2007, the Joint Commission has been working toward improving access to care for all patients at our accredited organizations through better communication, cultural competence, and patient- and family-centered care.

Transcultural Nursing Society

The Transcultural Nursing Society has developed a core curriculum in Transcultural Nursing that can be found at http://www.amazon.com/s/ref=nb_sb_noss?url=search-alias%3Dstripbooks&field-keywords=core+curriculum+for+transcultural+nursing

Douglas, M. K., Editor-in-Chief and Pacquiao, D. F., Senior Editor. (2010). *Core Curriculum for Transcultural Nursing and Health Care* is available here.

The Transcultural Nursing Society has also developed Standards for Culturally Competent Nursing Care and they can be found at Douglas, M. K., Pierce, J.U., Rosenkoetter, M., et al. (2011). Standards of Practice for Culturally Competent Care. *Journal of Transcultural Nursing,* 22(4), 318.

University of Michigan Health System: The Cultural Competency Division.

http://www.med.umich.edu/multicultural/ccp/index.htm

The Cultural Competency Division plays a vital role in implementing cultural competency in the UMHS and in promoting good community health care practices. This is an excellent website with links to numerous sites.

The Online Journal of Cultural Competence in Nursing and Healthcare

This journal's first issue appeared online in January 2011. It is a free quarterly peer-reviewed publication that provides a forum for discussion of the issues, trends, theory, research, evidence-based, and best practices in the provision of culturally congruent and competent nursing and healthcare. The address is http://www.ojccnh.org.

■ Internet Sources

American Institutes for Research. (2005). A Patient-Centered Guide to Implementing Language Access Services in Healthcare Organizations. Washington, DC: Office of Minority Health/U.S. Department of Health and Human Services. Retrieved from http://minorityhealth.hhs.gov/, August 2011.

Dirksen Congressional Center. (2011). Major Features of the Civil Rights Act of 1964, Public Law 88–352, §601, 78 Stat 252 (42 USC 2000d). Retrieved from http://www.congresslink.org/print_basics_histmats_civilrights-64text.htm, November 28, 2011.

The Joint Commission. (2010). Advancing Effective Communication, Cultural Competence, and Patient- and Family-Centered Care: A Roadmap for Hospitals. Oakbrook Terrace, IL: The Joint Commission. Retrieved from http://www.jointcommission.org/, July 2011.

United States Census Bureau. (2010a). American Community Survey Language Spoken at Home. Retrieved from http://factfinder2.census.gov/faces/tableservices/jsf/pages/productview.xhtml?pid=ACS_10_1YR_GCT1601.US01PR&prodType=table, April 11, 2012.

United States Census Bureau. (2010b). American Community Survey Language Spoken at Home. Retrieved from http://factfinder2.census.gov/faces/tableservices/jsf/pages/productview.xhtml?pid=ACS_10_1YR_B16002&prodType=table, April 11, 2012.

United States Census Bureau. (2010c) American Community Survey Language Spoken at Home. Retrieved from http://factfinder2.census.gov/faces/tableservices/jsf/pages/productview.xhtml?pid=ACS_10_1YR_B16001&prodType=tables, April 11, 2012.

■ References

American Institutes for Research. (2005). *A patient-centered guide to implementing language access services in healthcare organizations.* Washington, DC: Office of Minority Health/U.S. Department of Health and Human Services.

Civil Rights Act of 1964, Public Law 88–352, §601, 78 Stat 252 (42 USC 2000d).

Fadiman, A. (2001). *The spirit catches you and you fall down.* NY: Farrar, Straus, and Giroux.

Flores, G. (2006). Language barriers to health care in the United States. *New England Journal of Medicine,* 355(3), 229–231.

Smedley B. D., A. Y. Stith, and A. R. Nelson. (2004). *Unequal treatment: confronting racial and ethnic health disparities in health care.* Institute of Medicine Report. Washington, DC: National Academy Press.

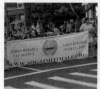

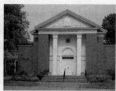

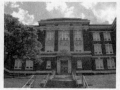

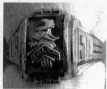

Figure 2-1   **Figure 2-2**   **Figure 2-3**   **Figure 2-4**

Chapter *2*

Cultural Heritage and History

Samoans, remember your culture.

◼ Objectives

1. Explain the factors that contribute to heritage consistency—culture, ethnicity, religion, and socialization.
2. Explain acculturation themes.
3. Determine and discuss sociocultural events that may influence the life trajectory of a given person.
4. Explain the factors involved in the cultural phenomena affecting health.

The image of a banner (Figure 2–1) was photographed at the International Parade in Honolulu, Hawaii, on March 13, 2011. It admonished Samoans—"remember YOUR culture"—a searing message for each of us to hear. This banner deeply resonated in me and made me aware of how important it is for me to know my culture and heritage—for all of us to know our culture and heritage. The opening images for this chapter depict critical aspects of the heritage I am a member of and are examples of the places and icons that were a part of my socialization as a child and teenager in the New England, American society of the mid-1950s. Figure 2–2 is that of Temple Shalom, the synagogue my family belonged to in Salem, Massachusetts. Here, I learned to read and write Hebrew, the history of the Jewish people, and the norms and expectations of being a Jewish American. Figure 2–3 is my high school, where I learned the skills to advance in life and experienced the roller coaster ride of the teenaged years. Last, my class ring (Figure 2–4), a cherished icon—I graduated from Salem

19

(Massachusetts) High School in 1958. These are examples of the highlights of my socialization—the places and icons representative of my cultural heritage and history. What are the places and icons of your generation and culture? If you had to choose 4 images to blend together as cornerstones of your cultural heritage, what would you choose?

Who are *you*? What is *your* cultural, ethnic, and religious heritage? How and where were you socialized to the roles and rules of your family, community, and occupation? *Who* is the person next to you? What is this person's cultural, ethnic, and religious heritage? How and where was this person socialized to the roles and rules of his or her family, community, and occupation? Are you this person's health care provider, instructor, colleague, or supervisor? The foundation for cultural competency rests in the knowledge and understanding of heritage, not only of yours but also of others with whom you are interacting.

This second chapter presents an overview of the salient content and complex theoretical content related to one's heritage and its impact on health beliefs and practices. Two sets of theories are presented, the first of which analyzes the degree to which people have maintained their traditional heritage; the second, and opposite, set of theories relates to socialization and acculturation and the quasi creation of a melting pot or some other common threads that are part of an American whole. It then becomes possible to analyze health beliefs by determining a person's ties to his or her traditional heritage, rather than to signs of acculturation. The assumption is that there is a relationship between people with strong identities—either with their heritage or the level at which they are acculturated into the American culture—and their health beliefs and practices. Hand in hand with the concept of ethnocultural heritage is that of a person's ethnocultural history; the journey a person has experienced predicated on the historical sociocultural events that have touched his or her life directly or indirectly.

■ Heritage Consistency

Heritage consistency is a concept developed by Estes and Zitzow (1980, p. 1) to describe "the degree to which one's lifestyle reflects his or her respective tribal culture." The theory has been expanded in an attempt to study the degree to which a person's lifestyle reflects his or her traditional culture, such as European, Asian, African, or Hispanic. The values indicating heritage consistency exist on a continuum, and a person can possess value characteristics of both a consistent heritage (traditional) and an inconsistent heritage (acculturated). The concept of heritage consistency includes a determination of one's cultural, ethnic, and religious background (Figure 2–5). It has been found over time that the greater a given person identifies with his or her traditional heritage, that is, his or her culture, ethnicity, and religion, the greater the chance that the person's health and illness beliefs and practices may vary from those of the mainstream society and modern health care providers. For example, Estes and Zitzow observed that when people who identified highly with their tribal culture were treated for alcoholism by a medicine man, the outcome was more favorable than with treatment in the modern culture. Other research found that people with a high

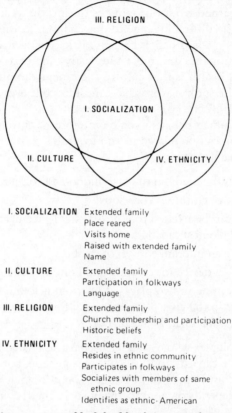

I. SOCIALIZATION	Extended family
	Place reared
	Visits home
	Raised with extended family
	Name
II. CULTURE	Extended family
	Participation in folkways
	Language
III. RELIGION	Extended family
	Church membership and participation
	Historic beliefs
IV. ETHNICITY	Extended family
	Resides in ethnic community
	Participates in folkways
	Socializes with members of same ethnic group
	Identifies as ethnic-American

Figure 2–5   Model of heritage consistency.

level of heritage consistency frequented health care sources not used by modern providers. The Heritage Assessment Tool, Appendix E, is a screening tool to assess for a person's level of heritage consistency and is a useful tool in research development.

Culture

The word *culture* showed 1,550,000,000 results on February 23, 2012, on the Internet. An overview of the content on selected sites, however, is certainly in harmony with the forthcoming discussion. There is no single definition of *culture*, and all too often definitions omit salient aspects of culture or are too general to have any real meaning. Of the countless ideas of the meaning of this term, some are of particular note. The classical definition by Fejos (1959, p. 43) describes culture as "the sum total of socially inherited characteristics of a human group that comprises everything which one generation can tell, convey, or hand down to the next; in other words, the nonphysically inherited traits we possess." Another way of understanding the concept of culture is to picture it as the luggage that each of us carries around for our lifetime. It is the sum of beliefs, practices, habits, likes, dislikes, norms, customs, rituals, and so forth that we learned from our families during the years of socialization. In turn, we transmit cultural luggage to our children. A third way of defining *culture* is the behaviors and beliefs characteristic of a particular social, ethnic, or age group (Dictionary.com, n.d.) and, lastly, one that is most relevant in areas of traditional health is that culture is a "metacommunication system," wherein not only the spoken words have meaning but everything else does as well (Matsumoto, 1989, p. 14).

All facets of human behavior can be interpreted through the lens of culture, and everything can be related to and from this context. Culture includes all the following characteristics:

1. Culture is the medium of personhood and social relationships.
2. Only part of culture is conscious.
3. Culture can be likened to a prosthetic device because it is an extension of biological capabilities.
4. Culture is an interlinked web of symbols.
5. Culture is a device for creating and limiting human choices.
6. Culture can be in two places at once—it is found in a person's mind and exists in the environment in such form as the spoken word or an artifact. (Bohannan, 1992, p. 12)

Culture is a complex whole in which each part is related to every other part. It is learned, and the capacity to learn culture is genetic, but the subject matter is not genetic and must be learned by each person in a family and social community. Culture also depends on an underlying social matrix, and included in this social matrix are knowledge, beliefs, art, law, morals, and customs (Bohannan, 1992, p. 13).

Culture is learned in that people learn the ways to see their environment—that is, they learn from the environment how to see and interpret what they see. People learn to speak, and they learn to learn. Culture, as the medium of our individuality, is the way in which we express ourselves. It is the medium of human social relationships, in that culture must be shared and creates social relationships. The symbols of culture—sound and acts—form the basis of all languages. Symbols are everywhere—in religion, politics, and gender; these are cultural symbols, the meanings of which vary between and within cultural groups (Bohannan, 1992, pp. 11–14). The society in which we live, and political, economic, and social forces tend to alter the way in which some aspects of a culture are transmitted and maintained. Many of the essential components of a culture, however, pass from one generation to the next unaltered. Consequently, our cultural background determines much of what we believe, think, and do, both consciously and unconsciously. In this way, culture and ethnicity are handed down from one generation to another. These classic definitions of *culture* continue to serve as a basis for understanding the term in the present time. In fact, the recent definition developed by the Joint Commission in 2010 defines **culture** as "integrated patterns of human behavior that include the language, thoughts, communications, actions, customs, beliefs, values, and institutions of racial, ethnic, religious, or social groups" (p. 91).

Ethnicity

The word *ethnicity* showed 23,600,000 results on February 23, 2012, on the Internet. A random exploration of selected sites did not provide information different from the classical information in the following discussion.

Cultural background is a fundamental component of one's ethnic background. Before we proceed with this discussion, though, we need to define some terms, so that we can proceed from the same point of reference. The classic reference defines *ethnic* as an adjective "of or pertaining to a social group within a cultural and social system that claims or is accorded special status on the basis of complex, often variable traits including religious, linguistic, ancestral, or physical characteristics" (Davies, 1976, p. 247). The contemporary definition applied by the Office of Minority Health is that of "a group of people that share a common and distinctive racial, national, religious, linguistic, or cultural heritage" (Office of Minority Health, 2001, p. 131). O'Neil (2008) described *ethnicity* as selected cultural and sometimes physical characteristics used to classify people into groups or categories considered to be significantly different from others.

The term *ethnic* has for some time aroused strongly negative feelings and is often rejected by the general population. One can speculate that the upsurge in the use of the term stems from the recent interest of people in discovering their personal backgrounds, a fact used by some politicians who overtly court "the ethnics." Paradoxically, in a nation as large as the United States and comprising as many different peoples as it does—with the American Indians being the only true native population—we find ourselves still reluctant to speak of ethnicity and ethnic differences. This stance stems from the fact that most foreign groups that come to this land often shed the ways of the "old country" and quickly attempt to assimilate themselves into the mainstream, or the so-called melting pot (Novak, 1973). Other terms related to *ethnic* include:

- Ethnicity: Identity with or membership in a particular racial, national, or cultural group and observance of that group's customs, beliefs, and language (Dictionary.com, n.d.)
- Ethnocentrism: (1) belief in the superiority of one's own ethnic group; (2) overriding concern with race
- Xenophobia: a morbid fear of strangers
- Xenophobe: a person unduly fearful or contemptuous of strangers or foreigners, especially as reflected in his or her political or cultural views

The behavioral manifestations of these phenomena occur in response to people's needs, especially when they are foreign born and must find a way to function (1) before they are assimilated into the mainstream and (2) in order to accept themselves. The people cluster together against the majority, who in turn may be discriminating against them.

Indeed, the phenomenon of ethnicity is "complex, ambivalent, paradoxical, and elusive" (Senior, 1965, p. 21). Ethnicity is indicative of the following characteristics a group may share in some combination:

1. Geographic origin
2. Migratory status
3. Race
4. Language and dialect
5. Religious faith or faiths
6. Ties that transcend kinship, neighborhood, and community boundaries
7. Traditions, values, and symbols
8. Literature, folklore, and music
9. Food preferences
10. Settlement and employment patterns
11. Special interest, with regard to politics, in the homeland and in the United States
12. Institutions that specifically serve and maintain the group
13. An internal sense of distinctiveness
14. An external perception of distinctiveness

There are at least 106 ethnic groups and more than 500 American Indian Nations in the United States that meet many of these criteria. People from every country in the world have immigrated to this country. Some nations, such as Germany, England, Wales, and Ireland, are heavily represented; others, such as Japan, the Philippines, and Greece, have smaller numbers of people living here (Thernstrom, 1980, p. vii). People continue to immigrate to the United States, with the present influx coming from Haiti, Mexico, South and Central America, India, and China.

Religion

The third major component of heritage consistency is religion. The word *religion* showed 170,000,000 results on February 23, 2012, on the Internet. Again, a random review of the material yielded information that was similar to existing data. One way to understand religion is that it is "the belief in a divine or superhuman power or powers to be obeyed and worshipped as the creator(s) and ruler(s) of the universe; it is a system of beliefs, practices, and ethical values." Religion is a major reason for the development of ethnicity (Abramson, 1980, pp. 869–875). Another way is to see religion as, "a set of beliefs concerning the cause, nature, and purpose of the universe, especially when considered as the creation of a superhuman agency or agencies, usually involving devotional and ritual observances, and often containing a moral code governing the conduct of human affairs and a specific fundamental set of beliefs and practices generally agreed upon by a number of persons or sects" (Dictionary.com, n.d.).

The Office of Minority Health has adopted the definition of *religion* as "a set of beliefs, values, and practices based on the teachings of a spiritual leader" (Office of Minority Health, 2001, p. 132). The practice of religion is revealed in numerous cults, sects, denominations, and churches. Ethnicity and religion are clearly related, and one's religion quite often determines one's ethnic group. Religion gives a person a frame of reference and a perspective with which to organize information. Religious teachings in relation to health help present a meaningful philosophy and system of practices within a system of social controls having specific values, norms, and ethics. These are related to health in that adherence to a religious code is conducive to spiritual harmony and health. Illness is sometimes seen as a punishment for the violation of religious codes and morals.

Religion plays a fundamental and vital role in the health beliefs and practices of many people. The following are general examples of the influences religion has on health practices:

1. Meditating
2. Being vaccinated
3. Being willing to have the body examined
4. Maintaining family viability
5. Hoping for recovery
6. Coping with stress
7. Caring for children.

Specific examples of a religious tradition and its influence on health include:

1. Judaism is rich in health-related proscriptions—from diet to activity to human relations and so forth.
2. The Catholic religion forbids abortion.
3. The Jehovah's Witnesses forbid blood transfusions.
4. The Mormons and Seventh Day Adventists prohibit the use of caffeine and tobacco.

An additional way of understanding the relationship of religion to health is to conceptualize religion as

1. particular churches or organized religious institutions;
2. a scholarly field of study; and
3. the domain of life that deals with things of the spirit and matters of "ultimate concern."

In addition, religious affiliation and membership benefit health by promoting healthy behavior and lifestyles in the following ways:

1. Regular religious fellowship benefits health by offering support that buffers and affects stress and isolation.
2. Participation in worship and prayer benefits health through the physiological effects of positive emotions.

3. Religious beliefs benefit health by their similarity to health promoting beliefs and personality styles.
4. Simple faith benefits health by leading to thoughts of hope, optimism, and positive expectation.
5. Mystical experiences benefit health by activating a healing bioenergy or life force or altered state of consciousness.
6. Absent prayer for others is capable of healing by paranormal means or by divine intervention (Levin, 2001, p. 9).

Unlike some countries, the United States does not include a question about religion in its census and has not done so for over 50 years. Religious adherent statistics in the United States are obtained from surveys and organizational reporting. However, it is also noteworthy that " 'we the people' of the United States now form the most profusely religious nation on earth" (Eck, 2001, p. 4). In 2006, Putnam and Campbell again found that Americans are a highly religious people. We have high rates of belonging, behaving, and believing, and when compared to other industrialized nations the United States ranks 7th in the rate of weekly attendance at religious services. Jordan, Indonesia, and Brazil are ahead of us. They also found that Mormons, Black Protestants, and Evangelicals are the most religiously observant groups in America; and that the deep south, Utah, and the Mississippi Valley are the most religious regions of the country (2010, pp. 7–23).

One source of religious preference is the Pew Forum on Religion and Public Life. (2011). The Forum delivers timely, impartial information on issues at the intersection of religion and public affairs. Table 2–1 illustrates the findings in the *Statistical Abstracts*, a government publication, regarding religious preferences in the United States (see Box 2–1).

Table 2-1   Self Described Religious Identification of the Adult Population: 2008

Religious Group	Estimate (In thousands (175,440 represents 175,440,000))
Christian	173,402
Jewish	2,680
Buddhist	1,189
Muslim	1,349
Hindu	582
Other Unclassified	1,030
No religion specified	34,169

Source: Adapted from U.S. Census Bureau, Statistical Abstract of the United States: 2012. Population. p. 61. Retrieved from http://www.census.gov/compendia/statab/ 11/28/11

Examples of Heritage Consistency

The factors that constitute heritage consistency are listed in Table 2–2. The following are examples of each factor:

1. The person's childhood development occurred in the person's country of origin or in an immigrant neighborhood in the United States of like ethnic group.

   The person was raised in a specific ethnic neighborhood, such as Italian, Black, Hispanic, or Jewish, in a given part of a city and was exposed to only the culture, language, foods, and customs of that group.

2. Extended family members encouraged participation in traditional religious and cultural activities.

   The parents sent the person to religious school, and most social activities were church-related.

3. The individual engages in frequent visits to the country of origin or returns to the "old neighborhood" in the United States.

   The desire to return to the old country or to the old neighborhood is prevalent in many people; however, many people, for various reasons, cannot return. The people who came here to escape religious persecution or whose families were killed during world wars or the Holocaust may not want to return to European homelands. Other reasons people may not return to their native country include political conditions in the homeland and lack of relatives or friends in that land.

Table 2–2   Factors Indicating Heritage Consistency

---

1. The person's childhood development occurred in the person's country of origin or in an immigrant neighborhood in the United States of like ethnic group.
2. Extended family members encouraged participation in traditional religious or cultural activities.
3. The individual engages in frequent visits to the country of origin or returns to the "old neighborhood" in the United States.
4. The individual's family home is within the ethnic community.
5. The individual participates in ethnic cultural events, such as religious festivals or national holidays, sometimes with singing, dancing, and special garments.
6. The individual was raised in an extended family setting.
7. The individual maintains regular contact with the extended family.
8. The individual's name has not been Americanized.
9. The individual was educated in a parochial (nonpublic) school with a religious or ethnic philosophy similar to the family's background.
10. The individual engages in social activities primarily with others of the same ethnic background.
11. The individual has knowledge of the culture and language of origin.
12. The individual possesses elements of personal pride about heritage.

---

4. The individual's family home is within the ethnic community of which he or she is a member.

   As an adult, the person has elected to live with family in an ethnic neighborhood.

5. The individual participates in ethnic cultural events, such as religious festivals or national holidays, sometimes with singing, dancing, and costumes.

   The person holds membership in ethno- or religious-specific organizations and primarily participates in activities with the groups.

6. The individual was raised in an extended family setting.

   When the person was growing up, there may have been grandparents living in the same household, or aunts and uncles living in the same house or close by. The person's social frame of reference was the family.

7. The individual maintains regular contact with the extended family.

   The person maintains close ties with members of the same generation, the surviving members of the older generation, and members of the younger generation who are family members.

8. The individual's name has not been Americanized.

   The person has restored the family name to its European original if it had been changed by immigration authorities at the time the family immigrated or if the family changed the name at a later time in an attempt to assimilate more fully.

9. The individual was educated in a parochial (nonpublic) school with a religious or ethnic philosophy similar to the family's background.

   The person's education plays an enormous role in socialization, and the major purpose of education is to socialize a person into the dominant culture. Children learn English and the customs and norms of American life in the schools. In the parochial schools, they not only learn English but also are socialized in the culture and norms of the religious or ethnic group that is sponsoring the school.

10. The individual engages in social activities primarily with others of the same religious or ethnic background.

    The major portion of the person's personal time is spent with primary structural groups.

11. The individual has knowledge of the culture and language of origin.

    The person has been socialized in the traditional ways of the family and expresses this as a central theme of life.

12. The individual expresses pride in his or her heritage.

    The person may identify him- or herself as ethnic American and be supportive of ethnic activities to a great extent.

It is not possible to isolate the aspects of culture, religion, and ethnicity that shape a person's worldview. Each is part of the other, and all three are united within the person. When one writes of religion, one cannot eliminate culture or ethnicity, but descriptions and comparisons can be made. Referring to Figure 2–5 and Figures 2–6A and 2–6B to assess heritage consistency can help determine ethnic group differences in health beliefs and practices. Understanding

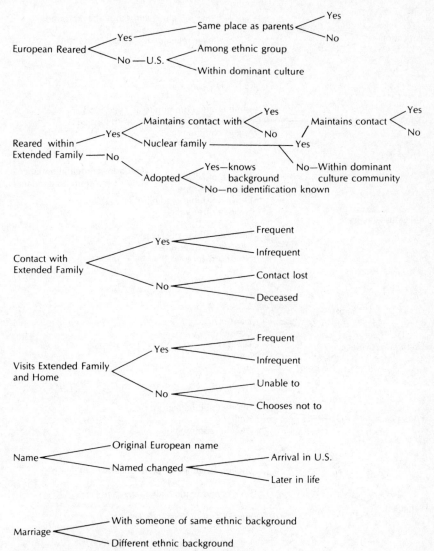

Figure 2-6A   Matrix of heritage consistency.

such differences can help enhance your understanding of the needs of patients and their families and the support systems that people may have or need.

■ Acculturation Themes

Several facets are relevant to the overall experience of acculturation. *Acculturation* is the broad term used to describe the process of adapting to and becoming absorbed into the dominant social culture. The overall process of acculturation into a new society is extremely difficult. Have you ever moved to a new community? Imagine moving to a new country and society where you

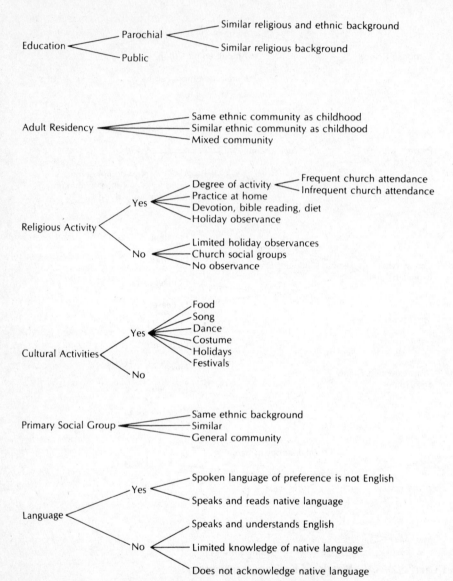

Figure 2–6B Matrix of heritage consistency, continued.

are unable to communicate, do not know your way around, and do not know know the "rules." The three facets to the process of overall acculturation are socialization, acculturation, and assimilation.

Socialization

Socialization is the process of being raised within a culture and acquiring the characteristics of that group. Education—be it pre-school, elementary school, high school, college, or a health care provider program—is a form of socialization. For many people who have been socialized within the boundaries of a "traditional culture" or a non-Western culture, modern American culture becomes a second cultural identity. Those who immigrate here, legally or illegally, from non-Western or non-modern countries may find socialization into the American culture, whether in schools or in society at large, to be an extremely difficult and painful process. They may experience biculturalism, which is a dual pattern of identification and one often of divided loyalty (LaFrombose, Coleman, & Gerton, 1993).

Understanding culturally determined health and illness beliefs and practices from different heritages requires moving away from linear models of process to more complex patterns of cultural beliefs and interrelationships.

Acculturation

While becoming a competent participant in the dominant culture, a member of the nondominant culture is always identified as a member of the original culture. The process of acculturation is involuntary, and a member of the nondominant cultural group is forced to learn the new culture to survive. Individuals experience second-culture acquisition when they must live within or between cultures (LaFrombose et al., 1993). *Acculturation* also refers to cultural or behavioral assimilation and may be defined as the changes of one's cultural patterns to those of the host society. In the United States, people assume that the usual course of acculturation takes three generations; hence, the adult grandchild of an immigrant is considered fully Americanized.

Assimilation

Acculturation also may be referred to as assimilation, the process by which an individual develops a new cultural identity. Assimilation means becoming in all ways like the members of the dominant culture. The process of assimilation encompasses various aspects, such as cultural or behavioral, marital, identification, and civic. The underlying assumption is that the person from a given cultural group loses this cultural identity to acquire the new one. In fact, this is not always possible, and the process may cause stress and anxiety (LaFrombose et al., 1993). Assimilation can be described as a collection of subprocesses: a process of inclusion through which a person gradually ceases to conform to any standard of life that differs from the dominant group standards and, at the same time, a process through which the person learns to conform to all the dominant group standards. The process of assimilation is considered complete when the foreigner is fully merged into the dominant cultural group (McLemore, 1980, p. 4).

There are four forms of assimilation: cultural, marital, primary structural, and secondary structural. One example of cultural assimilation is the ability to speak excellent American English. It is interesting to note that, according to the 2010 American Community Survey estimates, 79.4% of the American population over 5 years old speak only English; and 20.6% speak a language other than English (U.S. Census Bureau, 2010). Marital assimilation occurs when members of one group intermarry with members of another group. The third and fourth forms of assimilation, those of structural assimilation, determine the extent to which social mingling and friendships occur between groups. In primary structural assimilation, the relationships between people are warm, personal interactions between group members in the home, the church, and social groups. In secondary structural assimilation, there is nondiscriminatory sharing—often of a cold, impersonal nature—between groups in settings such as schools and workplaces (McLemore, 1980, p. 39).

The concepts of socialization, assimilation, and acculturation are complex and sensitive. The dominant society expects that all immigrants are in the process of acculturation and assimilation and that the worldview we share as health care practitioners is shared by our patients. Because we live in a pluralistic society, however, many variations of health beliefs and practices exist.

The debate still rages between those who believe that America is a melting pot and that all groups of immigrants must be acculturated and assimilated to an American norm, and those who dispute theories of acculturation and believe that the various groups maintain their own identities within the American whole. The concept of heritage consistency is one way of exploring whether people are maintaining their traditional heritage and of determining the depth of a person's traditional cultural heritage.

■ Ethnocultural Life Trajectories

Generational differences have been described as deep and gut-level ways of experiencing and looking at the cultural events that surround us. "The differences between generations—and the determination of who we are—are more than distinct ways of looking at problems and developing solutions for problems" (Hicks & Hicks, 1999, p. 4). Changes in the past several decades have created cultural barriers that openly or more subtly create misunderstandings, tensions, and often conflicts between family members, co-workers, and other individuals—as well as between patients and caregivers, especially in the practice of gerontology. The cycle of our lives is an ethnocultural journey and many of the aspects of this journey are derived from the social, religious, and cultural context in which we grew up. Factors that imprint our lives are the characters and events that we interacted with at 10 years of age, more or less (Hicks & Hicks, 1999, p. 25). Table 2–3 provides examples of seminal events that occurred from 1928–2001 and examples of workplace ethics, lifestyle, and social values of various generations.

One example of generational conflict between health care providers and patients is within institutional settings where the patients are cared for not only by people who are immigrants but also by those who are much younger and have limited knowledge as to what has been a patient's life trajectory. The patient may also be an immigrant who experienced a much different life trajectory than others of the same age and the caregivers. Imagine your life today and what it may have been like to live without a computer, a cell phone, an iPod, or an iPad. Many people may see today's commonplace objects as "strangers" rather than "friends," and could be "digital immigrants," not "digital natives."

Table 2-3 **Selected Seminal Sociocultural Events of the Past 75 Years, Workplace Ethos, Lifestyle, and Social Values**

Generation	Seminal Events	Workplace Ethos	Lifestyle	Social Values
The Silent Generation	The Great Depression	Traditional work ethic	Work first	Community service
	WWII	Employer loyalty	Conformist	Vote
b. 1928–1945	Hiroshima	Born to lead	Expect to lead	Family first
10:* 1938–1955	World's first electronic computer assembled	Conventional Believe in mission	Care for religion Buy decent home	
The Baby Boomers	Television— *I Love Lucy*	Money/work	Work/play hard	Reluctant community service
		Expect to lead	Religion acceptable	Vote only if convenient
b. 1946–1964		What do others think?	Buy most house you can	Family and friends
	TV dinners	Lip service to mission		
10: 1956–1974	Elvis Presley Marilyn Monroe Rosa Parks Sputnik			
Generation X	Kent State Watergate	Money/principle Lead and follow	Work/play hard Religion a hobby	I do not give Vote if you want to
	Nixon resigned	Independent and care what others think	Do I need a house?	Family and friends
b. 1965–1980	Vietnam Memorial Wall	Care about mission		
	HIV/AIDS epidemic	Principle/ satisfaction	Work hard if it does not interfere	May donate
	Challenger explosion	Lifestyle first	What is religion?	Vote privately
10: 1975–1990		Loyal to skills	Gentrify inner city	Friends are family
		Must have mission Individual first		

(continued)

Table 2-3 *continued*

Generation	Seminal Events	Workplace Ethos	Lifestyle	Social Values
Millennial Generation (First generation to come of age in new millennium)	Tiananmen Square	Principle/ satisfaction	Make others pay	Community service equals punishment
	Desert Storm	Lifestyle first	Comparative religions	Vote my issues
b. 1981–1992	President Clinton impeached	Must have a mission	Live with parents	Want extended families
	September 11, 2001	Individual first		
10: **1991–2001**	Afghanistan Iraq Hurricane Katrina			

*Generational names are the inherent work of popular culture. The names are derived from 1. a historic event, 2. rapid social or demographic change, or 3. a turn in the calendar. "10" marks the decade when a person turns 10. This is the decade (10–19 years of age) that influences a person's socio/cultural identity.

Sources: Taylor, P. and Keeter, S. (2010). MILLENNIALS A portrait of generation next: Confident. Connnected. Open to change. PEW RESEARCH CENTER. http://pewresearch.org/millennials/; Hicks, R., & Hicks, K. (1999). *Boomers, Xers, and other strangers.* Wheaton, IL: Tyndale House; Jennings, P. (1998). *The century.* Copyright 1998 by ABC Television.

■ Commingling Variables

Five commingling variables relate to this overall situation of social and generational divisions as they are potential sources of conflict:

1. **Decade of birth.** People's life experiences vary greatly, depending on the events of the decades in which they were born and the cultural values and norms of the times. People who tend to be heritage consistent—that is, have a high level of identification and association with a traditional heritage—tend to be less caught up in the secular fads of the time and popular sociocultural events.

2. **Generation in United States.** Worldviews differ greatly between the immigrant generation and subsequent generations, and people who score high as heritage consistent and mainstream people who may score low on the heritage consistency assessment and have been born into families who have resided in the United States for multiple generations.

3. **Class.** Social class is an important factor. The analysis of one's education, economics, and background is an important observation of people. There are countless differences among people predicated on class. The United States Department of Labor produces employment and wage estimates for over 800 occupations (Table 2–4). These are estimates of the number of people employed in certain occupations,

Table 2–4 May 2010 National Occupational Employment and Wage Estimates for Selected Major Occupational Groups

Major Occupational Group	Employment Estimate (number of employed)	Mean Annual Wage (dollars)
Management	6,022,860	105,400
Legal occupations	999,650	96,940
Computer and mathematical	3,283,950	77,230
Architecture and engineering	2,305,530	75,550
Health care practitioners and technical occupations	7,346,580	71,280
Registered nurses	2,655,020	67,720
Health care support occupations	3,962,930	26,920
Production occupations	8,236,130	33,770

Source: U.S. Department of Labor Statistics. Washington DC: United States Department of Labor. May 2010. National Occupational Employment and Wage Estimates. Retrieved from http://www.bls.gov/oes/current/oes_nat. htm#51-0000, February 23, 2012.

and estimates of the wages paid to them. Self-employed persons are not included in the estimates.

The unemployment rate in February 2011 was 9% (Bartash, 2011); in January 2008 it was 4.9% (U.S. Department of Labor). This has had an impact on the delivery of health care.

These figures, too, demonstrate the differences in economic class and play heavily in relation to issues of health care access and insurance coverage.

4. **Language.** There are frequent misunderstandings, as discussed in Chapter 1, when people who do not understand English must help and care for or take direction from English speakers. There are also countless conflicts when people who are hard of hearing attempt to understand people with limited English-speaking skills, and many cultural and social misunderstandings can develop.

5. **Education.** Increasing percentages of students have completed high school, from 69% in 1980 to 85.3% in 2009 (http://factfinder. census.gov/servlet/IPTable). "Every child in America deserves a world-class education." With these words, President Obama signed *A Blueprint for Reform: The Reauthorization of the Elementary and Secondary Education Act* in March, 2010. This blueprint challenges the nation to embrace education standards that would put America back on a path to global leadership in education. It provides incentives for states to adopt academic standards that prepare students to succeed in college and the workplace, and create accountability systems that measure student growth toward meeting the goal that all children graduate and succeed in college. It has three key priorities:

- **Raising standards** for all students—every student should graduate from high school ready for college and a career, regardless of income, race, ethnic or language background, or disability status

- **Better assessments**—the development and use of a new generation of assessments that are aligned with college- and career-ready standards
- **Effective teachers and principals**—to elevate the teaching profession to focus on recognizing, encouraging, and rewarding excellence (U.S. Department of Education, 2010).

■ Cultural Conflict

Hunter (1994) describes cultural conflicts as events that occur when there is polarization between two groups and the differences are intensified by the way they are perceived. The struggles are centered on the control of the symbols of culture. In the case of the conflict between the Lee family and the health care system, discussed in Chapter 1, the scope of the conflict is readily apparent and lends itself to further analysis. Hunter describes the fields of conflict as found in family, education, media and the arts, law, and electoral politics. Health care is a sixth field, and the conflict is between those who actively participate in traditional health care practices—that is, the practices of their given ethnocultural heritage—and those who are progressive and see the answers to contemporary health problems in the science and technology of the present.

When cultures clash, many misanthropic feelings, or "isms," can enter into a person's consciousness (Table 2–5). Just as Hunter proclaimed that the "differences" must be confronted, so, too, must stereotypes, prejudice, and discrimination. It is impossible to describe traditional beliefs without a temptation to stereotype, but each person is an individual; therefore, levels of heritage consistency differ within and between ethnic groups, as do health beliefs.

Another issue that manifests itself in this arena is prejudice. Prejudice occurs either because the person making the judgment does not understand the

Table 2–5 Common "Isms" Plus One Non-"Ism"

Belief	Definition
Racism	The belief that members of one race are superior to those of other races
Sexism	The belief that members of one gender are superior to the other gender
Heterosexism	The belief that everyone is or should be heterosexual and that heterosexuality is best, normal, and superior
Ageism	The belief that members of one age group are superior to those of other ages
Ethnocentrism	The belief that one's own cultural, ethnic, or professional group is superior to that of others; one judges others by one's "yardstick" and is unable or unwilling to see what the other group is really about—"My group is best!"
Xenophobia	The morbid fear of strangers

Source: American Nurses' Association. (1993). Proceedings of the invitational meeting, multicultural issues in the nursing workforce and workplace. Washington, DC: Author.

given person or his or her heritage, or because the person making the judgment generalizes an experience of one individual from a culture to all members of that group. Discrimination occurs when a person acts on prejudice and denies another person one or more of his or her fundamental rights.

■ Cultural Phenomena Affecting Health

Giger and Davidhizar (1995) have identified six cultural phenomena that vary among cultural groups and affect health care: time orientation, space, communication, social organization, biological variations, and environmental control.

Time Orientation

The viewing of time in the present, past, or future varies among cultural groups. Certain cultures in the United States and Canada tend to be future-oriented. People who are future-oriented are concerned with long-range goals and with health care measures in the present to prevent the occurrence of illness in the future. Others are oriented more to the present than the future and may be late for appointments because they are less concerned about planning to be on time. This difference in time orientation may become important in health care measures such as long-term planning and explanations of medication schedules.

Space

Personal space refers to people's behaviors and attitudes toward the space around themselves. Territoriality is the behavior and attitude people exhibit about an area they have claimed and defend or react emotionally to when others encroach on it. Both personal space and territoriality are influenced by culture, and thus different ethnocultural groups have varying norms related to the use of space.

Communication

Communication differences present themselves in many ways, including language differences, verbal and nonverbal behaviors, and silence. Language differences are possibly the most important obstacle to providing multicultural health care because they affect all stages of the patient-caregiver relationship.

Social Organization

The social environment in which people grow up and live plays an essential role in their cultural development and identification. Children learn their culture's responses to life events from the family and its ethnoreligious group. This socialization process is an inherent part of heritage—cultural, religious, and ethnic background.

Biological Variations

The several ways in which people from one cultural group differ biologically (i.e., physically and genetically) from members of other cultural groups constitute their biological variations; for example, body build and structure, including specific bone and structural differences between groups, such as the smaller stature of Asians and skin color, including variations in tone, texture, healing abilities, and hair follicles.

Environmental Control

Environmental control is the ability of members of a particular cultural group to plan activities that control nature or direct environmental factors. Included in this concept are the complex systems of traditional health and illness beliefs, the practice of folk medicine, and the use of traditional healers.

Figure 2–7 illustrates how a person, with a unique ethnic, religious, and cultural background, is affected by cultural phenomena. The discussions in

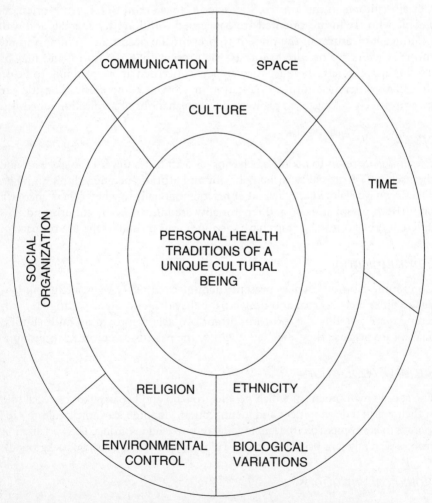

Figure 2–7 Personal health traditions of a unique cultural being.

Chapters 9 through 13 highlight these phenomena, and relevant examples are presented within the text and in tabular form. The examples used in the text to illustrate health traditions in different cultures are not intended to be stereotypical. With careful listening, observing, and questioning, the provider should be able to sort out the traditions of a given person. Table 2–6 suggests examples of etiquette relevant to each of the cultural phenomena.

This chapter has served as the foundation that delineates the multiple, interrelating phenomena that underlie the cultural conflict that occurs between health care providers and patients, many of whom have difficulty interacting with the health care providers and system. It has presented both classical and contemporary definitions and explanations relevant to the foundation of this conflict and sets the stage for further discussion.

Table 2–6 Examples of Etiquette as Related to Selected Cultural Phenomena

Time	Visiting	Inform person when you are coming
	Being on time	Avoid surprises
		Explain your expectations about time
	Taboo times	Ask people from other regions and cultures what they expect
		Be familiar with the times and meanings of person's ethnic and religious holidays
Space	Body language and distances	Know cultural and/or religious customs regarding contact, such as eye and touch, from many perspectives
Communication	Greetings	Know the proper forms of address for people from a given culture and the ways by which people welcome one another
		Know when touch, such as an embrace or a handshake, is expected and when physical contact is prohibited
	Gestures	Gestures do not have universal meaning; what is acceptable to one cultural group is taboo with another
	Smiling	Smiles may be indicative of friendliness to some, taboo to others
	Eye contact	Avoiding eye contact may be a sign of respect
Social organization	Holidays	Know what dates are important and why, whether to give gifts, what to wear to special events, and what the customs and beliefs are
	Special events	Know how the event is celebrated, the
	Births	meaning of colors used for gifts, and expected
	Weddings	rituals at home or religious services
	Funerals	

(continued)

Table 2-6 *continued*

Biological variations	Food customs	Know what can be eaten for certain events, what foods may be eaten together or are forbidden, and what and how utensils are used
Environmental control	Health practices and remedies	Know what the general *health* traditions are for person and question observations for validity

Source: Adapted from Dresser, N. (1996). *Multicultural manners.* New York: Wiley. Copyright © 1996 John Wiley & Sons, Inc. Reprinted by permission of John Wiley & Sons. Inc.

Explore 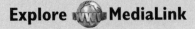 MediaLink

Go to the Student Resource Site at nursing.pearsonhighered.com for chapter-related review questions, case studies, and activities. Contents of the CULTURALCARE Guide and CULTURALCARE Museum can also be found on the Student Resource Site. Click on Chapter 2 to select the activities for this chapter.

Box 2–1: Keeping Up

The following resource will be helpful in maintaining current information related to religious participation.

   Pew Research Center http://pewresearch.org/topics/religion/

■ Internet Sources

Bartash, J. (2011). Digging Up U.S. Economic Trends Not Easy. Market Watch. Retrieved from http://www.marketwatch.com/story/forecast-for-us-economy-obscured-by-poor-weather-2011-02-06?reflink=MW_news_stmp, February 23, 2011.

culture. (n.d.). The American Heritage New Dictionary of Cultural Literacy, Third Edition. Dictionary.com. Retrieved from http://dictionary.reference.com/browse/culture, January 31, 2011.

ethnicity. (n.d.). The American Heritage New Dictionary of Cultural Literacy, Third Edition. Dictionary.com. Retrieved from http://dictionary.reference.com/browse/ethnicity, January 31, 2011.

O'Neil, D. (2008). Ethnicity and Race: An Introduction to the Nature of Social Group Differentiation and Inequality. San Marcos, CA: Palomar College. Retrieved from http://anthro.palomar.edu/ethnicity/Default.htm, February 18, 2008.

religion. (n.d.). The American Heritage New Dictionary of Cultural Literacy, Third Edition. Dictionary.com. Retrieved from http://dictionary.reference.com/browse/religion, January 31, 2011.

Taylor, P. and Keeter, S. (2011). MILLENNIALS: A Portrait of Generation Next: Confident. Connected. Open to change. Pew Research Center. Retrieved from http://pewresearch.org/millennials, February 23, 2011.

The Pew Forum on Religion and Public Life. (2011). U.S. Religious Landscape Survey. (2010). Recovered from http://religions.pewforum.org/, April 2011.

United States Census Bureau. (2012). Statistical Abstract of the United States. Population, p. 61. Retrieved from http://www.census.gov/compendia/statab/, November 28, 2011.

United States Census Bureau. (2010). American Community Survey Language Spoken at Home. Retrieved from http://factfinder2.census.gov/faces/tableservices/jsf/pages/productview.xhtml?pid=ACS_10_1YR_S1601&prodType=table, February 23, 2011.

United States Department of Education. (2007). No Child Left Behind – High School Facts at a Glance. Retrieved from http://www.ed.gov/about/offices/list/ovae/pi/hs/hsfacts.html, October 18, 2007.

United States Department of Education. (2010). A Blueprint for Reform: The Reauthorization of the Elementary and Secondary Education Act. Retrieved from http://www2.ed.gov/policy/elsec/leg/blueprint/blueprint.pdf, February 23, 2012.

United States Department of Health and Human Services. Fact Sheet – Your rights under Title VI of the Civil Rights Act. Retrieved from http://www.hhs.gov/ocr/generalinfo.html, July 15, 2007.

United States Department of Labor Statistics. (2010). National Occupational Employment and Wage Estimates. Washington, DC: United States Department of Labor. Retrieved from http://www.bls.gov/oes/current/oes_nat.htm#11-0000, February 23, 2012.

▪ References

Abramson, H. J. (1980). Religion. In S. Thernstrom (Ed.), *Harvard encyclopedia of American ethnic groups.* Cambridge: Harvard University Press.

American Heritage Dictionary. (1976). Boston: Houghton Mifflin.

American Nurses' Association. (1993). Proceedings of the invitational meeting, multicultural issues in the nursing workforce and workplace. Washington, DC: Author.

Bohannan, P. (1992). *We, the alien—An introduction to cultural anthropology.* Prospect Heights, IL: Waveland Press.

Carroll, J. (2003). *Harley-Davidson: The living legend.* Edison, NJ: Edison Books.

culture. (n.d.). *The American heritage new dictionary of cultural literacy, third edition.* Dictionary.com. Retrieved from http://dictionary.reference.com/browse/culture, January 31, 2011.

Davies, P. (Ed). (1976). *The American heritage dictionary of the English language,* Paperback edition. NY: Dell.

Dresser, N. (1996). *Multicultural manners.* New York: John Wiley & Sons, Inc.

Eck, D. L. (2001). *A new religious America: How a "Christian country" has become the world's most religious diverse nation.* San Francisco: Harper.

ethnicity. (n.d.). *The American heritage new dictionary of cultural literacy, third edition.* Dictionary.com. Retrieved from http://dictionary.reference.com/browse/ethnicity, January 31, 2011.

Estes, G., & Zitzow, D. (1980, November). *Heritage consistency as a consideration in counseling Native Americans*. Paper read at the National Indian Education Association Convention, Dallas, TX.

Fadiman A. (1997). *The spirit catches you and you fall down*. New York: Farrar, Straus, Giroux.

Fejos, P. (1959). Man, magic, and medicine. In L. Goldston (Ed.), *Medicine and anthropology*. New York: International University Press.

Giger, J. N., & Davidhizar, R. E. (1995). *Transcultural nursing assessment and intervention* (2nd ed.). St. Louis: Mosby-Year Book.

Hicks, R., & Hicks, K. (1999). *Boomers, Xers, and other strangers*. Wheaton, IL: Tyndale House.

Hunter, J. D. (1994). *Before the shooting begins—Searching for democracy in America's culture wars*. New York: Free Press.

LaFrombose, T., Coleman, L. K., & Gerton, J. (1993). Psychological impact of biculturalism: Evidence and theory. *Psychological Bulletin, 114*(3), 395.

Levin, J. (2001). *God, faith, and health*. New York: John Wiley & Sons.

Matsumoto, M. (1989). *The unspoken way*. Tokyo: Kodahsha International.

McLemore, S. D. (1980). *Racial and ethnic relations in America*. Boston: Allyn & Bacon.

Novak, M. (1973). How American are you if your grandparents came from Serbia in 1888? In S. Te Selle (Ed.), *The rediscovery of ethnicity: Its implications for culture and politics in America*. New York: Harper & Row.

Office of Minority Health. (2001). *National standards for culturally and linguistically appropriate services in health care*. Washington, DC: U.S. Department of Health and Human Services.

Putnam, R. D., & D. E. Campbell. (2010) *American grace: How religion divides and unites us*. New York: Simon and Schuster.

religion. (n.d.). *The American heritage new dictionary of cultural literacy, third edition*. Dictionary.com. Retrieved from http://dictionary.reference.com/browse/religion, January 31, 2011.

Senior, C. (1965). *The Puerto Ricans: Strangers then neighbors*. Chicago: Quadrangle Books.

The Joint Commission. (2010). *Advancing effective communication, cultural competence, and patient- and family-centered care: A roadmap for hospitals*. Oakbrook Terrace, IL: Author.

Thernstrom, S. (Ed.). (1980). *Harvard encyclopedia of American ethnic groups*. Cambridge: Harvard University Press.

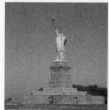 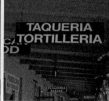 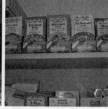 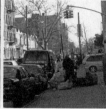

Figure 3-1   **Figure 3-2**   **Figure 3-3**   **Figure 3-4**

Chapter 3

Diversity

... Give me your tired, your poor,
Your huddled masses yearning to breathe free,
The wretched refuse of your teeming shore.
Send these, the homeless, tempest-tost to me,
I lift my lamp beside the golden door!

—*Emma Lazarus,* The New Colossus *(1886)*

■ Objectives

1. Describe the total population characteristics of the United States as presented in Census 2010.
2. Compare the population characteristics of the United States in 2000 and 2010.
3. Discuss the changes in points of origin of recent and past immigrants.
4. Discuss the meanings of terms related to immigration, such as *citizen, refugee, legal permanent resident, and naturalization.*
5. Discuss the facets of poverty.
6. Describe poverty guidelines.
7. Analyze the cycle of poverty.

The opening images for this chapter are representative of the demographic and socioeconomic diversity that exists in countless communities in this nation. The first figure, 3–1, is that of the Statue of Liberty—a reminder that most of the people who live in the United States of America are the descendants of immigrants or are themselves immigrants. Figures 3–2 and 3–3 depict places where people are able to purchase food and other necessities from their homelands—a Mexican market and other stores in San Juan Capistrano, California, and a shelf of canned goods in an Indian grocery store in Waltham, Massachusetts. Figure 3–4 depicts the poverty in this land of plenty—a homeless woman, guarding her cart of possessions while rummaging through the trash on a street in Brooklyn, New York. An infinite number of images could be placed in this chapter's opening. What comes to your mind when you think about the demographic diversity in your home community? What are your images of poverty and homelessness?

Health care providers are entangled in the revolutionary consequences of the enormous demographic, social, and cultural changes that have occurred in the United States. Many of these changes are playing a dramatic role both in the delivery of health care to patients, their families, and communities, and in the workforce and environment in which the provider practices. Table 3–1 demonstrates the growth of the emerging majority—people of color—that constituted 30.9% of the population in 2000; grew to 36.3% in the 2010 census (Humes, Jones, Ramirez, 2011 p. 6). The comments and data presented in this chapter are designed to provide you with an impression of the demographic features, derived from Census 2010 and other recent data from the Census Bureau and recent immigration, labor, and economic backgrounds of the American population.

Table 3–1   Population by Hispanic or Latino Origin and by Race for the United States: 2000 and 2010

Hispanic or Latino Origin and Race	2000	2010
Total population	281,421,906	308,745,538
	Percentage of Total Population	**Percentage of Total Population**
Hispanic or Latino	12.5	16.3
Not Hispanic or Latino	87.5	83.7
White alone	69.1	63.7
Race		
One race	97.6	97.1
White	75.1	72.4
Black or African American	12.3	12.6
American Indian and Alaska Native	0.9	0.9
Asian	3.6	4.8
Native Hawaiian and other Pacific Islander	0.1	0.2
Some other race	5.5	6.2
Two or more races	2.4	2.9

Source: Humes, et al. (2011). Overview of Race and Hispanic Origin: 2010. Census Briefs. p. 4. Retrieved from http://2010.census.gov/2010census/data/, June 26, 2011. p. 6.

In order to understand the profound changes that are taking place in the health care system, both in the delivery of services and in the profile of the people who are receiving and delivering services, we must look at the changes in the American population. The White majority is aging and shrinking; the Black, Hispanic, Asian, and American Indian populations are young and growing. It is imperative for those who deliver health care to be understanding of and sensitive to cultural differences, and the effect of the differences on a person's health and illness beliefs and practices and health care needs.

■ Census 2010

Every census adapts to the decade in which it is conducted. One of the most important changes to Census 2010 was the revision of the questions that were asked regarding race and Hispanic origin. The federal government considers race and Hispanic origin to be two separate concepts and the questions on race and Hispanic origin were asked of all people living in the United States. The changes were developed to reflect the country's growing diversity. The respondents were given the option of selecting one or more race categories to indicate their racial identities. A factor that presents confusion is that people were free to define themselves as belonging to many groups. However, the overwhelming majority of the population reported one race.

In 1997, the Office of Management and Budget established federal guidelines to collect and present data on race and Hispanic origin. Census 2010 adhered to the guidelines, and added "some other race." Data on race has been collected since the first census in 1790. The present categories are as follows:

1. **White**—refers to a person having origins in any of the original peoples of Europe, the Middle East, or North Africa. It includes people who indicated their race(s) as "White" or reported entries such as Irish, German, Italian, Lebanese, Arab, Moroccan, or Caucasian.
2. **Black or African American**—refers to a person having origins in any of the Black racial groups of Africa. It includes people who indicated their race(s) as "Black, African American, or Negro" or reported entries such as African American, Kenyan, Nigerian, or Haitian.
3. **American Indian or Alaska Native**—refers to a person having origins in any of the original peoples of North and South America (including Central America) and who maintains tribal affiliation or community attachment. This category includes people who indicated their race(s) as "American Indian or Alaska Native" or reported their enrolled or principal tribe, such as Navajo, Blackfeet, Inupiat, Yup'ik, Central American Indian groups, or South American Indian groups.
4. **Asian**—refers to a person having origins in any of the original peoples of the Far East, Southeast Asia, or the Indian subcontinent, including, for example, Cambodia, China, India, Japan, Korea, Malaysia, Pakistan, the Philippine Islands, Thailand, and Vietnam. It includes

people who indicated their race(s) as "Asian" or reported entries such as "Asian Indian," "Chinese," "Filipino," "Korean," "Japanese," "Vietnamese," and "Other Asian," or provided other detailed Asian responses.

5. **Native Hawaiian or Other Pacific Islander**—refers to a person having origins in any of the original peoples of Hawaii, Guam, Samoa, or other Pacific Islands. It includes people who indicated their race(s) as "Pacific Islander" or reported entries such as "Native Hawaiian," "Guamanian or Chamorro," "Samoan," and "Other Pacific Islander," or provided other detailed Pacific Islander responses.

6. **Some Other Race**—includes all other responses not included in the White, Black or African American, American Indian or Alaska Native, Asian, and Native Hawaiian or Other Pacific Islander race categories described above. Respondents reporting entries such as multiracial, mixed, interracial, or a Hispanic or Latino group (for example, Mexican, Puerto Rican, Cuban, or Spanish) in response to the race question are included in this category.

7. **Hispanic or Latino**—refers to a person of Cuban, Mexican, Puerto Rican, South or Central American, or other Spanish culture or origin regardless of race (Humes et al., 2011, p. 2).

These terms of classification will be used throughout this chapter and the text. The census does not break down the population by gender except to ask if the respondent is male or female. It questions neither gender preference nor if a person is abled or disabled. This text will follow census categories and not directly include the homosexual and diasabled populations in its discussions.

Total Population Characteristics

The 2010 census percentages are compared with the 2000 census percentages in Table 3–1. The figures demonstrate both the growth of the American population in general and the growth of people of color specifically. The changes are as follows:

Age. The age classification is based on the age of the person in complete years as of April 1, 2010. The age was derived from the date of birth information requested on the census form. It is critical to note the following points regarding age in 2010:

- The number of people under age 18 was 74.2 million (24% of the total population). Between 2000 and 2010, the population under the age of 18 grew at a rate of 2.6%.
- The population between 18 and 64 comprised 62.9% of the population.
- The younger working-age population, ages 18 to 44, represented 112.8 million persons (36.5%).
- The older working-age population, ages 45 to 64, made up 81.5 million persons (26.4%).

- The 65 and over population was 40.3 million persons (13%).
- The median age for the total population was 37.2 years. (Howden & Meyer, 2011, p. 1.)

American Indian, Aleut, and Eskimo Populations (Alone). The American Indian, Eskimo, and Aleut populations alone in the United States constituted 0.9% of the total population in 2010. The median age of the population was 27.7 years in 2000 and 31.0 years in 2010 (see Table 3–2).

Asian/Pacific Islander Population (Alone). Members of the Asian/Pacific Island communities made up 3.6% of the population in 2000 and 4.8% in 2010. The median age of the Asian/Pacific Island population was 32.5 years in 2000 and the Asian alone population in 2010 was 35.5 years.

Black Population (Alone). The Black population alone in the United States constituted 12.3% of the total population in 2000 and 12.6% in 2010. The median age of the Black population was 30.0 years in 2000 and 32.5 years in 2010.

Hispanic Population (of Any Race). Hispanic Americans (of any race) made up 12.5% of the total population in 2000 and 16.8% in 2010. The median age of the Hispanic population was 25.8 years in 2000 and 27.2 years in 2010.

White Population (Alone). In 2000, the White population in the United States constituted 72.1% of the total population and 63.2% in 2010. The median age of the population was 38.6 years in 2000 and 39.8 years in 2010 (U.S. Census Bureau, 2010).

The U.S. Census Bureau produces estimates of the resident population for the United States on an annual basis. It revises the estimates time series each year as final input data become available. These postcensal estimates from

Table 3–2   Median Ages of the Population, 2000 and 2010

Population Group	Median Age	
	2000 Census	2010 Census
American Indian alone	27.7 years	31.0 years
Asian alone	32.5 years	35.5 years
Black alone	30.0 years	32.5 years
Hispanic	25.8 years	27.2 years
White alone—not of Hispanic heritage	38.6 years	39.8 years
Native Hawaiian and other Pacific Islanders	26.8 years	28.6 years
2 or more races	19.8 years	19.7 years
Total Population	35.3 years	36.5 years

Source: U.S. Census Bureau. (2001). Retrieved from http://www.census.gov/popest/national/asrh/NC-EST2009-asrh.html, December 16, 2011; U.S. Census Bureau. (2010). American Community Survey. Retrieved from http://factfinder2.census.gov/faces/tableservices/jsf/pages/productview.xhtml?fpt=table, December 16, 2011.

April 1, 2000 through July 1, 2006 supersede all previous estimates produced since Census 2000. On March 30, 2007, the U.S. Census Bureau submitted to Congress the subjects it planed to address in the 2010 Census, which include gender, age, race, ethnicity, relationship, and whether you own or rent your home. It was estimated that the questions will take less than 10 minutes to complete. The 2010 Census was one of the shortest and easiest to complete since the nation's first census in 1790. There is also a yearly American Community Survey, which eliminates the need for a long-form questionnaire and provides key socioeconomic and housing data about the nation's rapidly changing population. The information required for the census was to be mailed in by April 1, 2010. A census enumerator interviewed the residents who did not submit their census forms during the months of May and June 2010. This measure was taken in order to ensure as complete a count as possible.

■ Immigration

Immigrants and their descendants constitute most of the population of the United States, and Americans who are not themselves immigrants have ancestors who came to the United States from elsewhere. The only people considered native to this land are the American Indians, the Aleuts, and the Inuit (or Eskimos), for they migrated here thousands of years before the Europeans (Thernstrom, 1980, p. vii).

Immigrants come to the United States seeking religious and political freedom and economic opportunities. The life of the immigrant is fraught with difficulties—going from an "old" to a "new" way of life, learning a new language, and adapting to a new climate, new foods, and a new culture. Socialization of immigrants occurs in American public schools, and Americanization, according to Greeley (1978), is for some a process of "vast psychic repression," wherein one's language and other familiar trappings are shed. In part, the concept of the melting pot has been created in schools, where children learn English, reject family traditions, and attempt to take on the values of the dominant culture and "pass" as Americans (Novak, 1973). This difficult experience, as noted and described by Greeley and Novak in the 1970s, continues today.

A citizen of the United States is a native-born, foreign-born child of citizens, or a naturalized person who owes allegiance to the United States and who is entitled to its protection. All persons born or naturalized in the United States, are citizens of the United States and of the state wherein they reside. A refugee is any person who is outside his or her country of nationality and who is unable or unwilling to return to that country because of persecution or a well-founded fear of persecution. Persecution or the fear thereof must be based on the alien's race, religion, nationality, membership in a particular social group, or political opinion. People with no nationality must generally be outside their country of last habitual residence to qualify as a refugee. Refugees are subject to ceilings by geographic area set annually by the president in consultation with Congress and are eligible to adjust to lawful permanent resident status after 1 year of continuous presence in the United States. A permanent resident alien is an alien admitted to the United States as a lawful permanent resident. A "green card" provides official immigration status (lawful permanent residency) in the United States. Immigrants are now referred to as Legal Permanent Residents; however, the Immigration and Nationality Act (INA) broadly defines an immigrant as "any alien in the United States, except one legally admitted under specific nonimmigrant categories." An illegal alien, or undocumented person, who entered the United States without inspection, for example, would be strictly defined as an immigrant under the INA but is not a Legal Permanent Resident. Legal Permanent Residents (LPRs) are legally accorded the privilege of residing permanently in the United States. **Naturalization** is the process by which United States citizenship is conferred upon foreign citizens or nationals after fulfilling the requirements established by Congress. Box 3–1 contains an

---

 Box 3–1

Sample Questions and Answers for the Naturalization Test

1. What is one responsibility that is only for United States citizens?
2. What is the supreme law of the land?
3. What do we call the first ten amendments to the Constitution?
4. How many amendments does the Constitution have?
5. Who makes federal laws?
6. What is the highest court in the United States?
7. How many justices are on the Supreme Court?
8. Under our Constitution, what powers belong to the states?
9. How old do citizens have to be to vote for President?
10. What did Susan B. Anthony do?

Answers

1. serve on a jury, vote in a federal election
2. the Constitution
3. the Bill of Rights
4. twenty-seven (27)
5. Congress, Senate and House (of Representatives), (U.S. or national) legislature
6. the Supreme Court
7. nine (9)
8. provide schooling and education, provide protection (police), provide safety (fire departments), give a driver's license, approve zoning and land use
9. eighteen (18) and older
10. fought for women's rights, fought for civil rights

Source: U.S. Department of Homeland Security. (2011). Learn about the United States: Quick Civics Lessons for the Naturalization Test. Retrieved from www.uscis.gov/citizenship, July 7, 2011.

example of the questions a person is asked when taking the examination for naturalization. They are able to obtain a civics book to study about our government and some history. The person is now also interviewed to determine English language competency and expected to meet other requirements.

In 2010, a total of 1,042,625 people became Legal Permanent Residents of the United States. The majority, 54%, already resided here. Among the LPRs, Mexico (13%), China (7%), and India (7%) were the leading countries of birth (Monger & Yankay, 2011, p. 1). In 1970, the highest percentage of people was from Europe whereas in 2010, people from Mexico, China, and India were the highest in percentage. In 2010, 619,913 people were naturalized. The largest percentage came from Asia (Lee, 2010, p. 2).

Table 3–3 lists the primary metropolitan areas for Legal Permanent Residents in 2010, and Table 3–4 lists the top 10 states where Legal Permanent

Table 3–3   Five Leading Legal Permanent Resident Flow Metropolitan Areas of Residence: 2010

1. New York, northern New Jersey–Long Island: 17.8%
2. Los Angeles–Long Beach–Santa Ana, California: 8.4%
3. Miami–Fort Lauderdale–Miami Beach, Florida: 6.7%
4. Washington, DC–Maryland–Virginia: 4.0%
5. Chicago–Naperville-Joliet, Illinois, Indiana, Wisconsin: 3.4%

Source: Monger, R., & Yankay, J. (2011). U.S. Legal Permanent Residents: 2010. p. 3. Washington, DC: Department of Homeland Security. Retrieved from http://www.dhs. gov/ximgtn/statistics/publications/index.shtm, May 24, 2011.

Table 3–4   Permanent Resident Flow by State of Residence: 2010

1. California	20.0%
2. New York	14.2%
3. Florida	10.3%
4. Texas	8.4%
5. New Jersey	5.5%
6. Illinois	3.6%
7. Massachusetts	3.0%
8. Virginia	2.7%
9. Maryland	2.5%
10. Georgia	2.4%
Other states	27.4%

Source: Monger, R., & Yankay, J. (2011). U.S. Legal Permanent Residents: 2010. Washington, DC: Department of Homeland Security. p. 4. Retrieved from http://www.dhs. gov/ximgtn/statistics/publications/index.shtm, May 24, 2011.

Residents are residing. Table 3–5 shows the leading 10 countries of origin for Legal Permanent Residents flow by country of birth in 2010. Table 3–6 compares selected characteristics of the native and foreign-born populations in 2005. The following are examples:

Table 3-5 Leading 10 Countries of Origin for Legal Permanent Resident Flow by Country of Birth: 2010

Country	Legal Permanent Residents (%)
1. Mexico	13.3
2. People's Republic of China	6.8
3. India	6.6
4. Philippines	5.6
5. Dominican Republic	5.2
6. Cuba	3.2
7. Vietnam	2.9
8. Haiti	2.2
9. Colombia	2.1
10. Korea	2.1

Source: Monger, R., & Yankay, J. (2011). U.S. Legal Permanent Residents: 2010. Washington, DC: Department of Homeland Security. p. 4. Retrieved from http://www.dhs. gov/ximgtn/statistics/publications/index.shtm, May 24, 2011.

Table 3-6 Selected Characteristics of the Native and Foreign-Born Populations: 2005–2009

Characteristic	Native Population	Foreign Born	Naturalized Citizens	Not a U.S. Citizen
Population	264.1 million	37.3 million	15.9 million	21.4 million
Median age	35.6 years	40.1	48.6 years	34.5 years
Asian	1.7%	23.5%	31.1%	17.9%
Hispanic	10.6%	47.0%	31.2%	58.7%
Population 25 years and older, less than high school	12.3%	32.2%	22.5%	40.7%
Speak language other than English	9.7%	84.2%	78.3%	88.7 %
Speak English less than well	2.0%	52.1%	38.8%	62.0%
Family poverty rates	8.9%	15.1%	8.7%	21.9%
Poverty status below 100% of poverty level	13.0%	16.4%	9.8%	21.3%
Renting household unit	31.1%	46.1%	31.1%	62.2%
Vehicle unavailable	8.1%	13.4%	11.5%	15.3%
No telephone service	4.2%	4.7%	2.5%	7.0%

Source: American Fact Finder. Selected Characteristics of the Native and Foreign-Born Population (2005–2009). American Community Survey. Retrieved from http://factfinder.census.gov/servlet/STTable?_bm=y&-geo_id=01000US&-qr_name=ACS_2009_5YR_G00_S0501&-ds_name=ACS_2009_5YR_G00_&-redoLog=false, July 7, 2011.

- Fewer foreign-born people are likely to have a vehicle than native-born residents.
- More foreign-born people are likely to graduate from high school than natives.
- More foreign-born people are likely to speak English less than well.
- More foreign-born people are likely to be unemployed.
- More foreign-born people are likely to earn less than natives.
- More foreign-born people are likely to live in poverty than natives.

There are estimated (as of 2007) to be 12 million undocumented people living in the United States. It is extremely difficult to count the number of people who are hiding because they are not documented. It is widely recognized that the population is growing by about 275,000 people each year. California is the leading state of residence for undocumented people. Other states include Texas, New York, and Florida.

There has been an effort by the government to tighten both immigration and travel access to the United States since the terrorist attacks in September 2001. On July 22, 2002, the Justice Department announced that it would use criminal penalties against immigrants and foreign visitors who fail to notify the government of change of address within 10 days. This requirement is not a new one, but it has not been strictly enforced. This will have an impact on at least 11 million people and visitors who stay in the United States for more than 30 days (Davis & Furtado, 2002, p. A2). In addition, this will have an impact on the health care system and on providers of health care both directly and indirectly. For example, it will be more difficult for people to work here and to visit family members who are ill. In addition, the passage of Proposition 187 in California in November 1994, and earlier laws relating to bilingual education in Texas, demonstrates that many citizens are no longer willing to provide basic human services, such as health care and education, to new residents in general and those who are undocumented specifically. Thus far, the implementation of these laws has been held up in the courts. Despite such efforts, however, it is evident that immigration to this country will continue. It is predicted that by the year 2020, immigration will be a major source of new people for the United States and will be responsible for whatever growth occurs in the United States after 2030. The United States will continue to attract about two-thirds of the world's immigrants, and 85% will be from Central and South America. Other immigration events are noted in Box 3–2.

On May 17, 2007, the U.S. president and a bipartisan group of senators reached bipartisan agreement on comprehensive immigration reform. The proposal included the following points:

1. Putting border security and enforcement first.
2. Providing tools for employers to verify the eligibility of the workers they hire.
3. Creating a temporary worker program.
4. No amnesty for illegal immigrants.

Box 3–2

Highlights of Immigration History: 1798–2007

Year	Event
1790	Naturalization Act passed
1798	Alien and Sedition Acts passed
1808	African slave trade prohibited
1819	First immigrant data collected
1824	Naturalization set at 2 years
1846	Potato famine in Ireland results in massive Irish influx
1862	Homestead Act opens land to immigrants
1870	Naturalization extended to Africans
1875	Federal government regulates immigration
1882–1943	Chinese Exclusion Act passed
1886	Statue of Liberty opens
1892	Ellis Island Immigration Station opens
1898	Immigrants classified by "race"
1903	Political radicals banned from entering the United States
	Call for rules governing entry into this country from Mexico
1907	Immigration Act to stem the flow of immigrants from Mexico
	1,004,756 people—a record—pass through Ellis Island
1908	"Gentleman's Agreement" restricts Japanese immigration
1910	Entrance barred to criminals, paupers, and the diseased
1917	Literacy required for immigrants over 16
1924	Annual racial quotas established; Border Patrol established
1940	Alien Registration Act—predecessor to the Green Card—passed
1942–1964	Bracero Program allows entry to temporary workers
1975	Vietnam War ends; Indochinese refugee program implemented
1980	Mariel boatlift from Cuba of 125,000 people occurs
1986	Amnesty for illegal aliens granted
1990	Ellis Island Immigration Museum opens
1996	Illegal Immigration Reform and Immigrant Responsibility Act of 1996 passed
1996	Personal Responsibility and Work Opportunity Reconciliation Act of 1996 passed
1996	Antiterrorism and Effective Death Penalty Act of 1996 passed
1999	Nursing Relief for Disadvantaged Areas Act of 1999 passed
2001	USA Patriot Act of 2001 passed
2002	Family Sponsor Immigration Act of 2002 passed
2002	Enhanced Security and Visa Entry Reform Act of 2002 passed
2003	Extension of the Special Immigrant Religious Worker Program passed
2003	Department of Homeland Security begins
2005	Disadvantaged Areas Reauthorization Act passed

(continued)

Box 3–2 *Continued*

Year	Event
2006	Secure Fence Act passed
2006	National Defense Authorization Act for Fiscal Year 2006 passed
2007	Failure of immigration reform

Sources: Lefcowitz, E. (1990). *The United States immigration history timeline.* New York: Terra Firma Press. Reprinted with permission; RapidImmigration. (2012). Significant Historic Dates in U.S. Immigration. Retrieved from http://www.rapidimmigration.com/1_eng_immigration_history.html, February 25, 2011; Homeland Security. (2010). Retrieved from http://www.dhsgov/index.shtm.

5. Strengthening the assimilation of new immigrants: the proposal declares that English is the language of the United States.
6. Establishing a merit system for future immigration.
7. Ending chain migration.
8. Clearing the family backlog in 8 years (Homeland Security, 2007).

This legislation did not pass, however, and will not be addressed until after the 2012 presidential election. As of this writing, the issue has not been resolved. Individual states have imposed their own laws regulating the residency of undocumented people but most of these laws have been struck down by the courts.

The need for strict enforcement of Title VI and the Culturally and Linguistically Appropriate Services (CLAS) standards becomes self evident when you realize the high numbers of people who do not understand and speak English, as seen in Table 3–6.

■ Poverty

There are countless ways to answer the question "What is poverty?" Poverty may be viewed through many lenses and from anthropological, cultural, demographic, economical, educational, environmental, historical, medical, philosophical, policy, political, racial, sexual, sociological, and theological points of view. The consequences of poverty are ubiquitous. They include, but are not limited to, battering, bullying, child abuse, gaming, obesity, spousal abuse, substance abuse, and violence. Poverty may also be viewed in a "holistic" way. Here, the physical, mental, and spiritual aspects of poverty are self-evident. Examples include, but are not limited to,

■ physical—substandard housing, no telephone or vehicle, limited access to health care;
■ mental—inadequate education, poor opportunity; and
■ spiritual—despair, the experience of being disparaged.

In 2005–2009, 39.5 million people, approximately 13.5% of the population, lived below the poverty level (American Fact Finder 2010). Poverty rates differ by age, gender, race, and ethnicity. For example, the rates of poverty in 2005–2009 were

- 25.1% for Blacks;
- 21.9% for Hispanics;
- 10.8% for non-Hispanic Whites;
- 18.6% for children under 18;
- 9.8% for adults over 65.

The federal government has an extensive history of efforts to improve the conditions of people living with limited incomes and material resources. Since the 1850s, there have been countless initiatives enacted to help citizens who were "poor." The programs described in Table 3–7 are examples of federal cash assistance programs available to low-income families.

Other ways of answering the question "what is poverty" include:

1. Using the description provided by the U.S. Bureau of Labor Statistics, which counts the poor and describes them by age, education, location, race, family composition, and employment status.
2. Using the federal government's definition of the poverty threshold. This poverty threshold, developed in 1965, is based on pretax income only, excluding capital gains, and does not include the value of

Table 3–7　Selected Examples of Federal Poverty Programs

Purpose	Program	Description
Cash aid	Temporary Assistance for Needy Families (TANF)	Basic cash aid through state Requires work
Food and nutrition	Food Stamps	Provides, depending on need, funding for food
	Special Supplemental Nutrition Program for Women, Infants, and Children (WIC)	Provides benefits for low-income mothers, infants, and children considered to be "at risk"
Medical	Medicaid	Provides payments to health care providers in full or in a co-pay for eligible low-income families and individuals, and for long-term care to those eligible who are aged or disabled
Housing	Section 8 Low-Income Housing Assistance	Provides rental assistance through vouchers or rental subsidies to eligible low-income families

Source: Nilsen, S. (2007). Poverty in America—Report to Congressional Requesters. Washington, DC: United States Government Accountability Office.

noncash benefits, such as employer-provided health insurance, food stamps, or Medicaid. The poverty-level figures are used by programs, such as Head Start, Low-Income Home Energy, and National School Lunch, to determine eligibility (U.S. Census Bureau, 2011).

3. Determining the poverty status, for people not living in families, by comparing the individual's income to his or her threshold. The poverty thresholds are updated annually to allow for changes in the cost of living using the Consumer Price Index (Bishaw & Macartney, 2010, p. 1).

The poverty threshold for an average family of four was $23,018 in 2011.

Table 3–8 lists the poverty weighted threshold for persons in a household for selected years.

The association between socioeconomic status and the health status of a person or family may be explained in part by the reduced access to health care among those with lower socioeconomic status. Income may be related to health because it

■ increases access to health care;

■ enables the person or family to live in a better neighborhood;

■ enables the person or family to afford better housing;

■ enables the person or family to reside in locations not abutting known environmentally degraded locations (heavy industrial pollution or known hazardous waste sites); and

■ increases the opportunity to engage in health promoting behaviors.

Health also may affect income by restricting the type and amount of employment a person may seek or by preventing a person from working.

Table 3–8 Poverty Weighted Average Thresholds for the Years 1986–2011 by Persons in Household

Year	First Person	Two Persons	Four Persons
1986	$5,572	$7,138	$11,203
1990	6,652	8,509	13,359
1994	7,547	9,661	15,141
1998	8,316	10,634	16,660
2002	9,183	11,756	18,392
2006	10,294	13,167	20,614
2010	11,139	14,218	22,314
2011	11,491	14,667	23,018

Sources: U.S. Census Bureau. Retrieved from http://www.census.gov/hhes/www/poverty/data/threshld/thresh86. html; http://www.census.gov/hhes/www/poverty/data/threshld/thresh90.html; http://www.census.gov/hhes/www/ poverty/data/threshld/thresh94.html; http://www.census.gov/hhes/www/poverty/data/threshld/thresh98.html; http:// www.census.gov/hhes/www/poverty/data/threshld/thresh02.html; http://www.census.gov/hhes/www/poverty/data/ threshld/thresh06.html; and http://wwwcensus.gov, April 12, 2012; Federal Register 63, no. 36. (1998, February 24), 9235–9238, and (2002, February 14), 6931–6933; U.S. Census Bureau. (2006, August 29).

There has been an increase in earning inequality over the last 25 years. The income for all races rose, then dipped, in this time period. For Blacks and Hispanics, it was much lower than for Whites and Asians and for people from the Pacific Islands. Much of this change and inequality was due to technological changes that increased income to highly skilled labor. At the same time, less skilled workers saw their wages decrease or stagnate. The other factors responsible for this phenomenon include

- globalization of the economy;
- decline in the real minimum wage;
- decline in unionization;
- increase in immigration; and
- increase in families headed by women (from 10% in 1970 to 18% in 1996 and 24.7% in 2000—households headed by women generally have lower incomes). In fact, in households headed by women, with no husband present, the percentage below the poverty level was 9.7% in 2009.

The following are compelling examples of the poverty in the United States:

- Nationally, 13.8% of the U.S. population was in poverty during the 5 years, 2006–2010, according to the estimate from the 5-year American Community Survey's data. (Bishaw, A. (2011) Areas With Concentrated Poverty: 2006–2010 American Community Survey Retrieved from http://www.census.gov/prod/2011pubs/acsbr10-17.pdf February 26, 2011).
- In 2009 alone, 43.6 million people were in poverty, up from 39.8 million in 2008—the third consecutive annual increase in the number of people in poverty.
- The poverty rate in 2009 (14.3%) was the highest poverty rate since 1994 but was 8.1 percentage points lower than the poverty rate in 1959, the first year for which poverty estimates are available.
- The number of people in poverty in 2009 (43.6 million) is the largest number in the 51 years for which poverty estimates have been published.
- Between 2008 and 2009, the poverty rate increased for children under the age of 18 (from 19.0% to 20.7%) and people aged 18 to 64 (from 11.7% to 12.9%), but decreased for people aged 65 and older (from 9.7% to 8.9%) (DeNavas-Walt, Proctor, & Smith, 2011, p. 14).

The poverty status of people between 2005 and 2009 for

- Blacks was 22.1%;
- Non-Hispanic Whites was 10.8%;
- American Indians and Alaska natives was 25.9%;

- Non-Hispanic Whites was 7.5%;
- Asians was 10.9%;
- Hispanics was 21.9%; and
- people 65 years old and over was 10.2% (Bishaw & Macartney, S. (2010)).

Cycle of Poverty

Poverty is more than the absence of money. One way of analyzing the phenomenon is by observing the effects of the "cycle of poverty," as illustrated in Figure 3–5. In this cycle, the person lives in a situation that may create poor intellectual and physical development and poor economic production, and in which the birth rate is high; this living situation in turn, causes numerous social problems and lower employment abilities, which creates insufficient salaries and a subsistence economy that often forces the person to reside in densely populated areas or remotely located rural areas where adequate shelter and potable

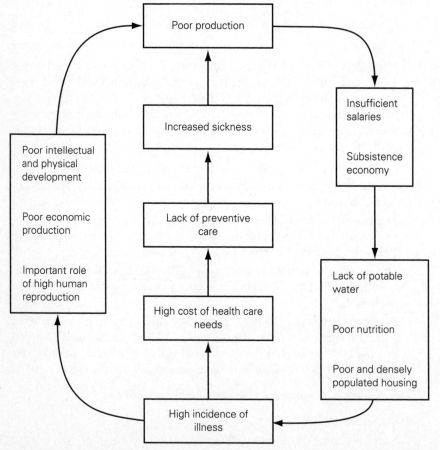

Figure 3–5 The Cycle of Poverty.

water are scarce, and the person suffers from chronically poor nutrition. These conditions all too often lead to high morbidity and accident rates, precipitating high health care costs, which, in turn, prevent the person from seeking health care services. Thus, there is an increase in sickness and poor production, in a cycle that has yet to be broken. Other barriers that are interrelated to this cycle are the lack of access to health care services, language issues, and transportation issues (Spector, 1979, pp. 148–152).

The issues of overcrowded housing, poor sanitation, inadequate nutrition, homelessness, and so forth that are part of the cycle of poverty have a profound and prolonged impact on the health status of people and in future generations.

This chapter has presented an overview of the major phenomena contributing to the profound diversity existing within the United States—demographic; population and immigration; and poverty. Additional issues will be explored in more depth in the chapters relating to each of the major population groups described in Census 2010.

Explore 🌐 MediaLink

Go to the Student Resource Site at nursing.pearsonhighered.com for chapter-related review questions, case studies, and activities. Contents of the CULTURALCARE Guide and CULTURALCARE Museum can also be found on the Student Resource Site. Click on Chapter 3 to select the activities for this chapter.

Box 3-3: Keeping Up

The following resources will be helpful in maintaining current information related to the demographics of your location, the United States, and your state; immigration issues and policies; and poverty:

United States Census 2010 http://2010.census.gov/2010census/

Department of Homeland Security http://www.dhs.gov/index.shtm

Poverty: United States Census Bureau http://www.census.gov/hhes/www/poverty/

■ Internet Sources

American Fact Finder. (2005–2009). Selected Characteristics of the Native and Foreign-Born Population. American Community Survey. Retrieved from http://factfinder.census.gov/servlet/STTable?_bm=y&-geo_id=01000US&-qr_name=ACS_2009_5YR_G00_S0501&-ds_name=ACS_2009_5YR_G00_&-redoLog=false, July 7, 2011.

Bishaw, A., & Macartney, S. (2010). Poverty: 2008 and 2009. U.S. Census Bureau American Community Survey Briefs. Retrieved from http://www.census.gov, July 7, 2011.

Bishaw, A. (2011). Areas With Concentrated Poverty: 2006–2010. American Community Survey. Retrieved from http://www.census.gov/prod/2011pubs/ac-sbr10-17.pdf, February 26, 2011.

DeNavas-Walt, C., Proctor, B. D., & Smith, J. C. (2010). Income, Poverty, and Health Insurance Coverage in the United States: 2009. U.S. Census Bureau. Retrieved from http://www.census.gov, July 7, 2011.

Howden, L. M., & Meyer, J. A. (2011). Age and Sex Composition: 2010. U.S. Census Bureau. Retrieved from http://2010.census.gov/news/releases/operations/cb11-cn147.html, May 30, 2011.

Humes, K. R., Nicholas, A. J., & Ramirez, R. (2011). Overview of Race and Hispanic Origin: 2010. Census Briefs. p. 4. Retrieved from http://2010.census.gov/2010census/data/, June 26, 2011.

Lee, J. (2011). Annual Flow Report U.S. Naturalizations: 2010. Washington, DC: U.S. Department of Commerce, Economics and Statistics Administration, Office of Homeland Security, Office of Immigration Statistics. Retrieved from http://www.dhs.gov/files/statistics/publications/gc_1302103955524.shtm, June 1, 2011.

Monger, R. & Yankay, J. (2011). U.S. Legal Permanent Residents: 2010 Annual Flow Report. Washington, DC: U.S. Department of Commerce, Economics and Statistics Administration, Office of Homeland Security, Office of Immigration Statistics. Retrieved from http://www.dhs.gov/files/statistics/publications/gc_1301497627185.shtm, June 1, 2011.

Nilsen, S. (2007). Poverty in America: Report to Congressional Requesters. Washington, DC: United States Government Accountability Office. Retrieved from www.gao.gov/cgi-bin/getrpt, July 21, 2007.

RapidImmigration. (2012). Significant Historic Dates in U.S. Immigration. Retrieved from http://www.rapidimmigration.com/1_eng_immigration_history.html, February 25, 2011).

U.S. Census Bureau. (2011). Preliminary Estimate of Weighted Poverty Thresholds for 2011. Retrieved from http://www.census.gov/hhes/www/poverty/data/threshld/index.html, April 12, 2011.

U.S. Census Bureau. (2010). American Community Survey. Retrieved from http://factfinder2.census.gov/faces/tableservices/jsf/pages/productview.xhtml?fpt=table, December 16, 2011.

U.S. Census Bureau. (2006). Current Population Survey. Annual Social and Economic Supplement. Last revised: August 29, 2006. Retrieved from http://pubdb3.census.gov/macro/032006/pov/new35_000.htm.

U.S. Census Bureau. (2001). Retrieved from http://www.census.gov/popest/national/asrh/NC-EST2009-asrh.html, December 16, 2011.

U.S. Department of Homeland Security. (2011). Learn about the United States: Quick Civics Lessons for the Naturalization Test 2011. Retrieved from www.uscis.gov/citizenship, July 7, 2011.

U.S. Department of Homeland Security. (2007). Press Release. Administration and Bipartisan Group of Senators Reach Bipartisan Agreement on Comprehensive Immigration Reform. Washington, DC: Department of Homeland Security. p. 1. Retrieved from http://www.dhs.gov/xnews/releases/pr_1179511978687.shtm, March 1, 2008.

United States Department of Homeland Security. (2007). United States History and Government Questions. Washington, DC: United States Citizenship and Immigration Services. Retrieved from http://www.uscis.gov/portal/site/uscis/menuitem.5af9bb95919f35e66f614176543f6d1a/?vgnextoid=12e596981298d010VgnVCM10000048f3d6a1RCRD&vgnextchannel=96719c7755cb9010VgnVCM10000045f3d6a1RCRD, March 1, 2008.

■ References

Davis, F., & Furtado, C. (2002, July 22). INS to enforce change-of-address rule. *Boston Globe*, p. A2.

Greeley, A. (1978). *Why can't they be like us? America's white ethnic groups.* New York: E. P. Dutton.

Lefcowitz, E. (1990). *The United States immigration history timeline.* New York: Terra Firma Press.

Novak, M. (1973). How American are you if your grandparents came from Serbia in 1888? In S. Te Selle (Ed.), *The rediscovery of ethnicity: Its implications for culture and politics in America.* New York: Harper & Row.

Spector, M. (1979). Poverty: The barrier to health care. In R. E. Spector (Ed.), *Cultural diversity in health and illness* (pp. 141–162). New York: Appleton, Century & Crofts.

Thernstrom, S. (Ed.). (1980). *Harvard encyclopedia of American ethnic groups.* Cambridge: Harvard University Press.

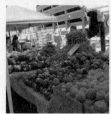 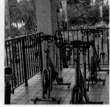 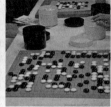 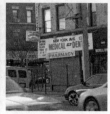

Figure 4-1　　　**Figure 4-2**　　　**Figure 4-3**　　　**Figure 4-4**

Chapter 4

Health and Illness

All things are connected. Whatever befalls the earth befalls the children of the earth.

—*Chief Seattle Suqwamish and Duwamish*

■ Objectives

1. Understand health and illness and the social determinants that affect them.
2. Reexamine and redefine the concepts of health and illness.
3. Understand the multiple relationships between health and illness.
4. Associate the concepts of good and evil and light and dark with health and illness.
5. Describe significant components of *Healthy People 2020*.
6. Analyze the concept of health disparities.
7. Analyze the Health Belief Model from both the provider and patient points of view.
8. Analyze the classical sick roles as described by Parsons, Alksen, and Suchman.
9. Analyze the natural history of the health-illness trajectory.

The opening images for this chapter represent—"The Four Corners of Health and Illness"—facets of health and illness in various stages along the health/illness continuum. Figure 4–1 is suggestive of maintaining health and the fresh, well-balanced food, especially fresh vegetables that must be included in a healthy diet. One of the greatest signs of a healthy person is that of being able to accomplish demanding physical challenges; in Figure 4–2, the bicycles are reminders of the workouts available at most gymnasiums and the notion of being fit. Figure 4–3 represents a resource from within the Asian-American communities—the game of Go. The game requires concentration and skill and is highly competitive. Figure 4–4 represents resources for primary care and over-the-counter remedies that may be used both for health maintenance and to restore health when everyday ailments occur.

There are countless images we can use to visualize comprehensive notions of health and illness. What do you do daily to maintain your health? Where do you go for help? What do you do when you experience a self-limiting ailment? How are ideas of health and illness reflected throughout the contemporary dominant culture in your family and home community? The community you work in? If you could pick four images relating to health and illness from your day-to-day experiences, what would they be?

■ Health

The answers to the question "What is health?" are not as readily articulated as you might assume. One response may be a flawless recitation of the World Health Organization (WHO) definition of *health* as a "state of complete physical, mental, and social well-being and not merely the absence of disease." This answer may be recited with great assurance—a challenge is neither expected nor welcomed but may evoke an intense dispute in which the assumed right answer is completely torn apart. Answers such as "homeostasis," "kinetic energy in balance," "optimal functioning," and "freedom from pain" are open to discussion. Experienced health care providers may be unable to give a comprehensive, acceptable answer to such a seemingly simple question. It is difficult to give a definition that makes sense without the use of some form of medical jargon. It is also challenging to define *health* in terms that a layperson can understand. (We lack skill in understanding "health" from the layperson's perspective.) It is not unusual to hear health care providers define health in a negative manner—"the absence of disease."

When you google *health*, the response on the World Wide Web is that there have been over 4.400 billion results as of February 29, 2012. One basic dictionary definition for the term is "health (helth) a state of physical, mental, and social well-being" (Dorland's Medical Dictionary, 2007).

As long ago as 1860, Florence Nightingale described health as "being well and using one's powers to the fullest extent." Health is "a condition of physical, mental, and social well-being and the absence of disease or other abnormal condition." It is not a static condition. Constant change and adaptation to stress result in homeostasis. René Dubos, often quoted in nursing education, says, "The states of health or disease are the expressions of the success or failure experienced by the organism in its efforts to respond adaptively to environmental challenges." Health can also be defined as high-level wellness, homeostasis (Mosby's Medical Dictionary, 2009).

These definitions—varying in scope and context—are essentially those that the student practitioner and educator within the health professions agree convey the meaning of *health*; albeit, the most widely used and recognized definition is that of WHO. Within the socialization process of the health care deliverer, the denotation of the word is that contained in the WHO definition. For other students, the meaning of the word *health* becomes clear through the educational experience.

In analyzing these definitions, we are able to discern subtle variations in denotation. In fact, the connotation does not essentially change over time. If this occurs in the denotation of the word, what of the connotation? That is, are health care providers as familiar with implicit meanings as with more explicit ones? Historically, Irwin M. Rosenstock (1966) commented that the health professions are becoming increasingly aware of the lack of clarity in the definition of *health*. This situation has not changed. Surely, this is a contemporary and an accurate thought on the educational process, which is indeed deficient. He concluded, "Whereas health itself is in reality an elusive concept, in much of research, the stages involved in seeking medical care are conceived as completely distinct" (p. 49). Furthermore, it may be argued that the connotation of health is most frequently seen as a 2-dimensional phenomenon—body and mind—with the larger emphasis on the body.

The framework of both education and research in the health professions continues to rely on the more abstract definitions of the word *health*. When taken in a broader context, health can be regarded not only as the absence of disease but also as a reward for "good behavior." In fact, a state of health is regarded by many people as the reward one receives for "good" behavior and illness as punishment for "bad" behavior. You may have heard something like "She is so good; no wonder she is so healthy" or a mother admonishing her child, "If you don't do such and such, you'll get sick." Situations and experiences may be avoided for the purpose of protecting and maintaining one's health. Conversely, some people seek out challenging, albeit dangerous, situations with the hope that they will experience the thrill of a challenge and still emerge in an intact state of health. Examples of such behavior include driving at high speeds, ongoing tobacco smoking, and not wearing seat belts.

Health can also be viewed as the freedom from and the absence of evil. In this context, health is analogous to day, which equals good light. Conversely, illness is analogous to night, evil, and dark. Illness, to some, is seen as a punishment for being bad or doing evil deeds; it is the work of vindictive evil spirits. In the modern education of health care providers, these concepts of health and illness are rarely if ever discussed, yet, if these concepts of health and illness are believed by some consumers of health care services, understanding these varying ideas is important for the provider. Each of us enters the health care community with our own culturally based concept of health. During the educational and socialization process in a health care provider profession—nursing, medicine, or social work—we are expected to shed these beliefs and adopt the standard definitions. In addition to shedding these old beliefs, we learn, if only by unspoken example, to view as deviant those who do not accept the prevailing, institutional connotation of the word *health*. In fact, you may agree, health tends to be defined as the absence of disease and not as a condition in its own right.

The following discussion illustrates the complex process necessary to enable providers to return to and appreciate our former interpretations of health, to understand the vast number of meanings of the word *health*, and to be aware of the difficulties that exist with definitions such as that of the World Health Organization.

How Do YOU Define Health?

You have been requested to describe the term *health* in your own words, and before you read further, jot down your definition of health. You may initially respond by reciting the WHO definition. What does this definition really mean? The following is a representative sample of actual responses:

1. Being able to do what I want to do.
2. Physical and psychological well-being: *physical* meaning that there are no abnormal functions with the body—all systems are without those abnormal functions that would cause a problem physically— and *psychological* meaning that one's mind is capable of a clear and logical thinking process and association.
3. Being able to use all of your body parts in the way that you want to—to have energy and enthusiasm.
4. Being able to perform your normal activities, such as working, without discomfort and at an optimal level.
5. The state of wellness with no physical or mental illness.
6. I would define health as an undefined term: it depends on the situations, individuals, and other things.

In the initial step of the unlocking process, it begins to become clear that no single definition fully conveys what health really is.[1] We can all agree on the WHO definition, but when asked "What does that mean?" we are unable to clarify or to simplify that definition. As we begin to perceive a change in the connotation of the word, we may experience dismay, as that emotional response accompanies the breaking down of ideas. When this occurs, we begin to realize that as we were socialized into the health care provider culture by the educational process our understanding of health changed, and we moved a great distance from our older cultural understanding of the term. The following list includes the definitions of *health* given by students at various levels of

---

[1]The unlocking process includes those steps taken to help break down and understand the definitions of both terms—*health* and *illness*—in a living context. It consists of persistent questioning: What is health? No matter what the response, the question "What does that mean?" is asked. Initially, this causes much confusion, but in classroom practice—as each term is written on the chalkboard and analyzed—the air clears and the process begins to make sense.

education and experience. The students ranged in age from 19-year-old college juniors to graduate students in both nursing and social work.

Junior Students (Age 18–19)

■ A system involving all subsystems of one's body that constantly works on keeping one in good physical and mental condition

Senior Students (Age 20–21)

■ Ability to function in activities of daily living to optimal capacity without requiring medical attention
■ Mental and physical wellness
■ The state of physical, mental, and emotional well-being

Graduate Students (Age 30+/−)

■ Ability to cope with stressors; absence of pain—mental and physical
■ State of optimal well-being, both physical and emotional
■ State of well-being that is free from physical and mental distress; I can also include in this social well-being, even though this may be idealistic
■ Not only the absence of disease but a state of balance or equilibrium of physical, emotional, and spiritual states of well-being

It appears that the definition becomes more abstract and technical as the student advances in the educational program. The terms explaining health take on a more abstract and scientific character with each year of removal from the lay mode of thinking. Can these layers of jargon be removed, and can we help ourselves once again to view heath in a more tangible manner?

In further probing this question, let us think back to the way we perceived health before our entrance into the educational program. I believe that the farther back we can go in our memory of earlier concepts of health, the better. Again, the question "What is health?" is asked over and over. Initially, the responses continue to include such terms and phrases as "homeostasis," "freedom from disease," or "frame of mind." Slowly, and with considerable prodding, we are able to recall earlier perceptions of health. Once again, health becomes a personal, experiential concept, and the relation of health to being returns. The fragility and instability of this concept also are recognized as *health* gradually acquires meaning in relation to the term *being* and is seen in a positive light and not as "the absence of disease."

This process of unlocking a perception of a concept takes a considerable amount of time and patience. It also engenders dismay that briefly turns to anger and resentment. You may question why the definitions acquired and mastered in the learning process are now being challenged and torn apart. The feeling may be that of taking a giant step backward in a quest for new terminology and new knowledge.

With this unlocking process, however, we are able to perceive the concept of health in the way that a vast number of health care consumers may perceive it.

The following illustrates the transition that the concept passed through in an unlocking process from the WHO definition to the realm of the health care consumer.

Initial Responses

- Feeling of well-being, no illness
- Homeostasis
- Complete physical, mental, and social well-being

Secondary Responses

- Frame of mind
- Subjective state of psychosocial well-being
- Ability to perform activities of daily living

Experiential Responses

Health becomes tangible; the description is illustrated by using qualities that can be seen, felt, or touched.

- Shiny hair
- Warm, smooth, glossy skin
- Clear eyes
- Shiny teeth
- Being alert
- Being happy
- Harmony between body and mind

Even this itemized description does not completely answer the question "What is health?" The words are once again subjected to the question "What does that mean?" and once again the terms are stripped down, and a paradox begins to emerge. For example, *shiny hair* may, in fact, be present in an ill person or in a person whose hair has not been washed for a long time, and a healthy person may not always have clean, well-groomed, lustrous hair. It becomes clear that, no matter how much we go around in a circle in an attempt to define *health*, the terms and meanings attributed to the state can be challenged. As a result of this prolonged discussion, we never really come to an acceptable definition of *health*, yet, by going through the intense unlocking process, we are able, finally, to understand the ambiguity that surrounds the word. We are, accordingly, less likely to view as deviant those people whose beliefs and practices concerning their own health and health care differ from ours.

Health Maintenance and Protection

Health can be seen from many other viewpoints, and many areas of disagreement arise with respect to how *health* can be defined. The preparation of health care providers tends to organize their education from a perspective of illness. Rarely (or superficially) does it include an in-depth study of the concept of health. The emphasis in health care delivery has shifted from acute care to preventive care. The need for the provider of health services to comprehend this concept is therefore crucial. As this movement for preventive health care continues to grow, to become firmly entrenched, and to thrive, multiple issues must be constantly addressed in answering the question "What is health?" *Unless the provider is able to understand health from the viewpoint of the patient, a barrier of misunderstanding is perpetuated.* It is difficult to reexamine complex definitions dutifully memorized at an earlier time, yet an understanding of health from a patient's viewpoint is essential to the establishment of comprehensive primary health care services inclusive of health maintenance and protection services because, as has been discussed, the perception of health is a complex psychological process. There tends to be no established pattern in what individuals and families see as their health needs and how they go about practicing their own health care.

Health maintenance and protection or the prevention of illness are by no means new concepts. As long as human beings have existed, they have used a multitude of methods—ranging from magic and witchcraft to present-day immunization and lifestyle changes—in an ongoing effort to maintain good health and prevent debilitating illness and death. Logic suggests that in order to maintain health we must prevent disease, and that is best accomplished by complying with immunization schedules, enforced by school policies; eating balanced meals, including avoiding salt and cholesterol; exercising regularly; and seeing a nurse practitioner, physician, or other health care provider once a year for a checkup. The annual ritual of visiting a health care provider has been extensively promoted by the health care establishment and is viewed as effective by numerous laypeople, primarily those who have access to these services. A provider's statement of good health is often required by a person seeking employment or life insurance. Furthermore, the annual physical examination has been advertised as the key to good health. A "clean bill of health" is considered essential for social, emotional, and even economic success. This clean bill of health is bestowed only by members of the health care profession. The general public has been conditioned to believe that health is guaranteed if a disease that may be developing is discovered early and treated with the ever-increasing varieties of modern medical technology. Although many people believe in and practice the annual physical and screening for early detection of a disease, there are some—both within and outside the health care professions—who do not subscribe to it. Preventive medicine grew out of clinical practice associated either with welfare medicine or with industrial or occupational medical practice. The approach of preventive medicine and health maintenance is the focus of health care practice in the United States among many segments of the population at large. However, countless disparities in overall health, and in access and utilization of the health care delivery system, exist and these will become increasingly evident as we progress through this text.

Healthy People 2020

In 1979, the Surgeon General's Report, *Healthy People: The Surgeon General's Report on Health Promotion and Disease Prevention* was published. This seminal report was followed by *Healthy People 1990: Promoting Health/Preventing Disease: Objectives for the Nation*—a series of concrete objectives for addressing national public health issues. A decade later, this document was followed by *Healthy People 2000: National Health Promotion and Disease Prevention Objectives*. These early documents presented the initiative for a national strategy for significantly improving the health of the American people in the decades preceding 2000 and the decades to follow. The documents recognized that lifestyle and environmental factors are major determinants in disease prevention and health promotion. They provided strategies for significantly reducing preventable death and disability, for enhancing quality of life, and for reducing disparities in health status among various population groups within our society. *Healthy People 2000: National Health Promotion and Disease Prevention and Objectives* was a statement of national opportunities, and was followed by *Healthy People 2010* that was adjusted to continue in this trajectory; *Healthy People 2020*, released in early 2011, has been designed to continue this momentum.

The *Healthy People* series provides science-based, 10-year national objectives for improving the health of all Americans. Over the past decades, *Healthy People* has established benchmarks and monitored progress in order to

1. encourage collaborations in different areas and disciplines,
2. guide individuals toward making informed health decisions, and
3. measure the impact of prevention activities.

The critical questions *Healthy People* addresses are

1. What makes some people healthy and others unhealthy?
2. How can we create a society in which everyone has a chance to live long healthy lives?

Healthy People 2020 is now exploring these questions by

1. developing objectives that address the relationship between health status and biology, individual behavior, health services, social factors, and policies and
2. emphasizing an ecological approach to disease prevention and health promotion.

The authors of *Healthy People* now view the determinants of health to be "the range of personal, social, economic, and environmental factors that influence health status." It is the interrelationships among the factors that determine the health status of a person and population, and poor health outcomes are often made worse by the interaction between individuals and their social and physical environment. It goes without saying that access to health services and the quality of health services can impact a given person's health. There are several barriers to health care services, such as cost, availability of health care resources, and lack of insurance.

Health equity is defined in *Healthy People 2020* as the "attainment of the highest level of health for all people. Achieving health equity requires valuing everyone equally with focused and ongoing societal efforts to address avoidable inequalities, historical and contemporary injustices, and the elimination of health and health care disparities" (Office of Disease Prevention and Health Promotion, 2011b).

Health disparities are defined in *Healthy People 2020* as

> a particular type of health difference that is closely linked with social, economic, and/or environmental disadvantage. They adversely affect groups of people who have systematically experienced greater obstacles to health based on their racial or ethnic group; religion; socioeconomic status; gender; age; mental health; cognitive, sensory, or physical disability; sexual orientation or gender identity; geographic location; or other characteristics historically linked to discrimination or exclusion. (Office of Disease Prevention and Health Promotion, 2011b)

During the past 2 decades of *Healthy People*, the overarching goals have focused on health disparities. In *Healthy People 2000*, this goal was to reduce health disparities among Americans. In *Healthy People 2010*, it was to eliminate, not just reduce, health disparities. In *Healthy People 2020*, that goal has been expanded even further "to achieve health equity, eliminate disparities, and improve the health of all groups" (Office of Disease Prevention and Health Promotion, 2011b).

Many dimensions of disparity exist in the United States, particularly in health and health care. If a health outcome, such as the incidence of a health problem, is seen in a greater or lesser extent between populations, there is a disparity. It is crucial to recognize that social determinants, which can also be viewed as "demographic disparities" have a profound impact on health outcomes of specific populations (Office of Disease Prevention and Health Promotion, 2011b). This situation will be further illustrated in the forthcoming chapters. In each of Chapters 9–12, there will be numerous examples of the existing health and demographic disparities.

The Health Belief Model

The Health Belief Model (Figures 4–5A and 4–5B) is useful for transitioning from a discussion of health to that of illness. It illustrates the patient's perceptions of health and illness and can be modified to reflect the viewpoint of health care providers. When implemented from the provider's viewpoint, the material provides a means of reinspecting the differences between professional and lay beliefs and expectations. Forging a link between the two helps one better understand how people perceive themselves in relation to illness and what motivates them to seek medical help and then follow that advice.

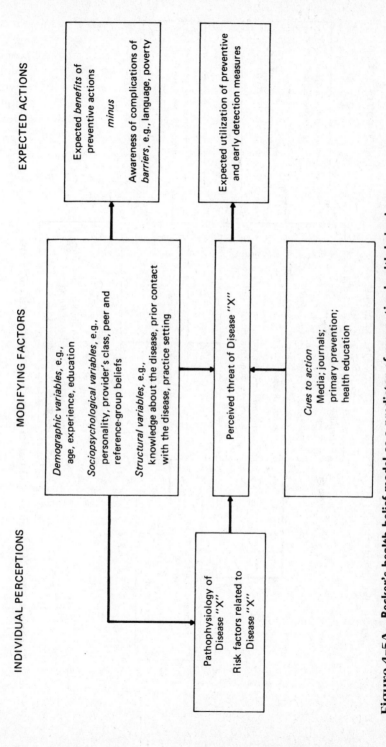

Figure 4-5A Becker's health belief model as a predictor of preventive health behavior.

Source: Becker, M. H. (1974). *The Health Belief Model and Personal Health Behavior.* Thorofare, NJ: B. Slack.

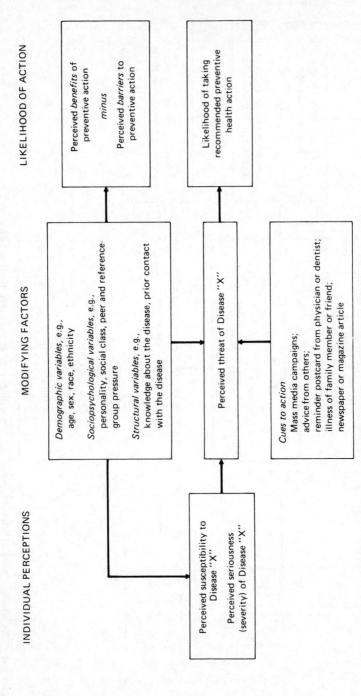

Figure 4–5B The health belief model from the patient's point of view.

Perceived Susceptibility. How susceptible to a certain condition do people consider themselves to be? For example, a woman whose family does not have a history of breast cancer is unlikely to consider herself susceptible to that disease. A woman whose mother and maternal aunt both died of breast cancer may well consider herself highly susceptible, however. In this case, the provider may concur with this perception of susceptibility on the basis of known risk factors.

Perceived Seriousness. The perception of the degree of a problem's seriousness varies from one person to another. It is in some measure related to the amount of difficulty the patient believes the condition will cause. From a background in pathophysiology, the provider knows—within a certain range—how serious a problem is and may withhold information from the patient. The provider may resort to euphemisms in explaining a problem. The patient may experience fear and dread by just hearing the name of a problem, such as cancer.

Perceived Benefits: Taking Action. What kinds of actions do people take when they feel susceptible, and what are the barriers that prevent them from taking action? If the condition is seen as serious, they may seek help from a doctor or some other significant person, or they may vacillate and delay seeking and using help. Many factors enter into the decision-making process. Several factors that may act as barriers to care are cost, availability, and the time that will be missed from work.

From the provider's viewpoint, there is a protocol governing who should be consulted when a problem occurs, when during that problem's course help should be sought, and what therapy should be prescribed.

Modifying Factors. The modifying factors shown in Figures 4–5A and 4–5B indicate the areas of conflict between patient and provider.

The variables of race and ethnicity are cited most often as complex problem areas when the provider is White and middle-class (or from one sociocultural economic class and the patient is from another) and the patient is a member of the emerging majority. The issues are complex and include overtones of personal and institutional racism. Such perceptions vary not only among groups but also among individuals.

Social class, peer group, and reference group pressures also vary between the provider and patient and among different ethnic groups. For example, if the patient's belief about the causes of illness is "traditional" and the provider's is "modern," an inevitable conflict arises between the 2 viewpoints. This conflict is even more evident when the provider either is unaware of the patient's traditional beliefs or is aware of the manifestation of traditional beliefs and practices and devalues them. Quite often, class differences exist between the patient and the provider. The reference group of the provider may well be that of the "technological health system," whereas the reference group of the patient may well be that of the "traditional system" of health care and health care deliverers.

Structural variables also differ when the provider and the patient see the problem from different angles. Often, each is seeing the same thing but is using different terms (or jargon) to explain it. Consequently, neither understands the other. Reference group problems also are manifested in this area, and the news and broadcast media are an important structural variable.

In summary, this section has attempted to deal solely with the concept of health. The multiple denotations and connotations of the word have been explored. A method for helping you tune in to your health has been presented, a transitional discussion illustrating the plethora of issues to be raised later in the text has been included, and an overview of *Healthy People 2020* has set the tone for the remainder of the text, and the Health Belief Model serves to provide a context for the discussion.

■ Illness

It is a paradox that the world of illness is the one that is most familiar to the providers of health care. It is in this world that the provider feels most comfortable and useful. Many questions about illness need to be answered:

- What determines illness?
- How do you know when you are ill?
- What prompts you to seek help from the health care system?
- At what point does self-treatment seem no longer possible?
- Where do you go for help? And to whom?

We tend to regard illness as the absence of health, yet we demonstrated in the preceding discussion that *health* is at best an elusive term that defies a specific definition. Let us look at the present issue more closely. Is illness the opposite of health? Is it a permanent condition or a transient condition? How do you know if you are ill?

When you google *illness*, the response on the World Wide Web is well over 37,500,000 results in 0.19 seconds (February 29, 2012). One basic dictionary definition for this term is an unhealthy condition of body or mind: SICKNESS (© 2005 by Merriam-Webster Incorporated). Another definition is found in Mosby's Medical Dictionary: unhealthy condition, an abnormal process in which aspects of the social, physical, emotional, or intellectual condition and function of a person are diminished or impaired compared with that person's previous condition" (Mosby's Medical Dictionary, 2009).

What is illness? A generalized response, such as "abnormal functioning of a body's system or systems," evolves into more specific assessments of what we observe and believe to be wrong. Illness is a sore throat, a headache, or a fever—the last one determined not necessarily by the measurement on a thermometer but by a flushed face; a warm-to-hot feeling of the forehead, back, and abdomen; and overall malaise. The diagnosis of intestinal obstruction is described as pain in the stomach (abdomen), a greater pain than that caused by "gas," accompanied by severely upset stomach, nausea, vomiting, and marked constipation.

Essentially, we are being pulled back in the popular direction and encouraged to use lay terms. We initially resist this because we want to employ professional jargon. (Why use lay terms when our knowledge is so much greater?) It is crucial that we be called to task for using jargon. We must learn to be constantly conscious of the way in which the laity perceive illness and health care.

Another factor emerges as the word *illness* is stripped down to its barest essentials. Many of the characteristics attributed to health occur in illness, too. You may receive a rude awakening when you realize that a person perceived as healthy by clinical assessment may then—by a given set of symptoms—define him- or herself as ill (or vice versa). For example, in summertime, one may see a person with a red face and assume that she has a sunburn. The person may, in fact, have a fever. A person recently discharged from the hospital, pale and barely able to walk, may be judged ill. That individual may consider himself well, however, because he is much better than when he entered the hospital—now he is able to walk! Thus, perceptions are relative and, in this instance, the eyes of the beholder have been clouded by inadequate information. Unfortunately, at the provider's level of practice, we do not always ask the patient, "How do you view your state of health?" Rather, we determine the patient's state of health by objective and observational data.

As is the case with the concept of health, we learn in nursing or medical school how to determine what illness is and how people are expected to behave when they are ill. Once these terms are separated and examined, the models that health care providers have created tend to carry little weight. There is little agreement as to what, specifically, illness is, but we nonetheless have a high level of expectation as to what behavior should be demonstrated by both the patient and the provider when illness occurs. We discover that we have a vast amount of knowledge with respect to the acute illnesses and the services that ideally must be provided for the acutely ill person. When contradictions surface, however, it becomes apparent that our knowledge of the vast gray area is minimal—for example, whether someone is ill or becoming ill with what may later be an acute episode. Because of the ease with which we often identify cardinal symptoms, we find we are able to react to acute illness and may have negative attitudes toward those who do not seek help when the first symptom of an acute illness appears. The questions that then arise are "What is an acute illness, and how do we differentiate between it and some everyday indisposition that most people treat by themselves?" and "When do we draw the line and admit that the disorder is out of the realm of adequate self-treatment?"

These are certainly difficult questions to answer, especially when careful analysis shows that even the symptoms of an acute illness tend to vary from one person to another. In many acute illnesses, the symptoms are so severe that the person experiencing them has little choice but to seek immediate medical care. Such is the case with a severe myocardial infarction, but what about the person who experiences mild discomfort in the epigastric region? Such a symptom could lead the person to conclude he or she has indigestion and to self-medicate with baking soda, an antacid, milk, or Alka-Seltzer. A person who experiences mild pain in the left arm may delay seeking care, believing the pain will disappear. Obviously, this person may be as ill as the person who seeks help during the onset of symptoms but will, like most people, minimize these small aches because of not wanting to assume the sick role.

The Sick Role

The seminal work of Talcott Parsons (1966) helps explain the phenomenon of "the sick role." In our society, a person is expected to have the symptoms viewed as illness confirmed by a member of the health care profession. In other words, the sick role must first be legitimately conferred on this person by the keepers of this privilege. You cannot legitimize your own illness and have your own diagnosis accepted by society at large. There is a legitimate procedure for the definition and sanctioning of the adoption of the sick role and it is fundamental for both the social system and the sick individual. Thus, illness is not only a "condition" but also a social role. Parsons describes 4 main components of the sick role:

1. "The sick person is exempted from the performance of certain of his/her normal social obligations." An example is a student or worker who has a severe sore throat and decides that he or she does not want to go to classes or work. For this person to be exempted from the day's activities, he or she must have this symptom validated by someone in the health care system, a provider who is either a physician or a nurse practitioner. The claim of illness must be legitimized or socially defined and validated by a sanctioned provider of health care services.

2. "The sick person is also exempted from a certain type of responsibility for his/her own state." For example, an ill person cannot be expected to control the situation or be spontaneously cured. The student or worker with the sore throat is expected to seek help and then to follow the advice of the attending physician or nurse in promoting recovery. The student or worker is not responsible for recovery except in a peripheral sense.

3. "The legitimization of the sick role is, however, only partial." When you are sick, you are in an undesirable state and should recover and leave this state as rapidly as possible. The student's or worker's sore throat is acceptable only for a while. Beyond a reasonable amount of time—as determined by the physician or nurse, peers, and the faculty or supervisors—legitimate absence from the classroom or work setting can no longer be claimed.

4. "Being sick, except in the mildest of cases, is being in need of help." Bona fide help, as defined by the majority of American society and other Western countries, is the exclusive realm of the physician or

nurse practitioner. A person seeking the help of the provider now not only bears the sick role but in addition takes on the role of patient. Patienthood carries with it a certain, prescribed set of responsibilities, some of which include compliance with a medical regimen, cooperation with the health care provider, and the following of orders without asking too many questions, all of which lead to the illness experience.

The Illness Experience

The experience of an illness is determined by what illness means to the sick person. Furthermore, *illness* refers to a specific status and role within a given society. Not only must illness be sanctioned by a physician for the sick person to assume the sick role, but it also must be sanctioned by the community or society structure of which the person is a member. Alksen, L., Wellin, E., Suchman, E., et al. (n.d.) divide this experience into four stages, which are sufficiently general to apply to any society or culture.

The first stage, onset, is the time when the person experiences the first symptoms of a problem. This event can be slow and insidious or rapid and acute. When the onset is insidious, the patient may not be conscious of symptoms or may think that the discomfort will eventually go away. If, however, the onset is acute, the person is positive that illness has occurred and that immediate help must be sought. This stage is seen as the prelude to legitimization of illness. It is the time when the person with a sore throat in the preceding discussion may have experienced some fatigue, a raspy voice, or other vague symptoms.

In the second stage of the illness experience, diagnosis, the disease is identified or an effort is made to identify it. The person's role is now sanctioned, and the illness is socially recognized and identified. At this point, the health care providers make decisions pertaining to appropriate therapy. During the period of diagnosis, the person experiences another phenomenon: dealing with the unknown, which includes fearing what the diagnosis will be.

For many people, going through a medical workup is an unfamiliar experience. It is made doubly difficult because they are asked and expected to relate to strange people who are doing unfamiliar and often painful things to their bodies and minds. To the layperson, the environment of the hospital or the provider's office is both strange and unfamiliar, and it is natural to fear these qualities. Quite often, the ailing individual is faced with an unfamiliar diagnosis. Nonetheless, the person is expected to follow closely a prescribed treatment plan that usually is detailed by the health care providers but that, in all likelihood, may not accommodate a particular lifestyle. The situation is that of a horizontal-vertical relationship, the patient being figuratively and literally in the former position, the professional in the latter.

During the third stage, patient status, the person adjusts to the social aspects of being ill and gives in to the demands of his or her physical condition.

The sick role becomes that of patienthood, and the person is expected to shift into this role as society determines it should be enacted. The person must make any necessary lifestyle alterations, become dependent on others in some circumstances for the basic needs of daily life, and adapt to the demands of the physical condition as well as to treatment limitations and expectations. The environment of the patient is highly structured. The boundaries of the patient's world are determined by the providers of the health care services, not by the patient. Herein lies the conflict.

Much has been written describing the environment of the hospital and the roles that people in such an institution play. As previously stated, the hospital is typically unfamiliar to the patient, who, nevertheless, is expected to conform to a predetermined set of rules and behaviors, many of which are unwritten and undefined for the patient—let alone by the patient.

The fourth stage—recovery—is generally characterized by the relinquishing of patient status and the assumption of prepatient roles and activities. There is often a change in the roles a person is able to play and the activities able to be performed once recovery takes place. Often, recovery is not complete. The person may be left with an undesirable or unexpected change in body image or in the ability to perform expected or routine activities. One example is a woman who enters the hospital with a small lump in her breast and who, after a surgery, returns home with only one breast. Another example is that of a man who is a laborer and enters the hospital with a backache and returns home after a laminectomy. When he returns to work, he cannot resume his job as a loader. Obviously, an entire lifestyle must be altered to accommodate such newly imposed changes.

From the viewpoint of the provider, this person has recovered. His or her body no longer has the symptoms of the acute illness that made surgical treatment necessary. In the eyes of the former patient, illness persists because of the inability to perform as in the past. So many changes have been wrought that it should come as no surprise if the person seems perplexed and uncooperative. Here, too, there is certainly conflict between society's expectations and the person's expectation. Society releases the person from the sick role at a time when, subjectively, the person may not be ready to relinquish it.

Table 4–1 is a tool designed for the assessment of the patient during the four stages of illness. Originally designed as a sociological measuring tool, the material has been altered here to meet the needs of the health care provider in achieving a better understanding of patient behavior and expectations. If the provider is able to obtain answers from the patient to all the questions raised in Table 4–1, understanding the patient's behavior and perspective and subsequent attempts to provide safe, effective care become easier.

Another method of dividing the illness experience into stages was developed by Edward A. Suchman (1965). He described the following five components:

1. **The symptom experience stage.** The person is physically and cognitively aware that something is wrong and responds emotionally.

Table 4–1   The Patient's Point of View: A Tool for the Personal Assessment of the Patient during the Four Stages of Illness

	Onset	Diagnosis	Patient Status	Recovery
The Personal Meaning of a Given Illness	1. What were your first symptoms of this illness? 2. What do you think was the extent of this health problem? 3. What do you believe caused this problem? 4. How did this illness fit with your image of health? 5. Did you see this as a life-threatening illness? 6. Why did you seek help? 7. From whom did you seek help? 8. Where did you go for help—initially and later?	1. Did you understand the diagnosis? 2. How did you interpret the diagnosis? 3. Did you understand the diagnostic procedures that were performed? 4. Could you adapt to this health problem? 5. What do others think about this problem?	1. Has your understanding of this health problem changed? 2. What are your short-term and long-term goals? 3. What motivated you to recover?	1. How will you know you have recovered? 2. Will you be able to return to your daily routine and activities? 3. Has your self-image changed? 4. Do you see yourself as more vulnerable or more resilient?
Reaction to a Given Illness	1. How do you react and relate to this problem? 2. Were you anxious, and how did you cope with your anxiety? 3. How did you express your anxiety? 4. Did you seek care before you visited a physician or other health care provider?	1. What medical treatment was prescribed? 2. Did you use any other forms of treatment for this problem?	1. How did you feel in the role of patient? 2. How did you relate to the health care providers?	1. Do you know if you will have permanent aftereffects from this health problem? 2. How did you adapt to your former roles?

Source: Adapted from Alksen, L., Wellin, E., Suchman, E., et al. (n.d.). *A conceptual framework for the analysis of cultural variations in the behavior of the ill.* Unpublished report. New York City Department of Health.

2. **The assumption of the sick role stage.** The person seeks help and shares the problem with family and friends. After moving through the lay referral system, seeking advice, reassurance, and validation, the person is temporarily excused from such responsibilities as work, school, and other activities of daily living as the condition dictates.

3. **The medical care contact stage.** The person then seeks out the "scientific" rather than the "lay" diagnosis, wanting to know the following: Am I really sick? What is wrong with me? What does it mean? At this point, the sick person needs some knowledge of the health care system, what the system offers, and how it functions. This knowledge helps the person select resources and interpret the information received.

4. **The dependent-patient role stage.** The patient is now under the control of the physician and is expected to accept and comply with the prescribed treatments. The person may be quite ambivalent about this role, and certain factors (physical, administrative, social, or psychological) may create barriers that eventually will interfere with treatment and the willingness to comply.

5. **The recovery or rehabilitation stage.** The role of the patient is given up at the recovery stage, and the person resumes—as much as possible—his or her former roles.

The Natural History of the Health-Illness Continuum

Lastly, a way of explaining both health and illness is to explore the dynamics of the natural history of the health-illness continuum (Figure 4–6). Here, it is possible to follow the continuum or trajectory of a healthy state through an illness that a person may experience. This summarizes the social science approaches that have been discussed to answer our fundamental questions—"What is health?" and "What is illness?"—and begins to shift our focus to the responses and experiences people have both to and with states of health and illness. The focus now begins to move to the active role the person plays in shaping and experiencing the course of a state of health and a given illness. For example, the *seemingly healthy* person who develops an illness may experience the following continuum: healthy state—he or she is carrying on activities of daily living, actively participating in family life, work, other activities and so forth; an illness—the symptoms of an illness may be acute, silent, or subtle in nature—occurs; the person may recover spontaneously or with treatment, or comeback and resume his or her life in an expected manner or resume his or her earlier stable status; or, the illness episode may be more severe, and the person may become unstable or experience the illness as a chronic condition; he or she may, over time, deteriorate; and at some point death occurs. The person may die with the onset of the acute phase or later in the continuum. The acute phase most often is treated in the home or an acute care setting, and the early phases of comeback and rehabilitation occur in one of these settings.

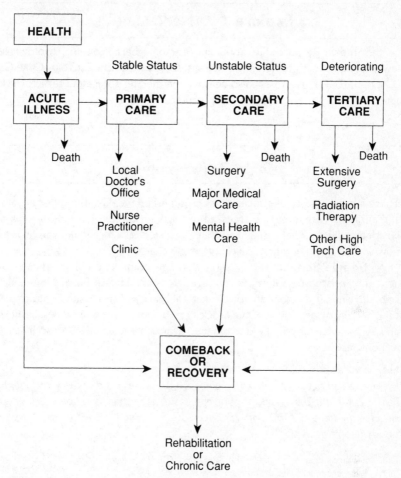

Figure 4–6   The natural history of the health-illness continuum.

The management of the chronic phase, except for acute episodes, is performed at home or in an institution that is either a rehabilitation facility or a long-term care institution. The illness may profoundly affect the lives of the ill and his or her family in the scope of day-to-day living and hopes for the future.

As you can see, there have been countless explanatory words and models developed over time to define *health*, *illness*, and the experiences of each. Each of these theories is valid; each of them is time-tested; each is relevant as we go forward in time and space.

In summary, this chapter has presented an introductory overview of the modern culture's perception of health and illness through countless lenses. The writings of a number of preeminent theorists and sociologists have been examined in terms of applicability to health care. Box 4-2 suggests resources that provide timely information.

Explore 🌐 MediaLink

Go to the Student Resource Site at nursing.pearsonhighered.com for chapter-related review questions, case studies, and activities. Contents of the CULTURALCARE Guide and CULTURALCARE Museum can also be found on the Student Resource Site. Click on Chapter 4 to select the activities for this chapter.

Box 4-2: Keeping Up

There are countless references that are published weekly, monthly, annually, and periodically that may be accessed to maintain currency in the domains of health and illness. There is also a wealth of historical articles that can now be downloaded at either a nominal charge or no charge.

Google Scholar (http://scholar.google.com/) is a search engine for literature related to countless topics, such as the Health Belief Model, sick role, the illness trajectory and/or the natural history of the health illness trajectory, and disparities. Many of the articles can be purchased from the publishers, and several articles may be downloaded at no charge as pdfs. It also links to dictionaries.

Healthy People 2020
Follow the progress of *Healthy People 2020*, review the history of *Healthy People 2000 and 2010*, and examine the evaluations that have been conducted on *Healthy People 2000 and 2010* on the following website: http://www.healthypeople.gov/hp2020/.

Office of Disease Prevention and Health Promotion. (2011b). *Healthy People 2020*. Rockville, MD: U.S. Department of Health and Human Service.

■ Internet Sources

Dorland's Medical Dictionary for Health Consumers. © 2007 by Saunders, an imprint of Elsevier, Inc. http://medical-dictionary.thefreedictionary.com/health

Mosby's Medical Dictionary, 8th edition. © 2009, Elsevier. http://medical-dictionary.thefreedictionary.com/health

Office of Disease Prevention and Health Promotion. (2011a). Healthy People 2020 Rockville, MD: U.S. Department of Health and Human Service. Retrieved from http://www.healthypeople.gov/hp2020/, January 11, 2011.

Office of Disease Prevention and Health Promotion. (2011b). Healthy People 2020 Rockville, MD: U.S. Department of Health and Human Service. Retrieved from http://www.healthypeople.gov/2020/about/disparities About.aspx, April 30, 2011.

■ References

Alksen, L., Wellin, E., Suchman, E., et al. (n.d.). *A conceptual framework for the analysis of cultural variations in the behavior of the ill.* Unpublished report (p. 2). New York: New York City Department of Health.

Becker, M. H. (1974). *The health belief model and personal health behavior.* Thorofare, NJ: B. Slack.

Kozier, B., Erb, G., Berman, A. J., & Burke, K. (2000). *Fundamentals of nursing concepts, process, and practice.* Upper Saddle River, NJ: Prentice Hall Health.

Mechanic, D. (1968). *Medical sociology* (p. 80). New York: Free Press of Glencoe.

National Center for Health Statistics (NCHS). (2007). *Health United States 2007.* Hyattsville, MD: Author.

Nightingale, F. (1860, 1946). (A fascimile of the first edition published by D. Appleton and Co.). *Notes on nursing—What it is, what it is not.* New York: Appleton-Century.

Parsons, T. (1966). Illness and the role of the physician: A sociological perspective. In W. R. Scott & E. H. Volkart (Eds.), *Medical care: Readings in the sociology of medical institutions* (p. 275). New York: John Wiley & Sons.

Rogers, M. (1989). Nursing: A science of unitary human beings. In Riehl-Sisca, J. (Ed.), *Conceptual Models for Nursing Practice* (3rd ed., pp. 181–188). Norwalk, CT: Appleton & Lange.

Rosenstock, I. M. (1966, July). Why people use health services. *Millbank Memorial Fund Quarterly, 44*(3), 94–127.

Suchman, E. A. (1965, fall). Stages of illness and medical care. *Journal of Health and Human Behavior, 6*(3), 114.

Unit

II

HEALTH
Domains

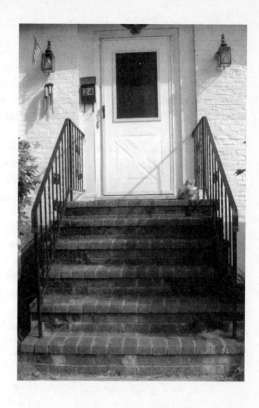

Unit II develops the "plot" of this book by providing background material for the central themes discussed in this text. Imagine climbing the stairs in the opening figure, and this unit will bring you to the fifth step. Chapters 5 and 6 will explore the concepts of HEALTH and will describe **traditional**[1] ways of maintaining, protecting, and restoring HEALTH and magico-religious traditions related to HEALING and HEALING practices. Chapter 7 will help you to explore your heritage and learn about the traditional HEALTH and HEALING beliefs and practices from your background.

■ HEALTH

HEALTH and the countless ways by which it is maintained, protected, and restored is the foundation of this text. *HEALTH* connotes the **balance** of a person, both within one's being—physical, mental, and spiritual—and in the outside world—natural, familial and communal, and metaphysical. The HEALTH Traditions Model is a method for describing beliefs and practices used to **maintain** through daily HEALTH practices, such as diet, activities, and clothing; to **protect** through special HEALTH practices, such as food taboos, seasonal activities, and protective items worn, carried, or hung in the home or workplace; and/or to **restore** through special HEALTH practices, such as diet changes, rest, special

[1]Tradition is the handing down of statements, beliefs, legends, customs, and information, from generation to generation, especially by word of mouth or by practice.

clothing or objects, **physical**, **mental**, and/or **spiritual** HEALTH. The accompanying image Figure II-1, *salud*, is a metaphor for HEALTH in countless ways. Here, it is whole and emerging from the shadows of early morning. Just as the sand sculpture is fragile, disappearing overnight, so, too, is HEALTH. It brings to mind the reality that HEALTH is finite, and each of us has the internal responsibility to maintain, protect, and restore our HEALTH; the reciprocal holds true for the external familial, environmental, and societal forces—they, too, must look after and safeguard our HEALTH. This book, in part, is a mirror that reflects the countless ways by which people are able to maintain, protect, and/or restore their HEALTH. Just as there is an interplay between a sand sculpture and the natural forces that can create and harm and destroy it, so, too, it is with HEALTH and the forces of the outside world.

ILLNESS is the imbalance of the person, both within one's being—physical, mental, and spiritual—and in the outside world—natural, familial and communal, and metaphysical. HEALING is the restoration of this balance. The relationships of the person to the outside world are reciprocal.

When these terms, HEALTH, ILLNESS, and HEALING, are used in small capitals in this text, it is to connote that they are being used holistically. When they are written in the general text font—health, illness, and healing—they are to be understood in the common way.

Chapter 8 will present an overview of the issues related to the modern, scientific, high-technology health care delivery system in general and will discuss why an analytical understanding of the modern allopathic philosophy relevant in this arena is so vital in regard to the development of a holistic philosophy of HEALTH, HEALING, and CULTURALCARE.

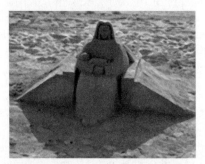

Figure II-1 Sand Sculpture—Postiquet Beach, Alicante, Spain.

The chapters in Unit II will present an overview of relevant historical and contemporary theoretical content that will help you to

1. Describe traditional aspects of HEALTH care.[2]
2. Describe traditional HEALTH care philosophies and systems.

[2]Small capital letters are used to differentiate traditional definitions of ILLNESS and HEALING from contemporary definitions.

3. Discuss various forms of HEALING practices.

4. Trace your family's beliefs and practices in
   a. Health/HEALTH maintenance,
   b. Health/HEALTH protection,
   c. Health/HEALTH restoration, and
   d. Curing/HEALING.

5. Discuss the interrelationships of sociocultural, public health, and medical events that have produced the crises in today's modern health care system.

6. Trace the complex web of factors that
   a. contribute to the high cost of health care,
   b. discuss ways of paying for health care services, and
   c. impede a person's passage through the health care system.

7. Describe common barriers to utilization of the health care system.

8. Compare and contrast the modern and traditional systems of health/ HEALTH care.

   As you proceed through this unit, you will encounter several activities that link Unit I to Unit II and will help the content resonate and come alive. These are activities in which several people may participate and share their experiences.

1. Re-answer questions 5–12 from Unit I, thinking of HEALTH rather than health. (Remember, when HEALTH is in small capital letters, it is to designate it as a holistic phenomenon, rather than dualistic, as is the common way it is defined.) They are the following questions:

   How do you define *HEALTH*?
   How do you define *ILLNESS*?
   What do you do to maintain your HEALTH?
   What do you do to protect your HEALTH?
   What do you do when you experience a noticeable change in your HEALTH?
   Do you diagnose your own HEALTH problems? If yes, how do you do so? If no, why not?
   From whom do you seek HEALTH care?
   What do you do to restore your HEALTH? Give examples.

2. To whom do you turn first when you are ILL? Where do you go next?

3. You have just moved to a new location. You do not know a single person in this community. How do you find health/HEALTH care resources?

4. Visit an emergency room in a large city hospital. Visit an emergency room in a small community hospital. Spend some time quietly observing what occurs in each setting.
   a. How long do patients wait to be seen?
   b. Are patients called by name—first name, surname—or number?
   c. Are relatives or friends allowed into the treatment room with the patient?

5. Determine the cost of a day of hospitalization in an acute care hospital in your community.
   a. How much does a room cost? How much is a day in the intensive care unit or coronary care unit? How much is time in the emergency room? How is a surgical procedure charged?
   b. How much is charged for diagnostic procedures, such as a computed tomography (CT) scan or an ultrasound? How much is charged for equipment, such as a simple intravenous (IV) setup?
   c. What are the pharmacy charges for medications such as "clot busters," antibiotics, cardiac medications, and so forth?
   d. How many days, or hours, are women kept in the hospital after delivery of a child? Is the newborn baby sent home at the same time? If not, why not? What is the cost of a normal vaginal delivery or cesarean section and normal newborn care?

6. Visit a homeopathic pharmacy or a natural food store and examine the shelves that contain herbal remedies and information about alternative or complementary HEALTH care.
   a. What is the cost of a variety of herbal remedies used to maintain HEALTH or to prevent common ailments?
   b. What is the cost of a variety of herbal remedies used to treat common ailments?
   c. What is the range of costs for the books and other reading and instructional materials sold in the store?

7. What does your faith tradition teach you in terms of how to maintain, protect, and/or restore your HEALTH?

8. Attend a service in a house of worship with which you are not familiar. Inquire of the clergyperson what is taught or done within the faith tradition to maintain, protect, and/or restore HEALTH.

9. Visit a HEALER other than a physician in your community.

10. Attend a HEALING service.

11. Explore other methods of HEALING, such as massage, herbal therapy, or prayer.

12. Explore birth and birthing practices and traditions in both your heritage and others' than those derived from your own sociocultural heritage.

13. Explore end-of-life beliefs and practices and mourning traditions in both your own heritage and of people from other sociocultural heritages.

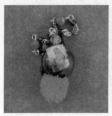 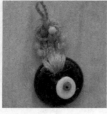 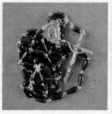 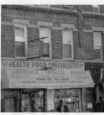

Figure 5-1   **Figure 5-2**   **Figure 5-3**   **Figure 5-4**

Chapter 5

HEALTH Traditions

You can do nothing to bring the dead to life; but you can do much to save the living from death.

—*B. Frank School (1924)*

■ Objectives

1. Describe traditional aspects of HEALTH care.
2. Describe the interrelated components of the HEALTH Traditions Model.
   a. Give examples of the traditional ways people maintain their physical, mental, and spiritual HEALTH.
   b. Give examples of the traditional ways people protect their physical, mental, and spiritual HEALTH.
   c. Give examples of the traditional ways people restore their physical, mental, and spiritual HEALTH.
3. Describe the factors that constitute traditional epidemiology.
4. Give examples of the choices that people have in health care.
5. Give examples of the traditional HEALTH care philosophies and systems.
6. Discover information available from the National Center for Complementary and Alternative Medicine.

The opening images in the chapter opener represent various methods people may use for the HEALTH—objects that may be used to protect, maintain, and/or restore physical, mental, or spiritual HEALTH and an example of a resource where some items may be purchased by people of many different heritages. These images contain items that are symbolic of the HEALTH Traditions Model and its themes, which will be discussed later in the chapter. Figure 5–1 is of a buck-eye with a small bead on top, red string, a red pompom, and an image of the Virgin of Guadalupe. It was purchased in a Mexican market in San Antonio, Texas. It is placed on an infant to protect his or her HEALTH. Figure 5–2 is a blue glass eye from Turkey. It may be pinned on clothing, pinned on a crib or bed, or hung in the home to protect the HEALTH of the baby, adult, or entire family. Figure 5–3, is rosary beads, symbolizes prayer and meditation methods used in both the spiritual maintenance and the maintenance and/or restoration of HEALTH. Figure 5–4 is a neighborhood health food store that sells numerous forms of HEALTH products such as herbs, tonics, and vegan items.

What are the sacred objects that you and your family may have hung in your home, placed on your bed, or worn? If you could pick four items from your heritage that are used to maintain or protect your HEALTH, what would they be? Do you know where the items can be purchased? Do you continue to use sacred objects to protect your HEALTH?

Health care providers have the opportunity to observe the most incredible phenomenon of life: health/HEALTH and the recovery, in most cases, from illness/HEALTH. In today's society, the healer is primarily thought by many to be the physician, and the other members of the health team all play a significant role in the maintenance and protection of HEALTH and the detection, and treatment of ILLNESS. However, human beings have existed, some sources suggest, for 2 million years. How, then, did the species *Homo sapiens* survive before the advent of the scientific methods and modern technology? What did the people of other times do to maintain, protect, and restore their health/HEALTH? It is quite evident that numerous forms of health/HEALTH care and healing/HEALING existed long before the technological methodologies that we apply today.

In the natural course of any life, a person can expect to experience the following set of events: He or she becomes ill/ILL; the illness/ILLNESS may be acute, with concomitant symptoms or signs, such as pain, fever, nausea, bleeding, depression, anxiety, or despair. On the other hand, the illness/ILLNESS may be insidious, with a gradual progression and worsening of symptoms, which might encompass slow deterioration of movement or a profound intensification of pain or desperation. Or the person may not experience symptoms, seek care for a routine ailment, and discover he or she has a near-fatal illness/ILLNESS.

If the illness/ILLNESS is mild, the person relies on self-treatment or, as is often the case, does nothing and gradually the symptoms disappear. If the illness/ILLNESS is more severe or is of longer duration, the person may consult expert help from a healer—usually, in contemporary times, a physician or nurse practitioner.

The person recovers or expects to recover. As far back as historians and interested social scientists can trace in the history of humankind, this phenomenon of recovery has occurred. In fact, it made very little difference what mode of treatment was used; recovery was expected and usual. It is this occurrence of natural recovery that has given rise to all forms of therapies and healing/HEALING beliefs and practices that attempt to explain a phenomenon that is natural. That is, one may choose to rationalize the success of a healing/HEALING method by pointing to the patient's recovery. Over the generations, natural healing/HEALING has been attributed to all sorts of rituals, including trephining (puncturing the skull), cupping, magic, leeching, and bleeding. From medicine man to sorcerer, the arts of maintaining, protecting, restoring health/HEALTH, and healing/HEALING have passed through succeeding generations. People knew the ailments of their time and devised treatments for them. In spite of ravaging plagues, disasters (both natural and those caused by humans), and pandemic and epidemic diseases, human beings as a species have survived!

This chapter explores the concepts of HEALTH and ILLNESS and the HEALTH Traditions Model; the choices people have in terms of folk medicine, natural, or magico-religious medicine; complementary and alternative methods of health/HEALTH maintenance, protection, and/or restoration; and other schools of health/HEALTH care in contemporary American society. Just as the understanding of health and illness is fundamental in the socialization process into the health care professions, the understanding of HEALTH and ILLNESS within the traditional context is fundamental to the development of CULTURAL COMPETENCY and the skills necessary to deliver CULTURALCARE.

■ HEALTH and ILLNESS

In this section, the "steps and bricks" of HEALTH and ILLNESS are going to be explored in greater depth. Once again, *HEALTH* is defined as "the balance of the person, both within one's beings—physical, mental, and spiritual—and in the outside world—natural, communal, and metaphysical, is a complex, interrelated phenomenon." On the other hand, *ILLNESS* is "the imbalance of one's being—physical, mental, and spiritual—and in the outside world—natural, communal, and meta-physical." When the terms *HEALTH* and *ILLNESS* are used in the remainder of this text, they denote the preceding definitions; small capitals are used to differentiate them from the terms *health* and *illness*, as defined in Chapter 4. *Health/HEALTH* and *illness/ILLNESS* are used in the text when there is an overlap between the terms.

The physical aspect of the person includes anatomical organs, such as the skin, skeleton, and muscles. It is our genetic inheritance, body chemistry, gender, age, and nutrition. The mind, mental, includes cognitive process, such as thoughts, memories, and knowledge. This includes emotional processes as feelings, defenses, and self-esteem. The spiritual facet includes both positive and negative learned spiritual practices and teachings, dreams, symbols, and stories; gifts and intuition; grace and protecting forces; and positive and negative metaphysical or innate forces. These facets are in constant flux and change over time, yet each is completely related to the others and related to the context of the person. The context includes the person's family, culture, work, community, history, and environment. There is also an overlap of the mental and spiritual facets of the person.

The person must be in a state of balance with the family, the community, and the forces of the natural world around him or her. This *balance* is what is perceived as HEALTH in a traditional sense and the way in which it is determined within most traditional cultures, as you will note in Chapters 9 through 13. ILLNESS, as stated, is the *imbalance* of one or all parts of a person (body, mind, and spirit); a person may be in a state of *imbalance* with the family, the community, or the forces of the natural world. The ways in which this *balance*, or harmony, is achieved, maintained, protected, or restored often differ from the prevailing scientific health philosophy of our modern societies. However, many of the traditional HEALTH-, ILLNESS-, and HEALING-related beliefs and practices exist today among people who know and live by the traditions of their own ethnocultural and/or religious heritage.

■ HEALTH Traditions Model

The HEALTH Traditions Model uses the concept of holistic HEALTH and explores what people do from a traditional perspective to maintain HEALTH, protect HEALTH or prevent ILLNESS, and restore HEALTH. HEALTH, in this traditional context, has nine interrelated facets, represented by

1. Traditional methods of maintaining HEALTH—physical, mental, and spiritual
2. Traditional methods of protecting HEALTH—physical, mental, and spiritual
3. Traditional methods of restoring HEALTH—physical, mental, and spiritual

The traditional methods of HEALTH maintenance, protection, and restoration require the knowledge and understanding of HEALTH-related resources from within a person's ethnocultural and religious heritage, and a reciprocal relationship exists between the person's needs and the available resources within the family and community to meet these needs. The methods may be used instead of or along with modern methods of health care. They are not alternative methods of health care because they are methods that are an integral part of a person's ethnocultural and religious heritage. Alternative, or complementary, medicine is a system of health care that persons may elect to use that is generic and not a part of his or her personal heritage. The burgeoning system of alternative medicine must not be confused with traditional HEALTH and ILLNESS beliefs and practices. In subsequent chapters of this book, traditional HEALTH and ILLNESS beliefs and practices are discussed, following (in part) the models (Figures 5-5 and 5-6). This model is two-dimensional in that it examines HEALTH as the internal perceptions of a person and addresses the ways by which a person can externally obtain the objects and/or substances necessary for his or her HEALTH. Tradition is the essential element in this model, and the model

	PHYSICAL	MENTAL	SPIRITUAL
MAINTAIN HEALTH	Proper clothing Proper diet Exercise/Rest	Concentration Social and Family support systems Hobbies	Religious worship Prayer Meditation
PROTECT HEALTH	Special foods and food combination Symbolic clothing	Avoid certain people who can cause illness Family activities	Religious customs Superstitions Wearing amulets and other symbolic objects to prevent the "Evil Eye" or defray other sources of harm
RESTORE HEALTH	Homeopathic remedies liniments Herbal teas Special foods Massage Acupuncture/ moxibustion	Relaxation Exorcism Curanderos and other traditional healers Nerve teas	Religious rituals—special prayers Meditation Traditional healings Exorcism

Figure 5-5 The nine interrelated facets of HEALTH (physical, mental, and spiritual) and personal methods of maintaining HEALTH, protecting HEALTH, and restoring HEALTH.

recognizes the fact that the role of tradition is fundamental. "When tradition is no longer adequate, human life faces the gravest crises" (Smith, 1991, p. 163). Given that the United States has been a melting pot, it has frequently weakened the traditions of immigrants during the processes of acculturation and assimilation, especially where health beliefs and practices are concerned. Many people relate that they "threw these practices away" when they came to the United States. Yet, for many people, modern medicine has not provided a compelling replacement. Examples of the barriers to modern health care are further explored in Chapter 8.

Traditional HEALTH Maintenance

The traditional ways of maintaining HEALTH are the active, everyday ways people go about living and attempting to stay well or HEALTHY—that is, ordinary

	PHYSICAL	MENTAL	SPIRITUAL
MAINTAIN HEALTH	Availability of Proper shelter, clothing, and food Safe air, water, soil	Availability of traditional sources of entertainment, concentration, and "rules" of the culture	Availability and promulgation of rules of ritual and religious worship Meditation
PROTECT HEALTH	Provision of the knowledge of necessary special foods and food combinations, the wearing of symbolic clothing, and avoidance of excessive heat or cold	Provision of the knowledge of what people and situations to avoid, family activities; Family activities	The teaching of: Religious customs Superstitions Wearing amulets and other symbolic objects to prevent the "Evil Eye" or how to defray other sources of harm
RESTORE HEALTH	Resources that provide Homeopathic remedies, liniments, Herbal teas, Special foods, Massage, and other ways to restore the body's balance of hot and cold	Traditional healers with the knowledge to use such modalities as: relaxation exorcism, storytelling, and/or Nerve teas	The availability of healers who use magical and supernatural ways to restore health: including religious rituals, special prayers, meditation, traditional healings, and/or Exorcism

Figure 5-6 The nine interrelated facets of HEALTH (physical, mental, and spiritual) and personal methods of maintaining HEALTH, protecting HEALTH and restoring HEALTH.

functioning within their family, community, and society. These include such actions as wearing proper clothing—boots when it snows and sweaters when it is cold, long sleeves in the sun, and scarves to protect from drafts and dust. Many traditional ethnic or religious groups may also prescribe garments, such as special clothing or head coverings. Many "special objects," such as hats to protect the eyes and face, long skirts to keep the body clean, down comforters to keep warm, special shoes for work and comfort, glasses to improve vision, and canes to facilitate walking, are used to maintain HEALTH, and they can be found in many traditional homes.

The food that is eaten and the methods for preparing it contribute to HEALTH. Here, too, one's ethnoreligious heritage plays a strong role in the determination of how foods are cooked, what combinations they may be eaten in, and what foods may be eaten. Foods are prepared in the home, and recipes from the family's tradition are followed. Traditional cooking methods do not use preservatives. Most foods are fresh and well prepared. Traditional diets are followed, and food taboos and restrictions are obeyed. Cleanliness of the self and the environment is vital. Hand washing and praying before and after meals are examples of necessary rituals.

Mental HEALTH in the traditional sense is maintained by concentrating and using the mind—reading and crafts are examples. There are countless games, books, music, art, and other expressions of identity that help in the maintenance of mental well-being. Hobbies also contribute to mental well-being.

The keys to maintaining HEALTH are, however, the family and social support systems. Spiritual HEALTH is maintained in the home with family closeness—prayer and celebrations. Rights of passage and kindred occasions are also family and community events. The strong identity with and connections to the "home" community are a great part of traditional life and the life cycle, as well as factors that contribute to HEALTH and well-being.

■ HEALTH Protection

The protection of HEALTH rests in the ability to understand the cause of a given ILLNESS or set of symptoms. Most of the traditional HEALTH and ILLNESS beliefs regarding the causation of ILLNESS differ from those of the modern epidemiological model. In modern epidemiology, we speak of viruses, germs, and other pathogens as the causative agents. In "traditional" epidemiology, factors such as the "evil eye," envy, hate, and jealousy may be the agents of ILLNESS.

Traditional Epidemiology

ILLNESS is most often attributed to the evil eye. The evil eye is primarily a belief that someone can project harm by gazing or staring at another's property or person (Maloney, 1976, p. 14). The belief in the evil eye is probably the oldest and most widespread of all superstitions, and it is found to exist in many parts of the world, such as southern Europe, the Middle East, and North Africa (Maloney, 1976, p. vi).

The evil eye is thought by some to be merely a superstition, but what is seen by one person as superstition may well be seen by another as religion. Various evil-eye beliefs were carried to this country by immigrant populations. These beliefs have persisted and may be quite strong among newer immigrants and heritage-consistent peoples (Maloney, 1976, p. vii).

The common beliefs in the evil eye assert that

1. The power emanates from the eye (or mouth) and strikes the victim.
2. The injury, be it illness or other misfortune, is sudden.

3. The person who casts the evil eye may not be aware of having this power.
4. The afflicted person may or may not know the source of the evil eye.
5. The injury caused by the evil eye may be prevented or cured with rituals or symbols.
6. This belief helps explain sickness and misfortune. (Maloney, 1976, p. vii)

The nature of the evil eye is defined differently by different populations. The variables include how it is cast, who can cast it, who receives it, and the degree of power it has. In the Philippines, the evil is cast through the eye or mouth; in the Mediterranean, it is the avenging power of God; in Italy, it is a malevolent force, like a plague, and is warded off by wearing amulets.

In different parts of the world, various people cast it: in Mexico—strangers; in Iran—kinfolk; and in Greece—witches. Its power varies, and in some places, such as the Mediterranean, it is seen as the "devil." In the Near East, it is seen as a deity and, among Slovak Americans, as a chronic but low-grade phenomenon (Maloney, 1976, p. xv).

Among Germans, the evil eye is known as *aberglobin* or *aberglaubisch*, and it causes preventable problems, such as evil, harm, and illness/ILLNESS. Among the Polish, the evil eye is known as *szatan*, literally, "Satan." Some "evil spirits" are equated with the devil and can be warded off by praying to a patron saint or guardian angel. *Szatan* also is averted by prayer and repentance and the wearing of medals and scapulars. These serve as reminders of the "Blessed Mother and the Patrons in Heaven" and protect the wearer from harm. The evil eye is known in Yiddish as *kayn aynhoreh*. The expression *kineahora* is recited by Jews after a compliment or when a statement of luck is made to prevent the casting of an evil spell on another's health/HEALTH. Often, the speaker spits three times after uttering the word (Spector, 1983, pp. 126–127).

Agents of disease may also be "soul loss," "spirit possession," "spells," and "hexes." Here, prevention becomes a ritual of protecting oneself and one's children from these agents. Treatment requires the removal of these agents from the afflicted person (Zola, 1972, pp. 673–679).

ILLNESS also can be attributed to people who have the ability to make others ILL—for example, witches and practitioners of voodoo. The ailing person attempts to avoid these people to prevent ILLNESS and to identify them as part of the treatment. Other "agents" to be avoided are "envy," "hate," and "jealousy." A person may practice prevention by avoiding situations that could provoke the envy, hate, or jealousy of a friend, an acquaintance, or a neighbor. The evil-eye belief contributes to this avoidance.

Another source of evil can be of human origin and occurs when a person is temporarily controlled by a soul not his or her own. In the Jewish tradition, this controlling spirit is known as *dybbuk*. The word comes from the Hebrew word meaning "cleaving" or "holding fast." A *dybbuk* is portrayed as a "wandering, disembodied soul which enters another person's body and holds fast" (Winkler, 1981, pp. 8–9).

Traditional practices used in the protection of HEALTH include, but are not limited to,

1. The use of protective objects—worn, carried, or hung in the home.
2. The use of substances that are ingested in certain ways and amounts or eliminated from the diet, and substances worn or hung in the home.
3. The practices of religion, such as the burning of candles, the rituals of redemption, and prayer.

Objects That Protect HEALTH

Amulets are sacred objects, such as charms, worn on a string or chain around the neck, wrist, or waist to protect the wearer from the evil eye or the evil spirits that could be transmitted from one person to another or have supernatural origins. For example, the *mano milagroso* (miraculous hand) (Figure 5–7) is worn by many people of Mexican origin for luck and the prevention of evil. A *mano negro* (black hand) (Figure 5–8) is placed on babies of Puerto Rican descent to ward off the evil eye. The *mano negro* is placed on the baby's wrist on a chain or pinned to the diaper or shirt and is worn throughout the early years of life.

Amulets may also be written documents on parchment scrolls, and these are hung in the home. Figure 5–9 is an example of a written amulet acquired in Jerusalem. It is hung in the home or workplace to protect the person, family, or business from the evil eye, famine, storms, diseases, and countless other dangers. Table 5–1 describes several practices found among selected ethnic groups to protect themselves from or to ward off the evil eye.

Bangles (Figure 5–10) are worn by people originating from the West Indies. The silver bracelets are open to "let out evil" yet closed to prevent evil from entering the body. They are worn from infancy, and as the person grows they are replaced with larger bracelets. The bracelets tend to tarnish and leave a black ring on the skin when a person is becoming ILL. When this

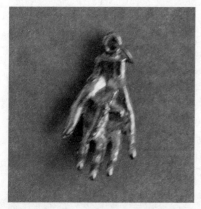

Figure 5-7 Mano milagroso.

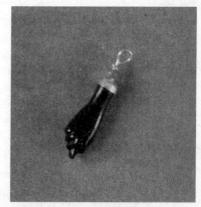

Figure 5-8 Mano negro.

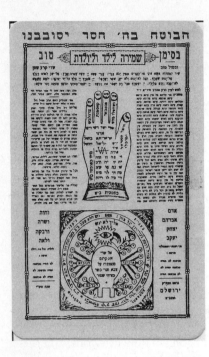

Figure 5-9 The Jerusalem amulet.
This amulet serves as protection
from pestilence, fire, bad wounds and
infection, the evil eye, bad decrees
and decisions, curses, witchcraft, and
from everything bad; to heal nervous
illness, weakness of body organs,
children's diseases, and all kinds of
suffering from pain; as a talisman
for livelihood for success, fertility,
honesty, and honor; and for charity,
love, mercy, goodness, and grace. It
also has the following admonition:
"Know before whom you stand—the
King of Kings, The Holy One, Blessed
be He."

Table 5-1 Practices to Ward Off the Evil Eye

Origin	Practices
Eastern European Jews	Red ribbon woven into clothes or attached to crib
Greece	Blue "eye" bead, crucifix, charms Phylacto—a baptismal charm placed on a baby Cloves of garlic pinned to shirt
Guatemala	Small red bag containing herbs placed on baby or crib
India	Red string worn on the wrist
India/Pakistan Hindus or Muslims	Copper plates with magic drawings rolled in them Slips of paper with verses from the Qur'an Black or red string around a baby's wrist
Iran	Child covered with amulets—agate, blue beads Children left filthy and never washed to protect them from the evil eye
Italians	Red ribbon worn on clothing The *corno* (horn) worn on a necklace
Mexico	Amulet or seed wrapped with red yarn
Philippines	Charms, amulets, medals
Puerto Rico	*Mano negro*

Table 5–1 Practices to Ward Off the Evil Eye (*continued*)

Origin	Practices
Scotland	Red thread knotted into clothing Fragment of Bible worn on body
Sephardic Jews	Blue ribbon or blue bead worn
South Asia	Knotted hair or fragment of Qur'an worn on body
Tunisia	Amulets pinned on clothing consisting of tiny figures or writings from the Qur'an Charms of the fish symbol—widely used to ward off evil

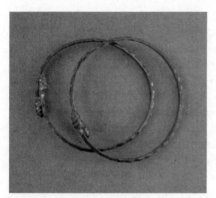

Figure 5–10 Bangles.

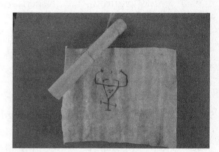

Figure 5–11 Talisman.

occurs, the person knows it is important to rest, to improve the diet, and to take other needed precautions. Many people believe they are extremely vulnerable to evil, even to death, when the bracelets are removed. Some people wear numerous bangles. When they move an arm, the bracelets tinkle. It is believed that this sound frightens away the evil spirit. Health care providers should realize that, when the bracelets are removed, the person experiences a great deal of anxiety.

In addition to amulets, there are talismans (Figure 5–11). A talisman is believed to possess extraordinary powers and may be worn on a rope around the waist or carried in a pocket or purse. The talisman illustrated in Figure 5–11 is a marionette, and it protects the wearer from evil. It is recommended that people who wear amulets or carry a talisman should be allowed to do so in health care institutions. The person who uses an amulet determines and interprets the meaning of the object.

Substances That Protect HEALTH

The second practice uses diet to protect HEALTH and consists of many different observances. People from many ethnic backgrounds eat raw garlic or onions

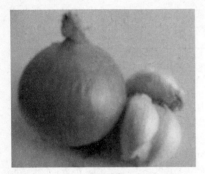

Figure 5-12 Garlic and onion.

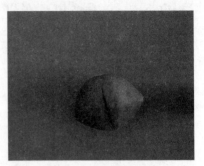

Figure 5-13 Chachayotel.

(Figure 5–12) in an effort to prevent ILLNESS. Garlic or onions also may be worn on the body or hung in the Italian, Greek, or Native American home. Chachayotel (Figure 5–13), a seed, may be tied around the waist by a Mexican person to prevent arthritic pain. Among traditional Chinese people, thousand-year-old eggs are eaten with rice to keep the body HEALTHY and to prevent ILLNESS. The ginseng root is the most famous of Chinese medicines. It has universal medicinal applications and is used preventively to "build the blood," especially after childbirth. Tradition states that, the more the root looks like a man, the more effective it is. Ginseng is also native to the United States and is used in this country as a restorative tonic (Figure 5–14).

Diet regimens also are used to protect HEALTH. It is believed that the body is kept in balance, or harmony, by the type of food one eats.

Traditionalists have strong beliefs about diet and foods and their relationship to the protection of HEALTH. The rules of the kosher diet practiced among Jewish people mandate the elimination of pig products and shellfish. Only fish with scales and fins are allowed, and only certain cuts of meat from animals

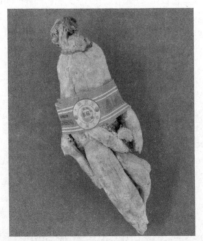

Figure 5-14 Ginseng root.

with a cleft hoof and that chew cud can be consumed. Examples of this kind of animal are cattle and sheep. Many of the dietary practices, such as the avoidance of pig products, are also adhered to by Muslims and the meats are halal, sanctioned by Islamic law. Jews also believe that milk and meat must never be mixed and eaten at the same meal.

In traditional Chinese homes, a balance must be maintained between foods that are *yin* or *yang*. These are eaten in specified proportions. In Hispanic homes, foods must be balanced as to "hot" and "cold." These foods, too, must be eaten in the proper amounts, at certain times, and in certain combinations. There are also foods that are consumed at certain times of the week or year and not during other times.

Spiritual Practices That Protect HEALTH

A third traditional approach toward HEALTH protection centers, in part, on religion. The words *spirituality* and *religion* are frequently used synonymously, but they are not the same. *Spirituality* connotes the way we orient ourselves toward the Divine, the way we make meaning out of our lives, the recognition of the presence of Spirit (breath) within us, a cultivation of a lifestyle consistent with this presence, and a perspective to foster purpose, meaning, and direction to life. It may find expression through religion, or religion may be a tool for finding one's spirit (Hopkins, E., Woods, L., Kelley, R., 1995, p. 11).

Religion is embedded in the life of many heritage-consistent traditional people in countless ways. For example, the religion's calendar gives order to people's lives by defining holidays in their season. A religion has sacred objects, spaces, and times; stipulates practices, such as dietary and wardrobe; teaches the rituals surrounding conception, pregnancy, birth, and the child's early life; and instructs how to bring babies into the world, and how to care for and remember the dead. It may also, in many cases, instruct how to protect ourselves from the envy of others and/or the evil eye (Leontis, A. 2009, p. 32). It strongly affects the way people choose to protect HEALTH, and it plays a strong role in the rituals associated with HEALTH protection. It dictates social, moral, and dietary practices that are designed to keep a person in balance. Many people believe that ILLNESS and evil are prevented by strict adherence to religious codes, morals, and practices. They view ILLNESS as a punishment for breaking a religious code. For example, I once interviewed a woman who believed she had cancer because God was punishing her for stealing money when she was a child. An example of a protective religious figure is the Virgin of Guadalupe (Figure 5–15), the patron saint of Mexico, who is pictured on medals that people wear or in pictures or icons hung in the home. She is believed to protect the person and home from evil and harm, and she serves as a figure of hope.

Religion and HEALTH

Religion helps to provide the believer with an ability to understand and interpret the events of the environment and life. Table 5–2 illustrates selected situations where religion and HEALTH intersect. Not every religious tradition

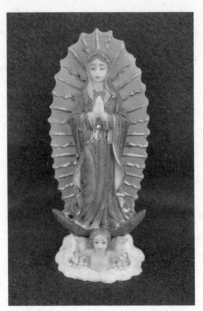

Figure 5-15   The Virgin of Guadalupe.

speaks to each situation. Most often, these situations are not overtly linked to HEALTH, but if thought through one can see their relationship. This discussion continues in Chapter 6.

Religion may, therefore, help provide the believer with an ability to understand and interpret the events of the environment and life.

HEALTH Restoration

HEALTH restoration in the physical sense can be accomplished by the use of countless traditional remedies, such as herbal teas, liniments, special foods and food combinations, massage, and other activities.

The restoration of HEALTH in the mental domain may be accomplished by the use of various techniques, such as performing exorcism, calling on traditional healers, using teas or massage, and seeking family and community support.

The restoration of HEALTH in the spiritual sense can be accomplished by healing rituals; religious healing rituals; or the use of symbols and prayer, meditation, special prayers, and exorcism. This will be further discussed in Chapter 6.

■ Health/HEALTH Care Choices

There are countless ways to describe and label health/HEALTH care beliefs, practices, and systems. "Health care" may be labeled as "modern," "conventional," "traditional," "alternative," "complementary," "allopathic," "homeopathic,"

Table 5-2 Selected Situations Where Religion and HEALTH Intersect

Physical	Mental	Spiritual
Agriculture—practices related to the planting, harvesting, and distributing of produce and meats	**Child rearing**—how, when and what children must be taught regarding rules of the given faith tradition	**Amulets and talismans**—sacred objects that may be worn, carried, or hung in the home
Blood—admonitions regarding the acceptance of blood transfusions	**Face**—how the essential part of the person must be safeguarded and that one must not compromise a person's face	**Beginning of life**—sacred ceremonies—baptism, circumcision, naming
Childbirth—numerous rituals and rites surrounding immediate birth		**Death**—rituals for funeral, burial, mourning, memorial services
Conception—prohibitions against birth control	**Familial relationships**—encourages close family bonds and respect for the elderly	**Dying**—confession, prayers
Death—the immediate care of the body after death	**Readings**—sacred readings developed to calm a person	**End-of-life care**—use of resuscitation and extreme care versus not using
Dietary practices—food prohibitions	**Sense of self and self in world**—answers to the questions: Who am I? and Why am I here?	**Forgiveness**—final words with family members and friends
Dying—care of the person in the final moments of life		**Pilgrimages**—visiting holy places such as shrines—sacred spaces
Exercise practices—physical daily care of the body	**Time**—weekly and seasonal festivals and holidays to set the rhythm of the year and keep person in balance	**Prayer times**—times of day when prayers are recited
Garments—special cloths and sacred clothes that must be worn at all times or for special occasions		**Prayer ways**—direction one faces, position of prayer, sacred garments that must be worn
Medications—admonitions to take prescribed medications		
Nature—respect for the sustainability of the earth and natural resources—stewardship		
Pregnancy—countless rules to be followed		
Specific maintenance & prevention practices—cleanliness—hand washing		

"folk," and so forth. The use of the word *traditional* to describe "modern health care" is, by definition, a misnomer. *Traditional* connotes a tradition—"The passing down of elements of a culture from generation to generation, especially by oral communication: *cultural practices that are preserved by tradition*," or "A mode of thought or behavior followed by a people continuously from generation to generation; a custom or usage" (American Heritage Dictionary of the English Language, 2011). The use of *traditional* to connote modern health care is a misnomer, as modern, allopathic, health care is a new science and has been passed down in writing for a relatively short amount of time, rather than orally over many generations.

There are also many reasons people may choose to use HEALTH care systems other than modern medical care. These include, but are not limited to, access issues, such as poverty, language, availability, and lack of insurance, and preference for familiar and personal care. *Traditional* here connotes HEALTH care beliefs and practices observed among peoples who steadfastly maintain their heritage and observe HEALTH care practices derived from their ethnocultural or religious heritage.

As stated earlier, in nearly every situation when a person becomes ill there is an expectation for the restoration of health/HEALTH, and the person usually recovers. As far back as historians and interested social scientists can trace in the extended history of humankind, the phenomenon of recovery has occurred. It made little difference what mode of treatment was used; health/HEALTH restoration was usual and expected. Established cultural norms have been attributed to the recovery from illness, and over time the successful methods for treating various maladies were preserved and passed down to each new generation within a traditional ethnocultural community. It is the occurrence of natural recovery that has given rise to all forms of therapeutic treatments, and the attempts to explain a phenomenon that is natural. Over the generations, natural recovery has been attributed to all sorts of rituals, including cupping, magic, leeching, and bleeding. Today, the people who are members of many different native, immigrant, and traditional cultural communities in the United States—American Indian, Black, Asian, European, and Hispanic—may continue to utilize the practices found within their tradition.

■ Folk Medicine

Folk medicine today is related to other types of medicine that are practiced in our society. It has coexisted, with increasing tensions, alongside modern medicine and was derived from academic medicine of earlier generations. There is ample evidence that the folk practices of ancient times have been abandoned only in part by modern health care belief systems, for many of these beliefs and practices continue to be observed today. Many may be practiced in secret, underground. Today's popular medicine is, in a sense, commercial folk medicine. Yoder (1972) describes two varieties of folk medicine:

1. Natural folk medicine—or rational folk medicine—is one of humans' earliest uses of the natural environment and utilizes herbs, plants, minerals, and animal substances to prevent and treat illnesses.

2. Magico-religious folk medicine—or occult folk medicine—is the use of charms, holy words, and holy actions to prevent and cure illnesses/ILLNESSES.

Natural Folk Medicine

Natural folk medicine has been widely practiced in the United States and throughout the world. In general, this form of prevention and treatment is found in old-fashioned remedies and household medicines. These remedies have been passed down for generations, and many are in common use today. Much folk medicine is herbal, and the customs and rituals related to the use of the herbs vary among ethnic groups. Specific knowledge and usages are addressed throughout this text. Commonly, across cultures, the herbs are found in nature and are used by humans as a source of therapy, although how these medicines are gathered and specific modes of use vary from group to group and place to place. In general, folk medical traditions prescribed the time of year in which the herb was to be picked; how it was to be dried; how it was to be prepared; the method, amount, and frequency of taking; and so forth.

In addition, an infinite number of maladies have, over the generations, cultivated an assortment of folk methods for thwarting or curing them. Boxes 5–1 and 5–2 describe these phenomena as related to cholera and choking. All too frequently, the practices consist of both natural and magico-religious forms.

Box 5–1

Choking

Choking, an often fatal mishap, occurs when air is prevented access to the lungs by compression or obstruction of the windpipe.

Folk Beliefs

It is widely believed that, throughout life, a person is at risk of all sorts of encounters with spirits and witches that may cause choking. The *alp* (incubus, nightmare) strangles people to death; the glacial demon springs on a boy's shoulders and strangles him to death; the poltergeist strangles a victim until he or she is half dead; witches pinch and attempt to strangle a person in bed; and *Naamah*, who is described in the Kabbala as a semi-human, deathless being, seduces men and strangles children in their sleep. If children are left outside on purpose, fairies strangle them, and mothers are warned to beware of the *striglas*, a wild and bad woman, who can catch hold of a baby and strangle it. It is widely believed that many activities, when undertaken by pregnant women, can cause the umbilical cord to be twisted around the unborn baby's neck, choking and strangling it to death.

Prevention

An expectant mother must avoid cords, such as by not wearing necklaces, or "wind string, yarn, or other material"; for that matter, she should "avoid seeing other women who do this" or stretching, and she is instructed never to "raise

(continued)

Box 5–1 *Continued*

her hands above her head," "hang up curtains," "sit with crossed legs," "scrub floors," or "walk through a hole in a fence."

The Catholic ritual of The Blessing of the Throats on Saint Blaise (3rd century) Day (February 3) is related to the prevention of choking. Two burning candles are crossed over the throat and the following prayer is recited: "May the Lord deliver you from the evils of the throat, and from every other evil." Other methods of prevention include the beliefs that

1. It is wise never to drink milk after eating choke-cherries.
2. One should not be eating while going over the threshold of a door.
3. If a person chokes without eating, it means that he or she told a lie, someone has told lies about the person, he or she is begrudging someone food, or the person's demise might entail choking on the gallows.

Treatment
Examples of advice regarding the treatment of choking include

1. If you swallow a fish bone, drink lemon juice or eat a biscuit; if you had choked in the early 1900s, you would have probably had to swallow a string with cotton on the end, which was pulled back up.
2. Swallow rice water or a raw egg.
3. Have someone pat or slap you hard between the shoulders.
4. Rub your nose.
5. Go on all fours and cough.

Choking is often a sign that foreshadows death, since it interrupts breathing and breath is the sign of life.

Sources: Thurston, H. (1955). Ghosts & poltergeists. *Journal of American Folklore Society, 68,* 97; Thompson, K. (1964). Body, boots, britches. *Journal of American Folklore Society, 77,* 305; Lee, K. (1951). Greek supernatural. *Journal of American Folklore Society, 64,* 309; Rivas, A. (1990). *Devotions to the saints* (p. 22). Los Angeles: International Imports; and UCLA Department of Folklore Archives.

 Box 5–2

Cholera

Cholera is an acute diarrheal, infectious disease caused by a bacterium. It is fatal 10% to 50% of the time.

Folk Beliefs
Cholera generates senses of mystery, fear, and dread; around the world, it was imagined in the form of a personified spirit and attributed to spiritual or human causes. The Eastern Europeans believed that a cat bringing home a baby stork after it fell out of the nest signaled the arrival of cholera, and Slavs saw cholera as a small woman with only one eye, one ear, and two long teeth.

Box 5–2 *Continued*

In India, cholera had many identities: the red flower mother and Marhai Devi, the goddess of cholera and the sister of the goddess Devi. In Italy, it was caused by the evil eye and/or an evil spirit, and in Sicily it was spread by rulers to get rid of people. In the American folk tradition, a change of the moon or a rainbow appearing in the west in the sign of the Twins signaled the arrival of cholera, and it was said that someone staring at a baby caused it. Others rationalized cholera outbreaks by regarding dead oak trees in the yard or foods—such as dried beans, green apples, green fruit, and food combinations such as cucumbers and ice cream—as the probable cause.

Prevention

Cholera was thought to be prevented by wearing wooden shoes to stop the seeping through of telluric poisons. A minister actually requested President Jackson to declare a day of fasting and prayer to halt a cholera epidemic. Fire and heat were popular methods, and when an epidemic hit Fort Riley, Kansas, in 1855 a physician burned barrels of pure tar beneath open hospital windows. Onions were a charm against cholera, and a bunch of onions could be hung in front of the threshold of the house. Tobacco smoke was found to slow the growth of many kinds of microbes, particularly those of Asiatic cholera.

Treatment

The range of homemade therapeutic remedies consisted of the use of a single agent, simple combinations, and some rather complex concoctions.

1. Simple substances—such as castor oil; nutmeg; camedative balsam, a patent medicine; wormwood tea; muskrat root; lettuce milk; dewberry or low blackberry—were praised by a 19th-century physician. Pyroligneous acid, used to cure hams, was also thought to cure cholera.
2. When the simple substances failed to halt the excessive diarrhea, herbal remedies were combined and/or used with popular patent medicines, such as calomel followed by castor oil; a teaspoon of wood ash was added to a cup of warm water; and nutmeg was added to milk. Powerful pills were rolled with red pepper and asafetida, or a large spoonful of pepper was added to a cup of boiled milk.
3. More elaborate concoctions contained such ingredients as turpentine, camphor, capsicum, cajeput, and tincture of flies or a combination of opium, charcoal, quinine, tobacco juice, and burning moxa.
4. A very exotic ritual consisted of chopping off the head of a black hen, ripping the gizzard from its body, and putting it into boiling water for a few minutes. The gizzard was discarded and the patient had to drink the boiling liquid.

Sources: Gifford, E. S. (1957, August). Evil eye in medicine. *Amer. J. Opth., 44*(2), 238; Lorenz, A. J. (1957). Scurvy in the gold rush. *Journal History of Medicine, 12,* 503; Koschi, B. *UCLA archive of California and western folklore,* unpublished, Cannon, UT, no. 3173; Erickson. (1941). Tarboro free press, *SFQ, 5,* 123; Karolevitz, R. F. (1967). *Doctors of the Old West* (p. 71). Seattle: Superior; Van-Ravenswaay. (1955). Pioneer medicine. In *Missouri, South Medical Journal, 48,* 36; Kell. (1965). Tobacco cures. *Journal of American Folklore Society, 78,* 106; VanWart. (1948). Native cures. *Canadian Medical Association Journal, 59*(342), 575; N. N., Collection, Hyatt, H. M. (1935). *Folklore from Adams County Illinois* (p. 433). New York, other materials in the archives of UCLA Folklore Department (2002).

Natural Remedies

The use of natural products, such as wild herbs and berries, accessible to healers developed into today's science of pharmacology. Early humankind had a wealth of knowledge about the medicinal properties of the plants, trees, and fungi in their environment. They knew how to prepare concoctions from the bark and roots of trees and from berries and wildflowers. Countless herbal preparations that were used many generations ago are in popular use today. Examples include purple foxglove, which contains the cardiotonic digitalis, that was used for centuries to slow the heart rate and feverfew, used to treat headaches.

Magico-Religious Folk Medicine

The magico-religious form of folk medicine has existed for as long as humans have sought to maintain, protect, and/or restore their HEALTH. It has now, in this modern age of science and technology, come to be labeled by some as "superstition," "old-fashioned nonsense," or "foolishness," yet for believers it may go so far on the continuum as to take the form of religious practices related to HEALTH maintenance, protection, restoration, and healing. Chapter 6 addresses these belief systems in more detail.

■ Health/HEALTH Care Philosophies

Two distinctly different health/HEALTH care philosophies determine the scope of health/HEALTH beliefs and practices: dualistic and holistic. Each of these philosophies espouses effective methods of maintaining, protecting, and restoring health/HEALTH, and the "battles for dominance" between the allopathic and homeopathic philosophies have been hard fought in this country (Starr, 1982) over the past century. One manifestation of these struggles is an emerging preference for homeopathic or holistic, complementary or alternative medicine among people from all walks of life.

The Allopathic (Dualistic) Philosophy, the dominant health care system in the United States is predicated on the allopathic philosophy. The word *allopathy* has two roots. One comes from the Greek meaning "other than disease" because drugs are prescribed on a basis that has no consistent or logical relationship to the symptoms. The second root of *allopathy* is derived from the German meaning "all therapies." Allopathy is a "system of medicine that embraces all methods of proven, that is, empirical science and scientific methodology is used to prove the value in the treatment of diseases" (Weil, 1983, p. 17). After 1855, the American Medical Association (AMA) adopted the "all therapies" definition of *allopathy* and has exclusively determined who can practice medicine in the United States. For example, in the 1860s the AMA refused to admit women doctors to medical societies, practiced segregation, and demanded the purging of homeopaths. Today, allopaths may show little or limited tolerance or respect for other providers of health care, such as homeopaths, osteopaths, and chiropractors, and for such traditional healers as lay midwives, herbalists, and American Indian medicine men and women (Weil, 1983, pp. 22–25). The allopathic health care system, the modern health care system, is further discussed in Chapter 8.

The Homeopathic (Holistic) Philosophy is the other health care philosophy in the United States. Homeopathic medicine was developed between 1790 and 1810 by Samuel C. Hahnemann in Germany and is extremely popular in much of Europe and other parts of the world. It is becoming, once again, more popular in the United States.

Homeopathy, or homoeopathy, comes from the Greek words *homoios* ("similar") and *pathos* ("suffering"). In the practice of homeopathy, the person, not the disease, is treated (Starr, 1982). This system has not been "tolerated" by the allopaths, yet it continues to thrive and is used by countless people. It espouses a holistic philosophy—that is, it sees health as a balance of the physical, mental, and spiritual whole. Homeopathic care encompasses a wide range of health care practices and is often referred to as "complementary medicine" or "alternative medicine." Complementary, alternative, unconventional, or unorthodox therapies are medical practices that do not conform to the scientific standards set by the allopathic medical community; they are not taught widely in the medical and nursing communities and are not generally available in the allopathic health care system, including the hospital settings. These include such therapies as acupuncture, massage therapy, and chiropractic medicine. Presently, this situation is changing, and the use of services such as acupuncture is more widespread in modern health care settings.

Table 5–3 demonstrates the health/HEALTH care choices, or pathways a person may follow when an illness occurs. The allopathic system comprises the conventional or familiar services within the dominant health care culture—acute care, chronic care, communtiy/public health care, psychiatric/mental health, rehabilitation, and so forth.

There are two types of care in the holistic system that are classified as complementary. These break down again into two categories, either alternative, or integrative, and traditional, or ethnocultural. Alternative therapies are

Table 5-3 Selected Examples of Health/HEALTH Care Choices.

Health Care Allopathic Conventional	HEALTH Care Homeopathic Complementary	
	Alternative (Integrative)	Traditional (Ethnocultural)
	Aromatherapy	Ayurveda
Acute care	Biofeedback	*Curanderismo*
Chronic care	Hypnotherapy	*Qi gong*
Community/public health	Macrobiotics	Reiki
Psychiatric/mental health	Massage therapy	*Santeria*
Rehabilitation	Reflexology	Voodoo

those that are not a part of one's ethnocultural or religious heritage, interventions neither taught widely in medical schools nor generally available in U.S. hospitals and other health care settings; traditional therapies are those that are part of one's traditional ethnocultural or religious heritage. In other words, a European American electing to use acupuncture as a method of treatment is seeking alternative treatment; a Chinese American using this treatment modality is using traditional medicine.

Homeopathic Schools

The period from 1870 through 1930 was when the allopathic health care model as we know it today was established. During the time that the roots of this system of health care were becoming firmly established, the ideas of the eclectic and other schools of medical thought were also prevalent.

Homeopathic Medicine. As stated earlier in this chapter, homeopathic medicine was developed between 1790 and 1810 by Samuel C. Hahnemann in Germany. In the practice of homeopathy, the person, not the disease, is treated. The practitioner treats a person by using minute doses of plant, mineral, or animal substances. The medicines are selected using the principle of the "law of similars." A substance that is used to treat a specific set of symptoms is the same substance that, if given to a healthy person, would cause the symptoms. The medicines are administered in extremely small doses. These medicines are said to provide a gentle but powerful stimulus to the person's own defense system, helping the person recover.

Homeopathy was popular in 19th-century America and Europe because it was successful in treating the raging epidemics of those times. In 1900, 20% to 25% of physicians were homeopaths. Due to allopathic efforts to wipe out the homeopaths beginning in 1906, the movement has dissipated. A small group of homeopaths still exists in the United States, however, and there are larger practices in India, Great Britain, France, Greece, Germany, Brazil, Argentina, and Mexico (Homeopathic Educational Services).

Osteopathic Medicine. Osteopathy, developed in 1874 by Dr. A. T. Still in Kirksville, Missouri, is the art of curing without the use of surgery or drugs. Osteopathy attempts to discover and correct all mechanical disorders in the human machine and to direct the recuperative power of nature that is within the body to cure the disease. Osteopathy is the knowledge of the structure, relation, and function of each part of the human body applied to the adjustment or correction of whatever interferes with the body's harmonious operation. As far back as 1921, George V. Webster described osteopathy as "the knowledge of the structure, relation and function of each part of the human body applied to the adjustment or correction of whatever interferes with the harmonious operation of the same." Furthermore, it claims that, if there is an unobstructed blood and nerve supply to all parts of the body, the effects of a disease will disappear (Dolgan, 2006). According to the American Association of Colleges of Osteopathic Medicine there are currently 26 colleges of osteopathic medicine in the United States, offering instruction at 34 locations in 25 states, that offer the doctor of osteopathic medicine (DO) degree.

Doctors of osteopathy (D.O.s) are fully qualified physicians who can practice in all areas of medicine and surgery. They, like medical doctors, have completed 4 years of medical school, 1 year of internship, and generally a further residency in a specialty area. They take the same course work as do medical doctors, often use the same textbooks, and often take the same licensing examinations. The lines of distinction between the medical doctor and the osteopath arise because the osteopath, in addition to using modern scientific forms of medical diagnosis and treatment, uses manipulation of the bones, muscles, and joints as therapy. Osteopaths also employ structural diagnosis and take into account the relationship between body structure and organic functioning when they determine a diagnosis. The osteopathic doctor has the same legal power to treat patients as a medical doctor (Dolgan, 2006).

Chiropractic.   Chiropractic is a health care profession that focuses on the relationship between the body's structure—mainly the spine—and its functioning. It is a controversial form of healing that has been in existence for over a century. It, too, adheres to a disease theory and a method of therapy that differ from allopathy. It was developed as a form of healing in 1895 in Davenport, Iowa, by a storekeeper named Daniel David Palmer, also known as a "magnetic healer." Palmer's theory underlying the practice of chiropractic was that an interference with the normal transmission of "mental impulses" between the brain and the body organs produced diseases. The interference is caused by misalignment, or subluxation, of the vertebrae of the spine, which decreases the flow of "vital energy" from the brain through the nerves and spinal cord to all parts of the body. The treatment consists of manipulation to eradicate the subluxation.

Chiropractic is practiced in two ways. One form is that of the "mixers," who use heat therapy, enemas ("colonic irrigation"), exercise programs, and other therapeutic practices. The other group, the "straight" chiropractors, who use only manipulation, disapprove of the practices of the "mixers." They believe that the other techniques are a form of allopathic medicine (Cobb, 1977).

Eclectic Medicine.   The word *eclectic* means "choosing," and it refers to choosing the means for treating disease. Methods and remedies are selected from all other systems. This school of medicine believes that nature has curative powers, and practitioners seek to remove the causes of disease through the natural outlets of the body. They treat the cause of disease, rather than the symptoms, and do not use bleeding, antimony, or poisons to treat diseases (School, 1924, pp. 1545–1546).

Hydrotherapy.   The use of water for the maintenance of health or the treatment of disease is one of the oldest known therapies. It is an ancient method of treatment that has been used to treat disease and injury by many different peoples. A German farmer, Vincent Priessnitz, reintroduced hydrotherapy in 1840. It includes the application of water, internally and externally, in any form at any temperature, with the belief that the water can have a very profound effect on the body (School, 1924, p. 1527). A popular form of hydrotherapy can be found in today's popular spa—*SPA* is an acronym for the Latin *salus per aquam*—"health by water."

There were also many popular theories of healing during this era that focused only on the mind. Some examples follow.

Mesmerism.   In the late 18th century, mesmerism was a popular form of healing by touch and was named for its founder, Friedrich Anton Mesmer. Mesmer believed that illness was a condition in which the body and mind of a person were influenced by a mysterious force emanating from another person. He further believed that the stars exerted an influence on people and that this force was the same as electricity and magnetism. Initially, he believed that stroking the body with magnets would bring about a cure for illness. He later modified this to the belief that touch alone could heal (School, 1924, p. 1592).

Hypnotism.   Hypnotism artificially creates a condition in which the person appears to be asleep and acts in obedience to the will of the operator as regards both motion and sensation. It was developed in 1841 by James Braid, an English surgeon (School, 1924, p. 1595).

Mind Cure.   Mind cure is the cure of disease by means of the mind alone, in which faith influences the cure of disease. Two prerequisites in faith healing are the desire to get well and faith in the treatment (School, 1924, p. 1598).

Christian Science.   The religious philosophy of scientism lies outside allopathic and most homeopathic philosophies and delivery systems. Christian Science, as a system of spiritual healing, was first explained in 1875 in Mary Baker Eddy's book *Science and Health with Key to the Scriptures.* Eddy introduced the term *Christian Science* to designate the scientific system of divine healing. Eddy's revelation consists of two parts:

1. The discovery of this divine science of mind-healing, through a spiritual sense of the Scriptures, and
2. The proof, by present demonstration, that the so-called miracles of Jesus did not specially belong to a dispensation now ended, but that they illustrated an ever-operative divine principle. (Eddy, 1875, p. 123: 16–27)

Eddy's own early research and experiments in homeopathy, allopathy, and diet preceded her discoveries about spiritual healing. Ultimately, she found that "a mental method produces permanent health" (Eddy, 1875, p. 79: 8–9).

Christian Scientists are free to choose the method of health care they feel is most effective. Their choice is not compelled by a church. Individuals and families make their own decisions. Christian Scientists, like others, grapple with the moral, social, and cultural implications of modern medical approaches and technological developments—including gene therapy, cloning, and artificial life support systems.

They are free to make their own choices on important social health matters, such as abortion, birth control, blood transfusions, and organ donations. Those who consider themselves Christian Scientists may have studied and practiced Christian Science for up to five generations. Or they may be reading *Science and Health* for the first time, for a better understanding of how spirituality is linked to health and well-being. Christian Scientists turn to the Bible and the pages of *Science and Health* for answers to humanity's deepest questions (Graunke, 2003).

National Center for Complementary and Alternative Medicine

The National Center for Complementary and Alternative Medicine (NCCAM) at the National Institutes of Health was founded in 1998 and is the federal government's lead agency for scientific research on complementary and alternative medicine, or CAM. The agency describes the different approaches to health care that are outside the realm of conventional medicine as either complementary or alternative. Conventional medicine is health care that is practiced by M.D.s or D.O.s and allied health professionals, such as registered nurses, physical therapists, and psychologists. The NCCAM differentiates between complementary and alternative medicine in that complementary medicine is used together with conventional medicine. An example of a complementary therapy is using aromatherapy to help lessen a patient's discomfort following surgery or while undergoing cancer therapies. Alternative medicine is used in place of conventional medicine. An example of an alternative therapy is using a special diet or medication to treat cancer instead of undergoing the surgery, radiation, or chemotherapy that has been recommended by a conventional doctor. The list of what is considered to be CAM changes continually, as the therapies that are proven to be safe and effective become adopted into conventional health care and as new approaches to health care emerge. The agency conducts ongoing research in many areas of complementary and alternative medicine.

The objectives of the NCCAM are to

1. explore complementary and alternative healing practices in the context of rigorous science,
2. train complementary and alternative medicine researchers, and
3. disseminate authoritative information to the public and professionals.

Tables 5–4 and 5–5 summarize selected findings of currently funded research projects.

Traditional, or Ethnocultural, Care

The following list describes selected traditional HEALTH care systems:

1. **Ayurvedic.** This 4,000-year-old method of healing originated in India and is the most ancient existing medical system that uses diet, natural therapies, and herbs. Its chief aim is longevity and quality of life. It formed the foundation of Chinese medicine.

Table 5-4 Selected Health Problems Studied by the National Center for Complementary and Alternative Medicine When CAM Is Utilized

Health Problem	Therapy
Arthritis, rheumatoid	Preparations made from botanicals (plants and their products, including herbs) • Vitamins and minerals in unconventional amounts • Other products taken by mouth, such as fish oil • Dietary approaches • Preparations applied to the skin, such as balms and liniments • Hydrotherapy • Items that are worn (for example, magnetic clothing or copper bracelets) • Mind-body therapies, such as relaxation techniques, meditation, prayer for health purposes, and tai chi • Whole medical systems, such as Ayurveda (a traditional medicine of India), traditional Chinese medicine, homeopathy, and chiropractic
Cancer	• Acupuncture to relieve neck and shoulder pain following surgery for head or neck cancer • Ginger as a treatment for nausea and vomiting caused by chemotherapy • Massage for the treatment of cancer pain • Mistletoe extract combined with chemotherapy for the treatment of solid tumors
Depression	St. John's wort for treating mild to moderate depression
Menopausal symptoms	• Six botanicals—black cohosh, red clover, dong quai root, ginseng, kava, and soy • Dehydroepiandrosterone (DHEA), a dietary supplement • Exercise • Paced respiration • Health education • Dietary supplements

Sources: NCCAM. (2005, 2007, and 2008). Retrieved from http://nccam.nih.gov/health/RA/; http://nccam.nih.gov/health/camcancer/; http://nccam.nih.gov/health/stjohnswort/sjwataglance.htm; http://nccam.nih.gov/health/menopauseandcam/, April 14, 2011.

2. *Curanderismo.* This traditional Hispanic (Mexican) system of HEALTH care originated in Spain and is derived, in part, from traditional practices of indigenous Indian and Spanish HEALTH practices.

3. *Qi gong.* This form of Chinese traditional medicine combines movement, meditation, and regulation of breathing to enhance the flow of qi (the vital energy), improve circulation, and enhance the immune system.

4. **Reiki.** This Japanese form of therapy is based on the belief that, when spiritual energy is channeled through a practitioner, the patient's spirit is healed, in turn healing the physical body.

Table 5-5   Selected Remedies Studied by the National Center for Complementary and Alternative Medicine

Remedy	Use
Black cohosh	• Rheumatism (arthritis and muscle pain) • Hot flashes • Night sweats • Vaginal dryness • Other symptoms that can occur during menopause • Menstrual irregularities and premenstrual syndrome • Induced labor
Echinacea	• Treat or prevent colds, flu, and other infections • Stimulate the immune system to help fight infections • Wounds and skin problems, such as acne or boils
Ginkgo	• Asthma • Bronchitis • Fatigue • Tinnitus • Improve memory • Prevent Alzheimer's disease and other types of dementia • Decrease intermittent claudication • Sexual dysfunction
St. John's wort	• Mental disorders and nerve pain • Balm for wounds, burns, and insect bites • Depression • Anxiety • Sleep disorders

Sources: NCCAM. (2004 and 2005). Retrieved from http://nccam.nih.gov/health/blackcohosh/; http://nccam.nih.gov/health/echinacea/; http://nccam.nih.gov/health/ginkgo/; http://nccam.nih.gov/health/stjohnswort/, April 14, 2011.

5. **Santeria.** This form of traditional HEALTH care is observed among the practitioners of a syncretic religion that comprises both African and Catholic beliefs, also called Santeria. This religion is practiced among Puerto Ricans and Dominicans.

6. **Voodoo.** This form of traditional HEALTH care is observed among the practitioners of a religion that is a combination of Christian and African Yoruba religious beliefs, called Voodoo.

The use of alternative therapies is growing rapidly. Astin (1998) reported that three theories have been offered to explain why people seek alternative care:

1. **Dissatisfaction.** Patients are not satisfied with allopathic care because it is seen as ineffective, it produces adverse effects, or it is impersonal, too costly, or too technological.

2. **Need for personal control.** The providers of alternative therapies are less authoritarian and more empowering, as they offer the patient the opportunity to have autonomy and control in their health care decisions.

3. **Philosophical congruence.** The alternative methods of therapy are compatible with the patients' values, worldview, spiritual philosophy, or beliefs regarding the nature and meaning of *health*/HEALTH and *illness*/ILLNESS. These therapies are now frequently used by patients with cancer, arthritis, chronic back or other pain, stress-related problems, AIDS, gastrointestinal problems, and anxiety.

Since 1990, Eisenberg and colleagues have studied the trends in the use of alternative medicine in the United States. They reported the results of a national survey of 1,539 subjects in 1993 and reported the findings of a 1997 survey in 1998. They found in 1991 that about a third of all American adults use some form of unconventional medical treatment; this number rose to 42.1% in 1997. A more recent study, in May 2004, CAM Use in America: Up Close, found that, in the United States, 40% of adults are using some form of CAM. The most frequent users in both the early studies were educated, upper-income White Americans in the 25–49 age group who were most likely to live on the West Coast. CAM use presently spans people of all backgrounds. However, according to the 2004 survey, some people are more likely than others to use CAM. Countless research studies regarding the use, efficacy, and costs of CAM are ongoing.

In 2007, adults in the United States spent $33.9 billion out of pocket on visits to CAM practitioners and purchases of CAM products, classes, and materials. Of this total expenditure, $22.0 billion was spent in self-care costs and $11.9 billion (35.2%) in practitioner costs. The major expenditures were for nonvitamin, nonmineral, natural products, $14.8 billion; yoga, tai chi, qi gong classes, $4.1 billion; homeopathic medicine, $2.9 billion; and relaxation techniques, $0.2 billion. National Health Iinformation Survey data indicate that the U.S. public makes more than 300 million visits to CAM providers each year and spends billions of dollars for these services, as well as for self-care forms of CAM. These expenditures, although a small fraction of total health-care spending in the United States, constitute a substantial part of out-of-pocket health care costs and are comparable to out-of-pocket costs for conventional physician services and prescription drug use. (Nahin, Barnes, Stussman, et al., 2009, p. 3)

It is difficult to sort out which aspects of complementary and traditional medicine have merit and which are a hoax. From the viewpoint of the patient, if he or she has faith in the efficacy of an herb, a diet, a pill, or a healer, it is not a hoax. From the viewpoint of the medical establishment, jealous of its territorial claim, the same herb, diet, pill, or healer is indeed a hoax if it is "scientifically" ineffective and prevents the person from using the method of treatment the physician-healer or other health care provider believes is effective.

The tensions between allopathic and homeopathic philosophies have been going on since the late 19th century. In this chapter, we have explored traditional ways of maintaining, protecting, and restoring HEALTH; the choices available to patients; and health/HEALTH care philosophies.

Explore 🌐 MediaLink

Go to the Student Resource Site at nursing.pearsonhighered.com for chapter-related review questions, case studies, and activities. Contents of the CULTURALCARE Guide and CULTURALCARE Museum can also be found on the Student Resource Site. Click on Chapter 5 to select the activities for this chapter.

Box 5–3: Keeping up

There are countless references that may be accessed to maintain currency in the domain of health. Suggested resources include, but are not limited to:

Homeopathic Educational Services http://www.homeopathic.com/

International Chiropractors Association http://www.chiropractic.org/

National Center for Complementary and Alternative Medicine http://nccam.nih.gov/

The Osteopathic Home Page http://osteohome.com/

UCLA online Archive of American Folkmedicine http://www.folkmed.ucla.edu/index.html

---

■ Internet Sources

American Heritage Dictionary of the English Language. (2011). Tradition. Retrieved from http://ahdictionary.com/word/search.html?q=tradition&submit.x=44&submit.y=23, March 4, 2011.

Christian Science Publishing Society. (2008). Writings of Mary Baker Eddy. Boston, MA: Author, p. 1. Retrieved from http://www.spirituality.com, April 25, 2011.

Dolgan, E. (2006). Addressing Osteopathy: The Osteopathic Home Page. Santa Monica, CA: Osteopathic Physicians, p. 1. Retrieved from http://www.osteohome.com/, April 25, 2011.

Eddy, M. B. (1875). Science and Health, p. 79: 8–9. Retrieved from http://www.spirituality.com/dt/toc_sh.jhtml, April 25, 2011.

Homeopathic Educational Services. Retrieved from http://www.homeopathic.com/, April 25, 2011.

National Center for Complementary and Alternative Medicine (NCCAM). (2011). Health Information. Washington, DC: National Institutes of Health. Retrieved from http://nccam.nih.gov/, April 25, 2011.

National Center for Complementary and Alternative Medicine (NCCAM). (2004). Herbs at a Glance: Blackcohosh. Washington, DC: National Institutes of

Health. Retrieved from http://nccam.nih.gov/health/blackcohosh/, April 14, 2011.

National Center for Complementary and Alternative Medicine (NCCAM). (2005). Herbs at a Glance: Echinacea. Washington, DC: National Institutes of Health, p. 1. Retrieved from http://nccam.nih.gov/health/echinacea/, April 14, 2011.

National Center for Complementary and Alternative Medicine (NCCAM). (2005). Herbs at a Glance: Ginkgo. Washington, DC: National Institutes of Health, p. 1. Retrieved from http://nccam.nih.gov/health/ginkgo/, April 14, 2011.

National Center for Complementary and Alternative Medicine (NCCAM). (2005). Herbs at a Glance: St. John's Wort. Washington, DC: National Institutes of Health, p. 1. Retrieved from http://nccam.nih.gov/health/St. John's Wort/, April 14, 2011.

National Center for Complementary and Alternative Medicine (NCCAM). (2005). Rheumatoid Arthritis and Complementary Medicine. Washington, DC: National Institutes of Health, p. 1. Retrieved from http://nccam.nih.gov/health/RA/, April 14, 2011.

National Center for Complementary and Alternative Medicine (NCCAM). (2007). Cancer and CAM. Washington, DC: National Institutes of Health, p. 1. Retrieved from http://nccam.nih.gov/health/camcancer/, April 14, 2011.

National Center for Complementary and Alternative Medicine (NCCAM). (2008). Menopausal Symptoms and CAM. Washington, DC: National Institutes of Health, p. 1. Retrieved from http://nccam.nih.gov/health/menopauseandcam/, April 14, 2011.

■ References

Astin, J. A. (1998, May 20). Why patients use alternative medicine: Results of a national study. *Journal of the American Medical Association, 279*(19), 1548–1553.

Cobb, A. K. (1977). Pluralistic legitimation of an alternative therapy system: The case of chiropractic. *Medical Anthropology, 6*(4), 1–23.

Eddy, M. B. (1875). *Science and health with key to the scriptures*. Boston: Christian Science Publishing.

Erickson. (1941). Tarboro free press, *SFQ, 5,* 123.

Gifford, E. S. (1957, August). Evil eye in medicine. *Amer. J. Opth., 44*(2), 238.

Graunke, K. (2003, January 8). Personal Interview. Boston, Massachusetts.

Hopkins, E., Woods, L., Kelley, R., et al. (1995). *Working with groups on spiritual themes*. Duluth, MN: Whole Person Associates.

Hyatt, H. M. (1935). *Folklore from Adams County Illinois* (p. 433). New York.

Karolevitz, R. F. (1967). *Doctors of the Old West* (p. 71). Seattle: Superior.

Kell. (1965). Tobacco cures. *Journal of American Folklore Society, 78,* 106.

Koschi, B. *UCLA archive of California and western folklore*, unpublished, Cannon, UT, no. 3173.

Lee, K. (1951). Greek supernatural. *Journal of American Folklore Society, 64,* 309.

Leontis, A. (2009). *Culture and customs of Greece*. Westport, CT: Greenwood Press.

Lorenz, A. J. (1957). Scurvy in the gold rush. *Journal History of Medicine, 12,* 503.

Maloney, C. (Ed.). (1976). *The evil eye*. New York: Columbia University Press.

Nahin, R. L., Barnes, P. M., Stussman, B. J., et al. (2009). *Costs of complementary and alternative medicine (CAM) and frequency of visits to CAM practitioners: United States, 2007.* National health statistics reports; no 18. Hyattsville, MD: National Center for Health Statistics.

Rivas, A. (1990). *Devotions to the saints* (p. 22). Los Angeles: International Imports.

School, B. F. (Ed.). (1924). *Library of health: Complete guide to prevention and cure of disease.* Philadelphia: Historical.

Smith, H. (1991, original 1958). *The world's religions.* San Francisco: Harper.

Spector, R. E. (1983). *A description of the impact of medicare on health–illness beliefs and practices of white ethnic senior citizens in central Texas* (pp. 126–127). Ph.D. diss. University of Texas at Austin School of Nursing. Ann Arbor, MI: University Microfilms International.

Starr, P. (1982). *The social transformation of American medicine* (pp. 79, 145). New York: Basic Books.

Thompson, K. (1964). Body, boots, britches. *Journal of American Folklore Society, 77,* 305.

Thurston, H. (1955). Ghosts & poltergeists. *Journal of American Folklore Society, 68,* 97.

Weil, A. (1983). *Health and healing.* Boston: Houghton Mifflin.

Winkler, G. (1981). *Dybbuk.* New York: Judaica Press.

Yoder, D. (1972). Folk medicine. In R. H. Dorson (Ed.), *Folklore and folklife* (pp. 191–193). Chicago: University of Chicago Press.

Zola, I. K. (1972). The concept of trouble and sources of medical assistance to whom one can turn with what. *Social Science and Medicine, 6,* 673–679.

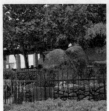 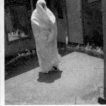 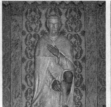 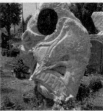

Figure 6-1   **Figure 6-2**   **Figure 6-3**   **Figure 6-4**

Chapter 6

HEALING Traditions

■ Objectives

1. Discover practices that were part of ancient forms of HEALING.
2. Distinguish ways that one's religion influences HEALING.
3. Identify saints related to HEALTH problems.
4. Discuss the various destinations and purposes of spiritual journeys.
5. Discuss the relationship of HEALING to today's health beliefs and practices.
6. Describe various forms of HEALING.
7. Differentiate rituals of birth and death among people of different religions.

The opening images for this chapter represent sacred places and shrines from selected destinations of pilgrimages or sacred practices. These are places where people may visit to seek HEALTH or HEALING. The images depicted here are locations that I have personally visited in the United States. Figure 6–1 is of the Kahuna Stones in Honolulu, Waikiki, O'hau, Hawaii. The ancient stones are part of the legends of Waikiki and the culture of the Hawaiian people. The stones are endowed with powers and are a source of HEALING. Figure 6–2 is the patio of a *Santero* in Los Angeles where a HEALING ceremony is being performed. Part of the ritual is a cleansing in a ring of fire. The Shrine of St. Peregrine for cancer sufferers, (Figure 6–3) in San Juan Capistrano, California, is a shrine people visit to pray for HEALING from cancer. Figure 6–4 is a gravestone in the Forever Hollywood cemetery in Los Angeles, California. A long lasting memorial has been placed there for the deceased person and is an integral part of the ritual mourning of survivors.

Are you having difficulties in your life that you would like to change? Are you seeking answers to questions that you cannot easily answer? Do you know about the HEALING traditions within your ethnoreligious heritage or the places you may visit to find the help you need? What are the HEALING practices within your family and ethnocultural heritage? What are the shrines, or sacred places, that are a part of your tradition or that you have visited? In the minds of countless people, shrines such as the ones in the chapter opener are an invaluable resource. If you could pick four images from your heritage that are related to HEALING, what would they be?

What is *HEALING*? What is the connotation of this word from a magico-religious or traditional perspective? What compels people to travel to shrines in the United States or in other parts of the world? Could it be that people who experience the need to seek consolation and solutions for overpowering events for which they cannot find rational answers turn to sources such as these holy shrines? The phenomenon of seeking HEALING is observed worldwide, and every religion and ethnic group offers substantive beliefs and practices in this genre. Are these examples of magic or of faith in a form of HEALTH care that is obtained from sources other than those that are conventional medicine? This chapter explores these questions by introducing a wide range of magico-religious and religious beliefs and practices regarding HEALING. It also discusses the traditions cross-culturally related to life cycle crises—birth, dying, and death—as these phenomena are closely linked to the beliefs and practices inherent in HEALING.

■ HEALING

The professional history of nursing was born with Florence Nightingale's knowledge (1860) that "nature heals." In more recent times, Blattner (1981) has written a text designed to help nurses assist patients in upgrading their lives in a holistic sense and in healing the person—body, mind, and spirit. Krieger (1979), in *The Therapeutic Touch*, has developed a method for teaching nurses how to use their hands to heal. Wallace (1979) has described methods of helping nurses diagnose and deliver spiritual care. She points out that the word *spiritual* is often used synonymously with *religion* but that the terms are not the same. If they are used synonymously as a basis for the health care and nursing assessment of needs, some of the patient's deepest needs may be glossed over. *Spiritual care* implies a much broader grasp of the search for meanings that goes on within every human life. In addition to answers to these questions from nursing raised in the introduction to this chapter, one is able to explore the concept from the classical and historical viewpoints of anthropology, sociology, psychology, and religion.

From the fields of anthropology and sociology come texts that describe rituals, customs, beliefs, and practices that surround healing. Shaw (1975, p. 121) contends that, "for as long as man has practiced the art of magic, he has sought to find personal immortality through healing practices." Buxton (1973) describes traditional beliefs and indigenous HEALING rituals in Mandari and relates the source of these rituals with how humans view themselves in relation to God and Earth. In this culture, the healer experiences a religious calling to become a healer. HEALING is linked to beliefs in evil and the removal of evil from the sick person. Naegele (1970, p. 18) describes healing in our society as a form of "professional practice." He asserts, however, that "healing is not wholly a professional monopoly and that there are several forms of nonprofessional healing such as the 'specialized alternatives.'" These include Christian Science and the marginally professional activities of varying legitimacy, such as chiropractic, folk medicine, and quackery. He states: "To understand modern society is to understand the tension between traditional patterns and self-conscious rational calculations devoted to the mastery of everyday life."

Literature from the field of psychology abounds with references to HEALING. Shames and Sterin (1978) describe the use of self-hypnosis to HEAL, and Progoff (1959), a depth psychologist, describes depth as the "dimension of wholeness in man." He has written extensively on how one's discovery of the inner self can be used for both HEALING and CREATION.

Krippner and Villaldo (1976, p. viii) contend that there is a "basic conflict between healing and technology" and that "the reality of miracles, of healing, of any significant entity that could be called God is not thought to be compatible with the reality of science." They further contend that healings are psychosomatic in origin and useful only in the sense of the placebo effect.

The literature linking religion to HEALING is bountiful. The primary source is the Bible (both the Old and New Testaments) and prayers. Bishop (1967, p. 45) discusses miracles and their relationship to healing. He states that the "miracles must be considered in relation to the time and place in which they occur." He further describes faith and its relationship to healing and states that "something goes on in the process of faith healing." He also points out that healing "is the exception rather than the rule." HEALING through faith generally is not accepted as a matter of plain fact, but it is an event to rejoice over.

Ford (1971, p. 6) describes healing of the spirit and methods of spiritual healing for spiritual illness. He describes suffering in 3 dimensions: body, mind, and spirit. He fully describes telotherapy—spiritual healing—which is both a means and an invitation. His argument is that full healing takes place only when there is agape love—divine love—and no estrangement from God. Russell (1937, p. 221) and Cramer (1923, p. 11) assert that healing is the work of God alone. Russell asserts that "God's will normally expresses itself in health," and Cramer focuses on the unity of human beings with God and claims that permanent health is truth, that healing is the gift of Jesus, and that it is a spiritual gift.

■ Ancient Forms of HEALING

ILLNESS was considered to be a crisis, and the people of ancient times developed elaborate systems of HEALING. The cause of an ILLNESS was attributed to the forces of evil, which originated either within or outside the body. Early forms of HEALING dealt with the removal of evil. Once a method of treatment was found effective, it was passed down through the generations in slightly altered forms.

If the source of sickness-causing evil was within the body, treatment involved drawing the evil out of the body. This may have been accomplished through the use of purgatives, which caused either vomiting or diarrhea, or by blood-letting: "bleeding" the patient or "sucking out" blood. (The barbers of medieval Europe did not originate this practice; bleeding was done in ancient times.) Leeching was another method used to remove corrupt humors from the body.

If the source of the evil was outside the body, there were a number of ways to deal with it. One source of external evil was witchcraft. In a community, there were often many people or a single person who was "different" from the other people. Quite often, when an unexplainable or untreatable illness occurred, it was these people who were seen as the causative agents. In such a belief system, successful treatment depended on the identification and punishment of the person believed responsible for the disease. (Certainly, the practice of scapegoating is in part derived from this belief.) It was believed that by removing or punishing the guilty person from the community, the disease would be cured. In some communities, the HEALERS themselves were seen as witches and the possessors of evil skills. How easy it was for ancient humankind to turn things around and blame the person with the skills to treat the disease for causing the disease!

Various rituals were involved in the treatment of ILL people. Often, the sick person was isolated from the rest of the family and community. In addition, it was customary to chant special prayers and incantations on the invalid's behalf. Sacrifices and dances often were performed in an effort to cure the ILLS. Often, the rituals of the healer involved reciting incantations in a language foreign to the ears of the general population ("speaking in tongues") and using practices that were strange to the observers. Small wonder, then, as superstition abounded, that at times the healers themselves were ostracized by the population.

Given that another cause of ILLNESS was believed to be the envy of people within the community, the best method, consequently, of preventing such an ILLNESS was to avoid provoking the envy of one's friends and neighbors. The treatment was to do away with whatever was provoking the envy—even though the act might have prevented a person from accomplishing a "mission in life," and the fear of being "responsible" might have been psychologically damaging.

Today, we tend to view the HEALING beliefs and methods of ancient people as "primitive," yet to fully appreciate their efficacy we need only make the simple observation that these methods in many forms exist today and have aided the survival of humankind.

■ Religion and HEALING

Religion plays a vital role in one's perception of HEALTH and ILLNESS. Just as culture and ethnicity are strong determinants in an individual's interpretation of the environment and the events within the environment, so, too, is religion. In fact, it is often difficult to distinguish between those aspects of a person's belief system arising from a religious background and those that stem from an ethnic and cultural heritage. Some people may share an ethnicity yet be of different religions; a group of people can share a religion yet have a variety of ethnic and cultural backgrounds. It is never safe to assume that all individuals of a given ethnic group practice or believe in the same religion. The point was embarrassingly driven home when I once asked a Mexican-American woman if she would like me to call the priest for her while her young son was awaiting a critical operation. The woman became angry with me. I could not understand why until I learned that she was a Methodist and not a Catholic. I had made an assumption, and I was wrong. She later told me that not all Chicanos are Catholic. After many years of hearing people make this assumption, she had learned to react with anger.

Religion strongly affects the way people interpret and respond to the signs and symptoms of ILLNESS. So pervasive is religion that the diets of many people are determined by their religious beliefs. Religion and the piety of a person determine not only the role that faith plays in the process of recovery but also in many instances the response to a given treatment and to the HEALING process. Each of these threads—religion, ethnicity, and culture—is woven into the fabric of each person's response to treatment and HEALING.

There are far too many religious beliefs and practices related to HEALING to include in this chapter. An introductory discussion of religious HEALING beliefs from the Judeo-Christian background, however, is possible.

The Old Testament does not focus on HEALING to the extent the New Testament does. God is seen to have total power over life and death and is the HEALER of all human woes. God is the giver of all good things and of all misfortune, including sickness. Sickness represented a break between God and humans. In Exodus 15:26, God is proclaimed the supreme HEALER ("I will put none of the diseases upon you which I put upon the Egyptians; for I am the Lord, your healer."). In a passage from Deuteronomy 32:39, it is stated "I kill, and I make alive. I have wounded and I heal." The traditionalist Jew believes that the "HEALING of illness comes from God through the mediation of His 'messenger,' the doctor." The Jew who is ill combines hope for a cure with faith in God and faith in the doctor (Ausubel, 1964, pp. 192–195). A prayer is recited for HEALING each Sabbath and other times throughout the week, and people are invited to submit or speak the names of people for whom they are petitioning for a restoration of their HEALTH.

The HEALING practices of the Roman Catholic tradition include a variety of beliefs and numerous practices of both a preventive and a HEALING nature. For example, St. Blaise, an Armenian bishop who died in A.D. 316 as a martyr, is revered as the preventer of sore throats. The blessing of the throats on his feast day (February 3) derives from the tradition that he miraculously saved the life of a boy by removing a fishbone he had swallowed (*Monthly Missalette*, 1980, p. 38).

The saints concerned with other aspects of ILLNESS include the following (Foy, 1980, pp. 305–313; Hallam, 1994):

Saint	Problem
St. Anthony of Padua	Barrenness
St. Odilia	Blindness
Our Lady of Lourdes	Bodily ills
St. Peregrine	Cancer
St. Francis de Sales	Deafness
St. Joseph	Dying
St. Vitus	Epilepsy
St. Raymond Nonnatus	Pregnancy
St. Lucy	Eye disease
St. Teresa of Avila	Headache
St. John of God	Heart disease
St. Roch	Being bedridden
St. Dymphna	Mental illness
St. Bruno	Possession

Many more saints could be included. I refer you to other sources for information, and I also recommend that you ask patients for information. I was caring for a young woman with terminal colon cancer. We began a conversation about St. Peregrine. She shared with me her belief in this saint, showed me a medal that she had carried with her, and expressed that she was comforted by sharing this information.

Spiritual Journeys

There are countless places in the United States and in this world where people make spiritual journeys, or pilgrimages, for the purpose of giving thanks or petitioning for favors. The shrines are related to magico-religious folk medicine and the use of charms, holy words, and holy actions. For example, at many shrines petitioners leave amulets or written petitions or light candles. Shrines range from small memorials—such as shrines that are created at the sites where accidents have occurred and people were killed to large, famous shrines where people who are part of a given religious tradition or a follower of a given healer may go to pray or petition at the site. In the United States, and throughout the world, people make pilgrimages to a number of shrines in search of special favors and HEALING. Shrines are not limited to any one-faith tradition, and they can be secular as well as religious. Over the years, I have visited many sacred shrines and have learned that they are indeed extraordinary places. The essentials that each of the shrines has in common are a feeling of peacefulness and serenity to the visitor; a calm, soothing atmosphere; and a place where petitions and/or objects are left when petitions for HEALING are made; or prayers have been answered, and people leave objects in gratitude. Most, but not all, have a source of water as part of the milieu, and it is a part of the tradition to take home water from the shrine.

The following are examples of shrines located in the United States.

The Tomb of Menachem Mendel Schneerson in Queens, New York, is a holy shrine where Jewish people from around the world gather to leave petitions and seek HEALING. People have reported healings when they visit his tomb (Figure 6–5).

The oldest shrine in the United States is the Shrine of Our Lady of La Leche, located in St. Augustine, Florida (Figure 6–6). The shrine was founded

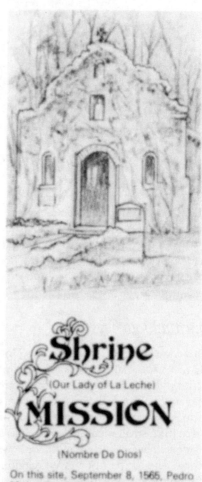

Figure 6-6   Shrine of Our Lady of La Leche.

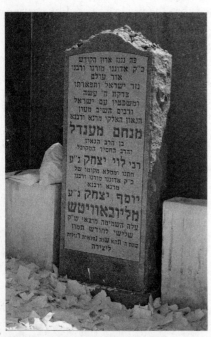

Figure 6-5   The Tomb of Menachem Mendel Schneerson in Queens, New York.

in 1620 by Spanish settlers as a sign of their love for the Mother of Christ. The shrine is visited by thousands of mothers to ask for the blessings of mother-hood, a safe and happy delivery, a healthy baby, and holy children. Countless letters can be read at the shrine attesting to the powers of Our Lady of La Leche (Informational brochure, 1953).

The Shrine of Our Lady of San Juan (Figure 6–7) is located in San Juan, Texas. This shrine houses a statue of the Virgin that was taken to

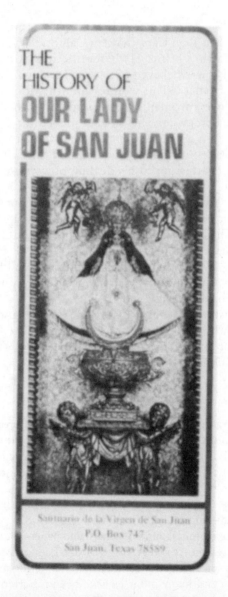

Figure 6–7   The Shrine of Our Lady of San Juan.

Mexico by Spanish missionaries in 1623. The statue was responsible for causing a miracle, and devotion to *La Virgin de San Juan* spread. The statue was taken to Texas in the 1940s after a woman claimed to have seen an image of the Virgin in the countryside around San Juan. The statue is presently housed in a beautiful new church, and pilgrims arrive daily to ask for HEALING and other favors. Countless letters are displayed attesting to the HEALING powers of this statue, and crutches and other artifacts are left at the church to attest to the miracles that happened there (Informational brochure, 1999).

The Shrine of St. Peregrine for cancer sufferers (Figure 6–8) is located in the Old Mission San Juan Capistrano in California. This statue is housed in a small grotto in the shrine. St. Peregrine was born in Italy in 1265 and died in 1345. He was believed to have miraculous powers against sickness and could cure cancer. This won for him the title "official patron for cancer victims." Once a woman was afflicted with cancer and a lady gave her a prayer to St. Peregrine. The woman prayed for 6 months, and her cancer was arrested. In gratitude for this, the woman had a statue of the saint placed in the mission. Today, the belief in this saint has spread, and countless documents attesting to his healing powers are on display in the mission.

Chimayo, New Mexico, is the home of the Shrine of our Lord of Esquipulas. The shrine was built between 1814 and 1816 and is visited by thousands of people each year. The shrine has been called the "Lourdes of America," and countless healings have been reported in this location (Figure 6–9). There is a hole in the shrine, and it is believed that eating the mud from this hole will cure many illnesses. The mud may also be mixed with water and rubbed on the body (Informational brochure, n.d.).

The National Shrine of Our Lady of the Snows (Figure 6–10) is located in Belleville, Illinois. It is a site that provides an atmosphere where people of all faiths have the opportunity to pray for HEALING and hope. There are numerous locations where petitions may be placed.

Other Shrines

The following are examples of sacred shrines located in Europe:

Three of the most revered and known shrines worldwide are located in France, Spain, and Portugal. Lourdes, in France, is believed to be a site where the Virgin Mary visited Bernadette Soubirous. In 1858, she observed a vision of St. Mary in a grotto. The Virgin was reported to have visited her several times. There have been 67 accepted miracle cures at this site, and countless— over 5 million a year—pilgrims go there (Lourdes, 2008).

Another famous shrine is found on a high and jiggered (saw-toothed) mountain near Barcelona, Spain. It is the Shrine of our Lady of Montserrat. Pilgrims have visited this site since the 13th century to venerate the miraculous statue of the Black Madonna, and many miracles have been reported here (Montserrat Shrine, 2008).

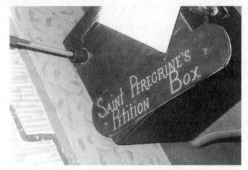

Figure 6-8 **The Shrine of St. Peregrine for cancer sufferers.**

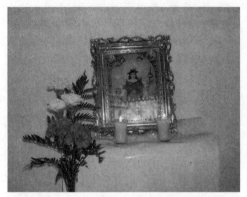

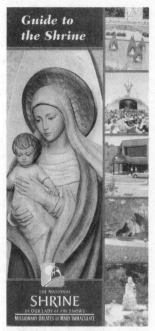

Figure 6-10 **The National Shrine of Our Lady of the Snows.**

Figure 6-9 **Shrine of our Lord of Esquipulas.**

One example of a present day petition is the following: "*Enagradecimiento por devolver la vida a neustro sobrino, I. G. R.* 14-9-01"; this translates to "Praise (or exaltation) for returning the life of our nephew." This brief note was found at the shrine. The immediate image was that of a couple making the difficult pilgrimage to Montserrat and placing this petition there. Note that the date is September 14, 2001—3 days after the attacks on the United States. Could it be that this person, the nephew, survived the attack on either the Pentagon or the World Trade Center? Could it be that the family sought and found a way to express their gratitude? The journey to Montserrat is difficult; the image this note evoked was one of sacrifice and homage.

Fatima is located in a small village in central Portugal, a short distance from Lisbon. It is a site of a shrine dedicated to the Virgin Mary. In 1917, 3 peasant children reported a vision of a woman who identified herself as the "Lady of the Rosary." The first national pilgrimage to the site occurred in 1927. Many miraculous cures have been reported at this site (Fatima, 2006).

One need only visit these remarkable places and bear witness to the display of faith that can be observed to begin to understand their important contributions in the complex areas of HEALING and faith.

Many people will not be fortunate enough to actually participate in a pilgrimage. However, there are countless websites that bring information and images to you. One such site, *El Nino Fidencio*, The *Curanderismo* Research Project from the University of Texas at Brownsville and Texas Southmost College, contains pertinent information about *El Nino Fidencio*. Fidencio Constantine, a folk curer, practiced in Nuevo Leon, Mexico from the early 1920s until his death in 1938, and is presently the central figure in a widespread curing cult. Twice each year, on the anniversaries of his birth and death, Espinazo (a town of about 300 population) is inundated by 10,000 to 15,000 people from Mexico and the United States who make pilgrimages in hopes of a cure and/or help from the *Niño* (The University of Texas at Brownsville and Texas Southmost College, 2006).

Believers combine elements of traditional Catholicism, Indian dances, herbology, and laying on of hands in effecting cures. It is believed that certain individuals receive the *Niño's* power to heal. They are called *Cajitas* or *Materias* (women) and *Cajones* (men)—"receptacles" of the *Niño's* power—and they cure in the name of *Niño Fidencio* and God. During the celebrations, they roam Espinazo curing all who wish a cure-blessing. There are several holy places in Espinazo where curing is conducted: Fidencio's tomb, temple, and deathbed; 2 trees; a cemetery hill; the hill of the bell; and the "charco" or mudpond, where Fidencio conducted baptisms to cure his patients. The pilgrimage to Espinazo has increased in popularity over recent years and extensive studies have been conducted in Espinazo (Gardner, 1992).

Table 6–1 summarizes the beliefs of people from several religious backgrounds with respect to health/HEALTH, healing/HEALING, and several events related to health care delivery. Remember, this is a summary, and you are urged

Table 6–1 Selected Religions' Responses to Health Events

Baha'i
"All healing comes from God."

Abortion	Forbidden
Artificial insemination	No specific rule
Autopsy	Acceptable with medical or legal need
Birth control	Can choose family planning method
Blood and blood products	No restrictions for use
Diet	Alcohol and drugs forbidden
Euthanasia	No destruction of life
Healing beliefs	Harmony between religion and science
Healing practices	Pray

Table 6-1 *continued*

Medications	Narcotics with prescription
	No restriction for vaccines
Organ donations	Permitted
Right-to-die issues	Life is unique and precious—do not destroy
Surgical procedures	No restrictions
Visitors	Community members assist and support

Buddhist Churches of America
"To keep the body in good health is a duty—
otherwise we shall not be able to keep our mind strong and clear."

Abortion	Patient's condition determines
Artificial insemination	Acceptable
Autopsy	Matter of individual practice
Birth control	Acceptable
Blood and blood products	No restrictions
Diet	Restricted food combinations
	Extremes must be avoided
Euthanasia	May permit
Healing beliefs	Do not believe in healing through faith
Healing practices	No restrictions
Medications	No restrictions
Organ donations	Considered act of mercy; if hope for recovery, all means may be taken
Right-to-die issues	With hope, all means encouraged
Surgical procedures	Permitted, with extremes avoided
Visitors	Family, community

Roman Catholicism
"The prayer of faith shall heal the sick, and the Lord shall raise him up."

Abortion	Prohibited
Artificial insemination	Illicit, even between husband and wife
Autopsy	Permissible
Birth control	Natural means only
Blood and blood products	Permissible
Diet	Use foods in moderation
Euthanasia	Direct life-ending procedures forbidden
Healing beliefs	Many within religious belief system
Healing practices	Sacrament of sick, candles, laying on of hands
Medications	May be taken if benefits outweigh risks
Organ donations	Justifiable
Right-to-die issues	Obligated to take ordinary, not extraordinary, means to prolong life
Surgical procedures	Most are permissible except abortion and sterilization
Visitors	Family, friends, priest
	Many outreach programs through church to reach sick

(continued)

Table 6–1   *continued*

Christian Science	
Abortion	Incompatible with faith
Artificial insemination	Unusual
Autopsy	Not usual; individual or family decides
Birth control	Individual judgment
Blood and blood products	Ordinarily not used by members
Diet	No solid food restrictions
	Abstain from alcohol and tobacco, some from tea and coffee (caffeine)
Euthanasia	Contrary to teachings
Healing beliefs	Accepts physical and moral healing
Healing practices	Full-time healing ministers
	Spiritual healing practiced
Medications	None
	Immunizations/vaccines to comply with law
Organ donations	Individual decides
Right-to-die issues	Unlikely to seek medical help to prolong life
Surgical procedures	No medical ones practiced
Visitors	Family, friends, and members of the Christian Science community and healers, Christian Science nurses
Church of Jesus Christ of Latter-day Saints	
Abortion	Forbidden
Artificial insemination	Acceptable between husband and wife
Autopsy	Permitted with consent of next of kin
Birth control	Contrary to Mormon belief
Blood and blood products	No restrictions
Diet	Alcohol, tea (except herbal teas), coffee, and tobacco are forbidden
	Fasting (24 hours without food and drink) is required once a month
Euthanasia	Humans must not interfere in God's plan
Healing beliefs	Power of God can bring healing
Healing practices	Anointing with oil, sealing, prayer, laying on of hands
Medications	No restrictions; may use herbal folk remedies
Organ donations	Permitted
Right-to-die issues	If death inevitable, promote a peaceful and dignified death
Surgical procedures	Matter of individual choice
Visitors	Church members (Elder and Sister), family, and friends
	The Relief Society helps members
Hinduism	
"Enricher, Healer of disease, be a good friend to us."	
Abortion	No policy exists
Artificial insemination	No restrictions exist but not often practiced

Table 6-1 *continued*

Autopsy	Acceptable
Birth control	All types acceptable
Blood and blood products	Acceptable
Diet	Eating of meat is forbidden
Euthanasia	Not practiced
Healing beliefs	Some believe in faith healing
Healing practices	Traditional faith healing system
Medications	Acceptable
Organ donations	Acceptable
Right-to-die issues	No restrictions
	Death seen as "one more step to nirvana"
Surgical procedures	With an amputation, the loss of limb is seen as due to "sins in a previous life"
Visitors	Members of family, community, and priest support

Islam
"The Lord of the world created me—and when I am sick, He healeth me."

Abortion	Not accepted
Artificial insemination	Permitted between husband and wife
Autopsy	Permitted for medical and legal purposes
Birth control	Acceptable
Blood and blood products	No restrictions
Diet	Pork and alcohol prohibited
Euthanasia	Not acceptable
Healing beliefs	Faith healing generally not acceptable
Healing practices	Some use of herbal remedies and faith healing
Medications	No restrictions
Organ donations	Controversial; must be discussed with family
Right-to-die issues	Attempts to shorten life prohibited
Surgical procedures	Most permitted
Visitors	Family and friends provide support

Jehovah's Witnesses

Abortion	Forbidden
Artificial insemination	Forbidden
Autopsy	Acceptable if required by law
Birth control	Sterilization forbidden
	Other methods; individual choice
Blood and blood products	Forbidden
Diet	Abstain from tobacco, moderate use of alcohol
Euthanasia	Forbidden
Healing beliefs	Faith healing forbidden

(continued)

Table 6–1 *continued*

Healing practices	Reading Scriptures can comfort the individual and lead to mental and spiritual healing
Medications	Accepted except if derived from blood products
Organ donations	Forbidden
Right-to-die issues	Use of extraordinary means is an individual's choice
Surgical procedures	Not opposed, but administration of blood during surgery is strictly prohibited
Visitors	Members of congregation and elders pray for the sick person

Judaism
"O Lord, my God, I cried to Thee for help and Thou has healed me."

Abortion	Therapeutic permitted; some groups accept abortion on demand; seek rabbinical consultation
Artificial insemination	Permitted
Autopsy	Permitted under certain circumstances
	All body parts must be buried together—seek rabbinical consultation
Birth control	Permissible, except with orthodox Jews—seek rabbinical consultation
Blood and blood products	Acceptable
Diet	Strict dietary laws followed by many Jews—milk and meat not mixed; predatory fowl, shellfish, and pork products forbidden; kosher products only may be requested
Euthanasia	Active euthanasia prohibited—passive euthanasia—not prolonging life may be acceptable—nutrition a basic need—not withheld—seek rabbinical consultation
Healing beliefs	Medical care expected
Healing practices	Prayers for the sick
Medications	No restrictions
Organ donations	Complex issue; some practiced—seek rabbinical consultation
Right-to-die issues	Right to die with dignity
	If death is inevitable, no new procedures need to be undertaken, but those ongoing must continue
Surgical procedures	Most allowed
Visitors	Family, friends, rabbi, many community services

Mennonite

Abortion	Therapeutic acceptable
Artificial insemination	Individual conscience; husband to wife
Autopsy	Acceptable
Birth control	Acceptable
Blood and blood products	Acceptable
Diet	No specific restrictions
Euthanasia	Not condoned
Healing beliefs	Part of God's work

Table 6-1 *continued*

Healing practices	Prayer and anointing with oil
Medications	No restrictions
Organ donations	Acceptable
Right-to-die issues	Do not believe life must be continued at all cost
Surgical procedures	No restrictions
Visitors	Family, community

Seventh-day Adventists

Abortion	Therapeutic acceptable
Artificial insemination	Acceptable between husband and wife
Autopsy	Acceptable
Birth control	Individual choice
Blood and blood products	No restrictions
Diet	Encourage vegetarian diet
Euthanasia	Not practiced
Healing beliefs	Divine healing
Healing practices	Anointing with oil and prayer
Medications	No restrictions
	Vaccines acceptable
Organ donations	Acceptable
Right-to-die issues	Follow the ethic of prolonging life
Surgical procedures	No restrictions
	Oppose use of hypnotism
Visitors	Pastor and elders pray and anoint sick person
	Worldwide health system includes hospitals and clinics

Unitarian/Universalist Church

Abortion	Acceptable, therapeutic, and on demand
Artificial insemination	Acceptable
Autopsy	Recommended
Birth control	All types acceptable
Blood and blood products	No restrictions
Diet	No restrictions
Euthanasia	Favor nonaction
	May withdraw therapies if death imminent
Healing beliefs	Faith healing: seen as "superstitious"
Healing practices	Use of science to facilitate healing
Medications	No restrictions
Organ donations	Acceptable
Right-to-die issues	Favor the right to die with dignity
Surgical procedures	No restrictions
Visitors	Family, friends, church members

Source: Adapted with permission from Andrews, M. M., & Hanson, P. A. (1995). Religion, culture, and nursing, In J. S. Boyle & M. M. Andrews (Eds.), *Transcultural concepts in nursing care* (2nd ed.) (pp. 371–406). Philadelphia: J. B. Lippincott. Used with permission.

not to generalize from this guide when relating to an individual patient and family. It is important to show respect, sensitivity, and an awareness and understanding of the different perspectives that may exist and to be able to convey to the patient and family your desire to understand their viewpoint on health care.

■ HEALING and Today's Beliefs

It is not an accident or a coincidence that today, more so than in recent years, we are not only curious but vitally concerned about the ways of HEALING that our ancestors employed. Some critics of today's health care system choose to condemn it, with more vociferous critics, such as Illich (1975), citing its failure to create a utopia for humankind. It is obvious to those who embrace a more moderate viewpoint that diseases continue to occur and that they outflank our ability to cure or prevent them. Once again, many people are seeking the services of people who are knowledgeable in the arts of HEALING and folk medicine. Many patients may elect, at some point in their lives, more specifically during an ILLNESS, to use modalities outside the medical establishment. It is important to understand the HEALERS.

Types of HEALING

A review of HEALING and spiritual literature reveals that there are 4 types of HEALING:

1. **Spiritual HEALING.** When a person is experiencing an illness of the spirit, spiritual HEALING applies. The cause of suffering is personal sin. The treatment method is repentance, which is followed by a natural healing process.

2. **Inner HEALING.** When a person is suffering from an emotional (mental) illness, inner HEALING is used. The root of the problem may lie in the person's conscious or unconscious mind. The treatment method is to heal the person's memory. The HEALING process is delicate and sensitive and takes considerable time and effort.

3. **Physical HEALING.** When a person is suffering from a disease or has been involved in an accident that resulted in some form of bodily damage, physical HEALING is appropriate. Laying on of hands and speaking in tongues usually accompany physical HEALING. The person is prayed over by both the leader and members of a prayer group.

4. **Deliverance, or exorcism.** When the body and mind are victims of evil from the outside, exorcism is used. In order to effect treatment, the person must be delivered, or exorcised, from the evil. The ongoing popularity of films such as *The Exorcist* gives testimony to the return of these beliefs. Incidentally, the priest who has lectured in my classes stated that he does not, as yet, lend credence to exorcisms; however, he was guarded enough not to discount it, either.

The people who HEAL, both in the past and in the present, often have been those who received the gift of HEALING from a "divine" source. Many receive this gift in a vision and have been unable to explain to others how they know what to do. Other HEALERS learned their skills from their parents. Most of the HEALERS with acquired skills are women, who subsequently pass their knowledge on to their daughters. People who use herbs and other preparations to remove the evil from the sick person's body are known as *herbalists*. Other HEALERS include bone setters and midwives, and although early humankind did not separate ILLS of the body from those of the mind, some HEALERS were more adept at solving problems by using early forms of "psychotherapy."

There are numerous HEALERS in the general population, some of whom are legitimate and some of whom are not. They range from housewives and priests to gypsies and "witches." Many people seek their services. There are numerous stylistic differences between the scope of practice of a modern health care practitioner and that of a traditional HEALER (Table 6–2). I have visited with several traditional healers. One man I visited was a *Santero*, a traditional HEALER from Puerto Rico. He enjoyed a reputation as a person who can "bring comfort to those most in need." I had an appointment for an interview but, when I arrived, he informed me that if I wanted to learn about his practice I had to "sit." I did.

Table 6–2 Comparisons: Traditional Homeopathic HEALER versus Modern Allopathic Physician

HEALER	Physician
1. Maintains informal, friendly, affective relationship with the entire family	1. Businesslike, formal relationship; deals only with the patient
2. Comes to the house, day or night	2. Patient must go to the physician's office or clinic, and only during the day; may have to wait for hours to be seen; home visits are rarely, if ever, made
3. For diagnosis, consults with head of house, creates a mood of awe, talks to all family members, is not authoritarian, has social rapport, builds expectation of cure	3. Rest of family usually is ignored; deals solely with the ill person and may deal only with the sick part of the person; authoritarian manner creates fear
4. Generally less expensive than the physician	4. More expensive than the healer
5. Has ties to the "world of the sacred"; has rapport with the symbolic, spiritual, creative, or holy force	5. Secular; pays little attention to the religious beliefs or meaning of an illness
6. Shares the worldview of the patient— that is, speaks the same language, lives in the same neighborhood, or lives in some similar socioeconomic conditions; may know the same people; understands the lifestyle of the patient	6. Generally does not share the worldview of the patient—that is, may not speak the same language, live in the same neighborhood, or understand the socioeconomic conditions; may not understand the lifestyle of the patient

He examined me by asking questions (history); examining my head and hands (palpation and observation); and casting cowrie shells (in-depth examination). He then told me a story, asked me to interpret it, and then, based on my interpretation, told me how to treat my "problem." I visited another *Santero* in Los Angeles in 2008 and was treated for a knee problem. He massaged my knee with a dark liquid, recited several incantations, and then I was wrapped in a large white sheet, placed in the center of his patio for a *limpia* (cleansing), and a circle was made around me with alcohol and that was then lit on fire (Figure 6–2). Of course, I relished the treatment, and my knee was actually better for a long time!

■ Ancient Rituals Related to the Life Cycle

Today, just as it did in antiquity, religion also plays a role in the rites surrounding both birth and death. Many of the rituals that we observe at the time of birth and death have their origins in the practices of ancient human beings. Close your eyes for a few moments and picture yourself living thousands and thousands of years ago. There is no electricity, no running water, no bathroom, and no plumbing. The nights are dark and cold. The only signs of the passage of time are the changing seasons and the apparent movement of the various planets and stars through the heavens. You are prey to all the elements, as well as to animals and the unknown. How do you survive? What sort of rituals and practices assist you in maintaining your equilibrium within this often hostile environment? It is from this milieu that many of today's practices sprang.

Generally speaking, 3 critical moments occur in the life of almost every human being: birth, marriage, and death (Morgenstern, 1966, p. 3). One needs to examine the events and rites that were attendant on birth and death in the past and to demonstrate how many of them not only are relevant to our lives today but also are still practiced. Rites related to marriage are not included in this text but certainly are related, in the long term, to a person's HEALTH.

Birth Rituals

In the minds of early human beings, the number of evil spirits far exceeded the number of good spirits, and a great deal of energy and time was devoted to thwarting these spirits. They could be defeated by the use of gifts or rituals or, when the evil spirits had to be removed from a person's body, with redemptive sacrifices. Once these evil spirits were expelled, they were prevented from returning by various magical ceremonies and rites. When a ceremony and an incantation were found to be effective, they were passed on through the generations. It has been suggested and supported by scholars that, from this primitive beginning, organized religion came into being. Today, many of the early rites have survived in altered forms, and we continue to practice them.

The power of the evil spirits was believed to endure for a certain length of time. The 3rd, 7th, and 40th days were the crucial days in the early life of a child and the new mother. Hence, it was on these days, or on the 8th day, that most of the rituals were observed. It was believed that, during this period, the newborn and the mother were at the greatest risk from the power of supernatural beings and thus in a taboo state. "The concept underlying taboo is that all things created by or emanating from a supernatural being are his, or are at least in his power" (Morgenstern, 1966, p. 31). The person was freed from this taboo by certain rituals, depending on the practices of a given community. When the various rites were completed and the 40 days were over, both the mother and child were believed to be redeemed from evil. The ceremonies that freed the person had a double character: They were partly magic and partly religious.

I have deliberately chosen to present the early practices of Semitic peoples because their beliefs and practices evolved into the Judaic, Christian, and Islamic religions of today. Because the newborn baby and mother were considered vulnerable to the threats of evil spirits, many rituals were developed to protect them. For example, in some communities, the mother and child were separated from the rest of the community for a certain length of time, usually 40 days. Various people performed precautionary measures, such as rubbing the baby with different oils or garlic, swaddling the baby, and lighting candles. In other communities, the baby and the mother were watched closely for a certain length of time, usually 7 days. (During this time span, they were believed to be intensely susceptible to the effects of evil—hence, close guarding was in order.) Orthodox Jews still refer to the seventh night of life as the "watch night" (Morgenstern, 1966, pp. 22–30).

The birth of a male child was considered more significant than that of a female, and many rites were practiced in observance of this event. One ritual sacrifice was cutting off a lock of the child's hair and then sprinkling his forehead with sheep's blood. This ritual was performed on the eighth day of life and may be practiced today among Muslims. In other Semitic countries, when a child was named, a sheep was sacrificed and asked to give protection to the infant. Depending on regional or tribal differences, the mother might be given parts of the sheep. It was believed that, if this sacrificial ritual was not performed on the seventh or eighth day of life, the child would die (Morgenstern, 1966, p. 87). The sheep's skin was saved, dried, and placed in the child's bed for 3 or 4 years as protection from evil spirits.

The practice of cutting a lock of a child's hair and the sacrifice of an animal served as a ceremony of redemption. The child could also be redeemed from the taboo state by giving silver—the weight of which equaled the weight of the hair—to the poor. Although not universally practiced, these rites are still observed in some form in some communities of the Muslim world.

Circumcision is closely related to the ceremony of cutting the child's hair and offering it as a sacrifice. Some authorities hold that the practice originated as a rite of puberty: a body mutilation performed to attract the opposite sex. (Circumcision was practiced by many peoples throughout the ancient world.) Other sources attribute circumcision to the concept of the sanctity of the male organ and claim that it was derived from the practice of ancestor worship. The Jews of ancient Israel, as today, practiced circumcision on the eighth day of life. The Muslims circumcise their sons on the seventh day in the tradition that Mohammed established. In other Muslim countries, the ritual is performed anywhere from the tenth day to the seventh year of life. Again, this sacrifice redeemed the child from being taboo in his early stages of life. Once the sacrifice was made, the child entered the period of worldly existence. The rite of circumcision was accompanied by festivals of varying durations. Some cultures and kinship groups feasted for as long as a week.

The ceremony of baptism is also rooted in the past. It, too, symbolically expels the evil spirits, removes the taboo, and is redemptive. It is practiced mainly among members of the Christian faith, but the Yezidis and other non-Christian sects also perform the rite. Water was thought to possess magical powers and was used to cleanse the body from both physical and spiritual maladies, which included evil possession and other impurities. Usually, the child was baptized on the 40th day of life. In some communities, however, the child was baptized on the eighth day. The 40th (or eighth) day was chosen because the ancients believed that, given performance of the particular ritual, this day marked the end of the evil spirits' influence (Morgenstern, 1966).

Some rituals also involved the new mother. For example, not only was she (along with her infant) removed from her household and community for 40 days, but in many communities she had to practice ritual bathing before she could return to her husband, family, and community. Again, these practices were not universal, and they varied in scope and intensity from people to people. Table 6–3 illustrates examples of birth-related religious rituals.

Table 6–3 Birth-Related Religious Rituals

Religion	Practice	Time	Method
Baptist (27 bodies)	Baptism	Older child	Immersion
Church of Christ	Baptism	8 years	Immersion
Church of Jesus Christ of Latter-day Saints (Mormons)	Baptism	8 years or older	Immersion
Eastern Orthodox	Baptism	Infants	Total immersion
Episcopalian	Baptism	Infant	
Friends (Quaker)	No baptism	Named	
Greek Orthodox	Baptism	40 days	Sprinkle or immersion
Islam	Circumcision	Seventh day	
Jewish	Circumcision	Eighth day	
Lutheran	Baptism	6–8 weeks	Pouring, sprinkling, immersion
Methodist	Baptism	Childhood	
Pentecostal	Baptism	Age of accountability	
Roman Catholic	Baptism	Infant	Pour water
Russian Orthodox	Baptism	Infant	Immerse 3 times
Unitarian	Baptism	Infant	

Extensions of Birth Rituals to Today's Practices

Early human beings, in their quest for survival, strove to appease and prevent the evil spirits from interfering with their lives. Their beliefs seem simple and naive, yet the rituals that began in those years have evolved into those that exist today. Attacks of the evil spirits were warded off with the use of amulets, charms, and the like. People recited prayers and incantations. Because survival was predicated on people's ability to appease evil spirits, the prescribed rituals were performed with great care and respect. Undoubtedly, this accounts in part for the longevity of many of these practices through the ages. For example, circumcision and baptism still exist, even when the belief that they are being performed to release the child from a state of being taboo may not continue to be held. It is interesting also that adherence to a certain timetable is maintained. For example, as stated, the Jewish religion mandates that the ritual of circumcision be performed on the eighth day of life as commanded by Jewish law in the Bible.

The practice of closely guarding the new mother and baby through the initial hours after birth is certainly not foreign to us. The mother is closely watched for hemorrhage and signs of infection; the infant initially is watched for signs of choking or respiratory distress. This form of observation is very intense. Could factors such as these have been what our ancestors watched for? If early human beings believed that evil spirits caused the frequent complications that surrounded the birth of a baby, it stands to reason that they would seek to control or prevent these complications by adhering to astute observation, isolation, and rituals of redemption. In fact, in our present times, it is not unusual to observe women using ancient practices to facilitate pregnancy, ensure a safe pregnancy, labor and delivery; and employ traditional ways of protecting both herself and her newborn child. Table 6–4 lists birth rites from selected nations.

Death Rituals

It was believed that the work of evil spirits and the duration of their evil— whether it was 7 or 40 days—surrounded the person, family, and community at the time of and after death. Rites evolved to protect both dying and dead persons and the remaining family from these evil spirits. The dying person was cared for in specific ways (ritual washing), and the grave was prepared in set ways (storing food and water for the journey after death). Further, rituals were performed to protect the deceased's survivors from the harm believed to be rendered by the deceased's ghost. It was believed that this ghost could return from the grave and, if not carefully appeased, harm surviving relatives (Morgenstern, 1966, pp. 117–160).

Countless ethnocultural and religious differences can be found in the ways we observe dying, death, and mourning. Table 6–5 displays a sampling of the ways death is talked about at various locations in the United States. The expressions for death have been collected over several years of randomly reading the local newspapers' death notices. It is interesting to observe the regional

Table 6-4   Cross-Cultural Guide to Birth Rites from Selected Nations

National Origin of Your Client/Family	Rites You May Observe Before, When, and/or After Birth
Afghanistan (population 89% Muslim)	Use of traditional birth attendant (dais) Breast-feeding nearly universal BCG[a] at birth
Albania (population 70% Muslim, 20% Orthodox, 10% Catholic)	BCG at birth
Algeria (population 99% Muslim)	Father not present at delivery Baby wrapped in swaddling clothes Breast-feeding common, BCG at birth
Australia (population 76% Christian)	Physician delivers, father usually present Breast-feeding BCG at birth
Bahrain (population 100% Muslim)	BCG at birth
Bangladesh (population 83% Muslim, 16% Hindu, 1% other)	Mother prays postpartum, remains indoors up to 40 days Only husband visits Objects placed over door to prevent evil spirits Breast-feeding BCG at birth
Belize (population 90% Christian)	Fifty percent of children born out of wedlock Christened before visitors allowed, to prevent evil eye Bottle-feeding preferred BCG at birth
Brazil (population 70% Catholic, 30% other)	Fathers not present during labor and delivery Forty-day rest period for mother Short-term breast-feeding BCG at birth
Cambodia	Seek prenatal care at 5 to 6 months of pregnancy
Kampuchea (population 95% Buddhist)	Do not compliment newborn to prevent evil spirits Breast-feeding BCG at birth
Chad (population 44% Muslim)	Female circumcision BCG at birth
China (population 97% atheist and eclectic)	Fathers do not come into labor and delivery Newborn considered 1 year at birth Breast-feeding

Table 6–4 *continued*

National Origin of Your Client/Family	Rites You May Observe Before, When, and/or After Birth
Cuba (population 85% Catholic)	Avoid loud noises and looking at deformed people when pregnant Stay home for 41 days Breast-feeding BCG at birth
Egypt (population 94% Muslim)	Sugar water and foods offered after 40 days Newborn swaddled Celebration held on seventh day of life
Ethiopia (population 45% Muslim, 35% Ethiopian Orthodox, 20% animist and other)	Pregnancy is a dangerous time because of evil eye Unfulfilled cravings may cause miscarriage Mother confined 14–40 days postpartum Father may not attend labor and delivery
France (population 90% Catholic)	BCG at birth
Germany (population predominantly Christian)	Breast-feeding BCG at birth
Greece (population 98% Greek Orthodox)	Amulets may be placed on baby or crib BCG at 5–6 years
Haiti (population 80% Catholic, 10% Protestant, 10% Voodoo)	Avoid exposure to cold air during pregnancy May bury placenta beneath the doorway to the home or burn it Infants named after a 1-month confinement Nutmeg, castor oil, or spider webs may be placed on umbilical stump; bellybands may be used
India (population 83% Hindu, 11% Muslim, 6% other)	Cravings during pregnancy are satisfied Birth of son may be festively celebrated BCG at birth
Indonesia (population 88% Muslim)	Many children valued Breast-feeding BCG at birth
Iran (population 98% Muslim)	May place amulets on baby or in room BCG at birth
Iraq (population 97% Muslim)	Fertility of five children rewarded May place amulets on baby or in room BCG at birth
Ireland (population 94% Catholic)	BCG at birth Baptism at 40 days

(continued)

Table 6-4 *continued*

National Origin of Your Client/Family	Rites You May Observe Before, When, and/or After Birth
Israel (population 80% Jewish)	Orthodox Jews do not allow men into labor and delivery Newborn vulnerable to evil during the first week of life—amulets used Male circumcision on eighth day of life
Italy (population 99% Catholic)	Grandmother may want to give grandson his birth bath Amulets and/or medals may be placed on the baby or in room
Japan (population 84% Buddhist)	Midwives may be used Mother may stay confined up to 100 days Mother may not shower or wash hair for a week
Jordan (population 95% Muslim)	Mother has a 40-day confinement postpartum Males are circumcised on the seventh day Infant rubbed with salt and oil after birth and swaddled
Korea (South) (population 72% Buddhist and Confucianist, 28% Christian)	Father not present at birth Mother avoids exposure to cold and does not drink cold liquids Breast-feeding
Kuwait (population 85% Muslim)	Breast-feeding Amulets used to prevent evil eye BCG at $3^1/2$–4 years
Laos (population 85% Buddhist)	Newborns not complimented to avoid evil spirits Colostrum believed to cause diarrhea BCG at birth
Malaysia (population 58% Muslim, 30% Buddhist, 8% Hindu)	Many birth taboos Amulets used Breast-feeding BCG at birth
Mali	BCG at birth
Mexico (population 97% Catholic)	Avoid cold air Be active to have a small, easy-to-deliver baby Coin may be strapped to navel to keep it attractive
Morocco (population 99% Muslim)	BCG at birth
Netherlands	Home births common

Table 6–4 *continued*

National Origin of Your Client/Family	Rites You May Observe Before, When, and/or After Birth
Nigeria (population 50% Muslim)	Traditional birth attendants are frequently used BCG at birth
Norway (population 94% Lutheran)	Kangaroo care (baby is carried in a "pocket" that the mother wears) Father may attend delivery Breast-feeding
Pakistan (population 97% Muslim)	Traditional birth attendants BCG at birth
Philippines (population 83% Catholic, 9% Protestant, 5% Muslim)	Symbolic unlocking ritual performed during labor Showers and bathing prohibited for 10 days postpartum New mother dresses in warm clothing BCG at birth
Portugal (population 97% Catholic)	Midwives Mother may consume chicken soup or melted butter after delivery to help uterus return to normal
Russia	Breast-feeding May use amulets
Sweden (population 94% Lutheran)	Low infant mortality rate Breast-feeding
Thailand (population 95% Buddhist)	Mother keeps warm to increase milk supply BCG at birth
Tunisia (population 98% Muslim)	Use of henna to decorate body before going into labor BCG at birth
Vietnam (population 60% Buddhist, 13% Confucianist, 12% Taoist, 3% Catholic, 12% other)	Some type of blossom may be used during labor to symbolically open the cervix Mother drinks only warm liquids during labor Child 1 year old at birth BCG at birth

[a]Bacillus Calmette-Guérin (BCG) vaccine is used routinely to prevent tuberculosis. The vaccine is not used in the United States, but it is administered in countless other countries.

Source: Adapted from Geissler, E. M. (1994). *Pocket guide: Cultural assessment.* St. Louis, MO: Mosby. Used with permission. This material was published in the Pocket Guide to Cultural Assessment, Elaine Marie Geissler, Copyright Elsevier (1994).

Table 6-5 **Ways of Expressing Death, from Bangor, Maine; Boston, Massachusetts; Dallas, Houston, and San Antonio, Texas; Des Moines, Iowa; Elk Horn, Iowa; Los Angeles, California; Honolulu, Hawaii; and New York City**

Expression	Location	Religion[a]
Left this world entirely too early	Boston	Not listed
"Nothing" (only the name of the person, family, and funeral details)	New York, Dallas, Boston, Los Angeles	Catholic, Episcopalian
. . . found her way over the rainbow	New York	Not listed
Ushered into his heavenly home	St. Albans, West Virginia	Baptist
Departed this life	Durham, North Carolina	Church of Christ
Passed away	New York, Dallas, Boston, Houston, Elk Horn, Los Angeles	Catholic, Jewish, Baptist, Church of Christ
Died	New York, Dallas, Boston, San Antonio, Bangor, Houston, Des Moines	Baptist, Catholic, Congregational, Christian
Died peacefully	Houston, Bangor, Los Angeles, Boston	Catholic, Episcopalian, Jewish
Suddenly	New York	
Passed away peacefully	Houston, Los Angeles	
Entered into the arms of his Lord	San Antonio	Catholic
Went to be with her heavenly father	Houston	
Went to be with her (his, our) Lord	San Antonio	Catholic
Went home to be with God	Houston	
Sunrise . . . sunset . . .	Houston	Methodist
Departed this life	Dallas, Houston	Baptist
Passed from this life	Houston	
Passed into a new life . . . called home to be with her Lord	Boston	A.M.E. Church
Deceased	Dallas	Baptist
Expired	Houston	
Unexpectedly	Boston, Bangor	
With his Lord	Houston	
Entered into rest	Boston, San Antonio	Jewish, Catholic
Went to the next room	Honolulu	

[a]Most death notices do not list the religion of the deceased, and it is difficult to tell unless the funeral is held in a church or synagogue.

differences in expressions and that in some locations deaths are merely listed by the person's name and in other locations the event of death evokes comments such as "sunrise . . . sunset" and "departed this life." Table 6–6 is a guide to death rites from selected nations. Table 6–7 lists beliefs that people from different religious backgrounds may have regarding death. Finally, Table 6–8 lists selected cultural traditions in after-death rituals and mourning.

Table 6-6   Cross-Cultural Guide to Death Rites from Selected Nations

National Origin of Your Client/Family	Rites When Death Occurs
Afghanistan (population 89% Muslim)	Muslim rites: Body generally remains at home—cared for, washed, wrapped in white cloth Mullah often in attendance Friends and family visit Buried in 24 hours Ceremony held 2 days after burial and is followed by a meal
Albania (population 70% Muslim, 20% Orthodox, 10% Catholic)	Muslim rites
Algeria (population 99% Muslim)	Muslim rites
Australia (population 76% Christian)	Cremation and burial both practiced Grieving may be reserved—crying with no wailing
Bahrain (population 100% Muslim)	Muslim rites
Bangladesh (population 83% Muslim, 16% Hindu, 1% other)	Muslim rites
Belize (population 90% Christian)	Demonstrative in grief May have spectacular funerals
Burma (population 85% Buddhist)	May prefer quality rather than quantity of life Dying person may be helped to recall past good deeds Cremation may be preferred
Cambodia	Buddhist beliefs as discussed earlier
Kampuchea (population 95% Buddhist)	White clothing worn during 3-month mourning period Some mourners shave their heads
Chad (population 44% Muslim)	Muslim rites
China (population 97% atheist and eclectic)	Initial burial in a coffin; after 7 years, body is exhumed and cremated, and the urn is reburied in a tomb
Cuba (population 85% Catholic)	Family and friends stay with body through night Burial in 24 hours May have holy hour every night for 9 consecutive days

(continued)

Table 6-6 *continued*

National Origin of Your Client/Family	Rites When Death Occurs
Egypt (population 94% Muslim)	Muslim rites
Ethiopia (population 45% Muslim, 35% Ethiopian Orthodox, 20% Animist and other)	Muslim rites Loud wailing may be a normal grief reaction
France (population 90% Catholic)	Chrysanthemums used exclusively for funerals
Germany (population predominantly Christian)	Crying in private is expected Cremation may be selected
Greece (population 98% Greek Orthodox)	May isolate dying person and withhold truth Death at home important Person buried; exhumed in 5 years and bones reburied in urn or vault Widow wears dark mourning clothes for rest of life
Haiti (population 80% Catholic, 10% Protestant, 10% Voodoo)	Burial in 24 hours White clothing represents death
India (population 83% Hindu, 11% Muslim, 6% other)	Non-Hindus ought not touch body; wash body themselves Cremation is preferred Reincarnation is a Hindu belief
Indonesia (population 88% Muslim)	Muslim rites
Iran (population 98% Muslim)	Muslim rites Mourning may be loud, obvious, and expressive
Iraq (population 97% Muslim)	Muslim rites
Ireland (population 94% Catholic)	Practice of watching or "waking" the dead originates from keeping vigil to keep evil spirits away from the deceased—now a religious ritual
Israel (population 83% Jewish)	Relatives remain with dying person Eyes must be closed at death Body is never left alone Buried in ground in 24 hours except if Sabbath (Saturday)
Italy (population 99% Catholic)	Before death, fatal diagnosis is not discussed with patient and family
Japan (population 84% Buddhist)	Control public expressions of grief
Jordan (population 95% Muslim)	Muslim rites
Korea (North) (population 95% atheist)	Confucian funeral—elaborate Chief mourner and relatives weep
Korea (South) (population 72% Buddhist and Confucianist, 28% Christian)	Buddhists accept death as birth into another life

Table 6–6 *continued*

National Origin of Your Client/Family	Rites When Death Occurs
	Family members observe last breath; may respond with loud wailing and display intense emotion
Kuwait (population 85% Muslim)	Muslim rites
Laos (population 85% Buddhist)	Beliefs in reincarnation White flowers or candles may be placed in the deceased's hands Cremation and burial are practiced
Lebanon (population 75% Muslim)	Muslim rites
Libya	Muslim rites
Malaysia (population 58% Muslim, 30% Buddhist, 8% Hindu)	Muslim rites
Mali	Muslim rites
Mexico (population 97% Catholic)	Family members stay with dying person around the clock Grief may be expressive "Day of the Dead" celebrated in November
Morocco (population 99% Muslim)	Muslim rites
Netherlands	Active euthanasia permitted under certain circumstances
Nigeria (population 50% Muslim)	Muslim rites
Norway (population 94% Lutheran)	Close family members stay with person; no one should die alone Cremation and/or burial
Oman	Muslim rites
Pakistan (population 97% Muslim)	Muslim rites
Philippines (population 83% Catholic, 9% Protestant, 5% Muslim)	Muslim rites Protect person from knowing prognosis Emotional grief may occur after death
Portugal (population 97% Catholic)	Widow wears black and never remarries Visits grave frequently
Russia	Family is told of serious illness and decides if patient should know
Sweden (population 94% Lutheran)	Quiet and open grief acceptable Dying person not left alone Body usually not viewed after death

(continued)

Table 6-6 *continued*

National Origin of Your Client/Family	Rites When Death Occurs
Thailand (population 95% Buddhist)	Belief in reincarnation
Tunisia (population 98% Muslim)	Muslim rites
Vietnam (population 60% Buddhist, 13% Confucianist, 12% Taoist, 3% Catholic, 12% other)	Death at home preferred Body washed and wrapped in white sheets Burial in ground

Source: Adapted from Geissler, E. M. (1994). *Pocket guide: Cultural assessment.* St. Louis, MO: Mosby. This material was published in the Pocket Guide to Cultural Assessment, Elaine Marie Geissler, Copyright Elsevier (1994). Adapted from Lipson, J. G., Dibble, S. L., & Minarik, P. A. (1996). *Cultural and nursing care: A pocket guide.* San Francisco: UCSF Nursing Press. Used with permission.

Table 6-7 Religious Groups and Death Beliefs

Religious Group	Is There a Heaven?	What Is Heaven Like?	Belief in Resurrection?	Recognition of Friends and Relatives	Is Cremation Allowed?
Assemblies of God	Heaven is a real place	A pleasant place	Of the body	Yes	Not encouraged
Baha'is	Heaven designates spiritual proximity to God	An eternal spiritual evolution of the soul	Spiritual	Yes	No
Baptists	A place where the redeemed go	Filled with mansions and golden streets	Physical	Yes	Allowed but not encouraged
Buddhists	Numerous heavens	It has no independent existence	No future time is foreseen	See living friends and relatives but are not seen	Preferred
Churches of Christ	Dwelling place of God and future residence of the righteous	A realm of peace and love	Consciousness leaves body at death and takes rebirth until enlightened	Yes	Permitted
Hindus	A relative plane of existence to which souls go to after death	Dwellers in heaven enjoy long life and are free from thirst, hunger, and old age	Liberation of the soul	Visions	Most common method for disposing of body

Table 6–7 *continued*

Religious Group	Is There a Heaven?	What Is Heaven Like?	Belief in Resurrection?	Recognition of Friends and Relatives	Is Cremation Allowed?
Jews	Place where anxiety and travail are ended	Quiet, peaceful intellectual activity takes place	Yes, some only in soul	Yes	Not practiced
Lutherans	Believe in heaven	Nature unknown	Physical	Yes	Yes
Mormons	There are 3 "degrees of glory"	Places of continuing growth and progress	Yes	Yes	Yes, but not encouraged
Muslims	Several layers, usually 7	A garden	Describe afterlife as physical pains and pleasures	Some believe families are reunited	Not practiced
Roman Catholics	A condition: eternal full-ness of life	Supreme happiness flowing from intimacy with God	Physical	Entire community together	Disposal of body does not affect afterlife
Seventh-day Adventists	A being in the presence of God	Will be located in the renewed earth	Glorified body will be resurrected for life to come	Yes	No objection
United Methodists	Heaven exists	Being in the presence of God	Body and spirit	Yes	Yes

Source: Adapted from Johnson, C. J., & McGee, M. G. (Eds.). (1991) . *How different religions view death and afterlife.* Philadelphia: The Charles Press.

Table 6–8 Cultural Traditions in Mourning and After-Death Rituals

Religion of Your Patient/Family	Rituals You May Observe When Death Occurs
American-Indian religions	Beliefs and practices vary widely Seeing an owl is omen of death
Buddhism	Believe in impermanence Last-rite chanting at bedside Cremation common Pregnant women should avoid funerals to prevent bad luck for baby

(*continued*)

Table 6-8   *continued*

Religion of Your Patient/Family	Rituals You May Observe When Death Occurs
Catholicism	Obligated to take ordinary, not extraordinary, means to prolong life Sacrament of the sick Autopsy, organ donation acceptable Burial usual
Christian Science	Euthanasia contrary to teachings Do not seek medical help to prolong life Do not donate body parts Disposal of body and parts decided by family
Hinduism	Seen as opposite of birth—a passage—expect rebirth Autopsy, organ donation—acceptable Religious prayers chanted before and after death Men and women display outward grief Cremation common; ashes disposed of in holy rivers Thread is tied around wrist to signify a blessing—do not remove
Islam	Euthanasia prohibited Organ donation acceptable Autopsy only for medical or legal reasons Body washed only by Muslim of same gender
Jehovah's Witnesses	Euthanasia forbidden Autopsy acceptable if legally necessary Donations of body parts forbidden Burial determined by family preference
Judaism	Autopsy, organ donation not acceptable Euthanasia prohibited Life support not mandated Body ritually washed Burial as soon as possible Seven-day mourning period
Mormonism	Euthanasia not practiced Promote peaceful and dignified death Organ donation—individual choice Burial in "temple clothes"
Protestantism	Organ donation, autopsy, and burial or cremation usually individual decisions Prolonging life may have restrictions Euthanasia—varies
Seventh-day Adventism	Prefer prolonging life Euthanasia—no Autopsy, organ donation acceptable Disposal of body and burial—individual decisions

Source: Adapted from Lipson, J. G., Dibble, S. L., & Minarik, P. A. (1996). *Cultural and nursing care: A pocket guide.* San Francisco: UCSF Nursing Press. Used with permission.

Expressions of death and death rituals are also found in objects and memorial stones. Figures 6–11 to 6–16 depict several objects and memorial stones that may be used.

- Masks (Figure 6–11) represent methods people use to hide from the "Angel of Death." Masks may also be placed on the face of the deceased. The mask is from Colombia.
- Candles (Figure 6–12) are used by many people after a death as a way of lighting the way for the soul of the deceased.
- Jade stone (Figure 6–13), from China, is placed in orifices of the body to block the entrance of evil spirits after death.
- Ghost money, from China (Figure 6–14), is burned to send payments to a deceased person and to ensure his or her well-being in the afterlife.
- Elaborate grave markings, such as this one, marking the burial site of Johnny Ramone in the Forever Hollywood cemetery, Los Angeles, California (Figure 6–15).
- Monument in the Valley of the Temples, Honolulu, Hawaii. Food has been left for the deceased (Figure 6–16).

Intersections of HEALTH, HEALING, and RELIGION

There are several areas in which there is an intersection of HEALTH, HEALING, and RELIGION. The following are examples of additional spiritual/religious factors that link with the myriad of facets that have been described earlier in this chapter and in Chapter 5. One's religious affiliation may be seen as providing many links in a complex chain of life events. Religious affiliation frequently provides a background for a person regarding HEALTHY behavior and contributes to HEALTH. Participation in religious practices provides social support and this in turn brings HEALTH. In addition, religious worship may create positive emotions; this, too, contributes to HEALTH. Table 6–9 illustrates several of these intersections, which must be known by health care providers.

This chapter has been no more than an overview of the topics introduced. The amount of relevant knowledge could fill many books. The issues raised here are those that have special meaning to the practice of nursing, medicine, and health care delivery. We must be aware (1) of what people are thinking that may differ from our own thoughts and (2) that sources of help exist outside the modern medical community. As the beliefs of ethnic communities are explored in later chapters, the text discussions will attempt to delineate who are specifically recognized and used as HEALERS by the members of the communities, and will describe some of the forms of treatment used by each community.

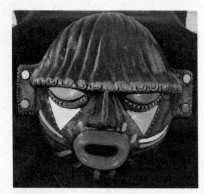

Figure 6-11   Mask.

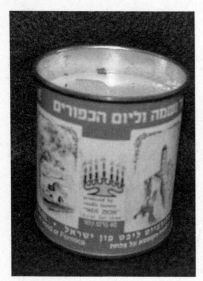

Figure 6-12   Candle.

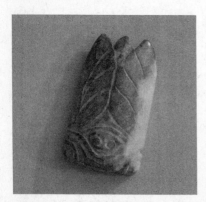

Figure 6-13   Jade stone.

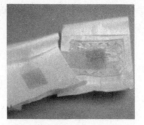

Figure 6-14   Ghost money.

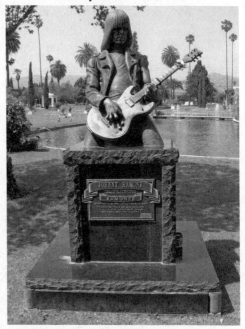

Figure 6-15   Forever Hollywood—Johnny Ramone.

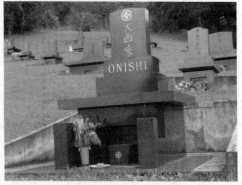

Figure 6-16   Valley of the Temples—Food at grave Honolulu, Hawaii.

Table 6-9   **Areas of Intersection Between the Provision of Health Care and HEALTH, HEALING, and RELIGION**

Communication	Spirituality and religion begin in silence; however, the need for adequate interpreters has been addressed, but it is also imperative to have available to people the members and leaders of their faith community who can reach out and interpret what is happening in regard to a health crisis at a deeper and spiritual level for the patient and family.
Gender	Understand the "rules" for gender care; in many faith traditions— for example, among Orthodox Jews and Muslims—care must be gender-specific, and people may be forbidden to be touched by someone of the opposite gender.
Manners	Religious and elderly people may be extremely sensitive as to the manner in which they are addressed—never call a person by their given name unless given permission to do so.
Modesty	Religious and elderly people may be extremely modest and modesty *must* be safe-guarded at all times.
Diet	There are many food taboos predicated by one's religion and consideration must be given to see that improper foods are not served to patients.
Objects	Sacred objects, such as amulets and statues, must be allowed in the patient's space and all precautions must be observed to safeguard them and when a person wears an amulet, every effort must be made to protect this amulet and permit the patient to wear it.
Social organization	Spirituality or a religious background contributes many positive factors to the health care situation; collaboration with the leaders of a faith community can result in strongly positive outcomes for a patient and family.
Space	Space must be defined and allocated for the patient's and family's private use.
Time	Health care providers must be knowledgeable about sacred time— for example, what day the patient and family observe as a day of rest—Friday for Muslims; Friday sunset until Saturday sunset for Jews; Saturday for Seventh-day Adventists; and Sunday for Christians; calendars must be posted that note holidays for all the faith traditions of people served within a given institution; meetings should not be held on these dates; Appendix B contains a list of religious holidays that do not occur on the same date each year; clergy within the faith tradition *must* be contacted to provide the dates for the holidays on a yearly basis; major meetings should not be scheduled on holidays.

Explore 🌐 MediaLink

Go to the Student Resource Site at nursing.pearsonhighered.com for chapter-related review questions, case studies, and activities. Contents of the CULTURALCARE Guide and CULTURALCARE Museum can also be found on the Student Resource Site. Click on Chapter 6 to select the activities for this chapter.

■ Internet Sources

Fatima, A Grace for Mankind. (2006). Retrieved from http://www.ewtn.com/fatima and http://sacredsites.com/europe/portugal/fatima.html, April 25, 2011.

Kukaniloko Birth Stones. (2010). Retrieved from http://www.hawaiiweb.com/oahu/sites_to_see/kukaniloko_birth_stones.htm, April 25, 2011.

Lourdes, France. (2008). Numerous links to information and history of the site. Retrieved from http://www.sacred-destinations.com/france/lourdes, April 25, 2011.

Montserrat Shrine, Spain. (2008). Retrieved from http://www.sacred-destinations.com/spain/montserrat-shrine, April 25, 2011.

The University of Texas at Brownsville and Texas Southmost College. (2006). *El Nino Fidencio, Curanderismo Research Project*. Brownsville, Texas. Retrieved from http://vpea.utb.edu/elnino/fidencio.html, April 26, 2011.

Welcome to El Santuario de Chimayo, (2010). Author. Retrieved from http://www.elsantuariodechimayo.us/indexAlt.html, March 5, 2012.

■ References

Ausubel, N. (1964). *The book of Jewish knowledge*. New York: Crown.

Bishop, G. (1967). *Faith healing: God or fraud?* Los Angeles: Sherbourne.

Blattner, B. (1981). *Holistic nursing*. Englewood Cliffs, NJ: Prentice Hall.

Buxton, J. (1973). *Religion and healing in Mandari*. Oxford: Clarendon.

Cramer, E. (1923). *Divine science and healing*. Denver: The Colorado College of Divine Science.

Ford, P. S. (1971). *The healing trinity: Prescriptions for body, mind, and spirit*. New York: Harper & Row.

Foy, F. A. (Ed.). (1980). *Catholic almanac*. Huntington, IN: Our Sunday Visitor.

Gardner, D. (1992). *Niño Fidencio: A heart thrown open*. Santa Fe: Museum of New Mexico Press.

Geissler, E. M. (1994). *Pocket guide: Cultural assessment*. St. Louis: Mosby.

Geissler, E. M. (1998). *Pocket guide: Cultural assessment* (2nd ed.). St. Louis: Mosby.

Hallam, E. (1994). *Saints*. New York: Simon & Schuster.

Illich, I. (1975). *Medical nemesis: The expropriation of health*. London: Marion Bogars.

Informational brochure. (1953). Shrine of Our Lady of La Leche, St. Augustine, FL (personal visit, 1999).

Informational brochure. (1999). Shrine of the Blessed Virgin Mary, Christ of the Hills Monastery, Blanco, TX (personal visit, 1997).

Informational brochure. (n.d.). Shrine of our Lord of Esquipulas, Chimayo, New Mexico.

Johnson, C. J., & McGee, M. G. (Eds.). (1991). *How different religions view death and afterlife*. Philadelphia: Charles Press.

Krieger, D. (1979). *The therapeutic touch*. Englewood Cliffs, NJ: Prentice Hall.

Krippner, S., & Villaldo, A. (1976). *The realms of healing*. Millbrae, CA: Celestial Arts.

Lipson, J. G., Dibble, S. L., & Minarik, P. A. (1996). *Cultural and nursing care: A pocket guide*. San Francisco: UCSF Nursing Press.

Monthly Missalette, 15(13) (1980, February), 38.

Morgenstern, J. (1966). *Rites of birth, marriage, death and kindred occasions among the Semites*. Chicago: Quadrangle Books.

Naegele, K. (1970). *Health and healing*. San Francisco: Jossey-Bass.

Nightingale, F. (1860, 1946). (A facsimile of the first edition published by D. Appleton and Co.). *Notes on nursing—What it is, what it is not*. New York: Appleton-Century.

Progoff, I. (1959). *Depth psychology and modern man*. New York: McGraw-Hill.

Russell, A. J. (1937). *Healing in his wings*. London: Methuen.

Shames, R., & Sterin, C. (1978). *Healing with mind power*. Emmaus, PA: Rodale Press.

Shaw, W. (1975). *Aspects of Malaysian magic*. Kuala Lumpur, Malaysia: Nazibum Negara.

Wallace, G. (1979, November). Spiritual care—A reality in nursing education and practice. *The Nurses Lamp, 5*(2), 1–4.

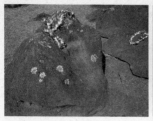 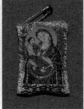 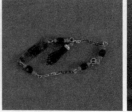 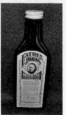

Figure 7-1   **Figure 7-2**   **Figure 7-3**   **Figure 7-4**

Chapter *7*

Familial HEALTH Traditions

As modern medicine becomes more impersonal, people are recalling with some wistfulness old country cures administered by parents and grandparents over the generations.

—*F. Kennet (1976)*

■ Objectives

1. Trace your family's heritage.
2. Describe your and your family's beliefs and practices in
   a. Health/HEALTH maintenance,
   b. Health/HEALTH protection,
   c. Health/HEALTH restoration, and
   d. Curing/HEALING.
3. Compare and contrast the difference and similarities between you and your peers in respect to beliefs and practices in
   a. Health/HEALTH maintenance,
   b. Health/HEALTH protection,
   c. Health/HEALTH restoration, and
   d. Curing/HEALING.

The opening images for this chapter depict a place and objects symbolic of items used to maintain, protect, and restore HEALTH in a family setting. A baby is born—a new life begins. The child may go home with birth parents, foster parents, or adoptive parents and to a nuclear, an extended, same gender, or a single-parent family with parents who have lived in this country for many generations or are immigrants, who are heritage consistent or heritage inconsistent. The family may use objects and remedies that were used in earlier generations or elect to use today's remedies for the maintenance, protection, and restoration of the family's health/HEALTH. Figure 7–1 is of the Birthing Stones in Kukaniloko, central Oahu, Hawaii. The stones are on sacred grounds where the chief of Oahu was to be born. Today, the traditional Native Hawaiian woman may go there to recite prayers for a healthy baby and leave a floral lei on the stones. Figure 7–2 is that of a *phylacto*—a small beaded cushion-like object that may be pinned on a baby's shirt for protection. It is the Greek custom for the godparent to buy this item and pin it on a newborn baby before he or she is baptized. Figure 7–3 is a beaded bracelet with a small black hand made of jet, worn to protect the Hispanic child from the evil eye. Figure 7–4 is Father John's Medicine—a remedy that has been used to treat coughs and colds since 1855. It contains neither alcohol nor drugs and continues to be available.

What are your traditional HEALTH beliefs and practices? What are your family's traditional HEALTH beliefs and practices? What family stories have been passed to you from your parents and grandparents? If you could choose 4 ways to present the HEALTH traditions from your or your family's heritage, what would they be?

Given the now apparent difficulty of defining *health/HEALTH* and *illness/ILLNESS*, it can be assumed that you may have little or no working knowledge of personally practiced "folk medicine," or traditional medicine, within your own family, or you may come from a family where traditional HEALTH and ILLNESS beliefs and practices constitute a significant part of your daily life.

In addition to exploring the already described questions regarding the definitions of *health* and *illness*, it is beneficial to your understanding to describe how you maintain, protect, and/or restore your *health/HEALTH*. Common forms of self-medication and treatment are the use of aspirin for headaches and colds and occasional vitamin supplements. Initially, one may admit to using tea, honey, and lemon and hot or cold compresses for headaches and minor aches and pains. For the most part, however, we tend to look to the health care system for the prevention and treatment of illness.

There is an extremely rich tradition in the United States related to self-care. This includes the early use of patent medicines. Throughout most of their history, patent medicines enjoyed a free existence and were very popular with the people of the times. Some of the most popular medicines of the early 20th century contained alcohol; others contained opium and cocaine. This increased their popularity, and the practice continued until passage of the Food, Drug, and Cosmetic Act of 1938. Today, as our lives become more complex and the health care system becomes more complicated, costly, and difficult to access, we see a return to self-care and an increasing use of traditional and homeopathic health care systems (see Chapters 5 and 6).

■ Familial Health/HEALTH Traditions

We are now ready for a transition, and it is time to resume climbing the steps to CULTURALCOMPETENCY. The foundation—a discussion of heritage, an overview of demographic issues, an exploration of terms such as *health* and *illness*, and a discussion of HEALTH and ILLNESS as they relate to religion and spirituality—has been presented and what remains is the ascent! Before you read on, ask yourself the following questions regarding your health/HEALTH beliefs and practices:

- Again, what remedies and/or methods do you use to maintain, protect, and restore your health/HEALTH?
- Do you know the health/HEALTH and illness/ILLNESS beliefs and practices that were or are a part of your heritage?
- Were you ever thought to be seriously ill/ILL?
- What did your familial caregiver do to take care of you?
- Did he or she consult someone in your own ethnic or religious community to find out what was wrong?

It has been mentioned earlier in this text that the first step for developing CULTURALCOMPETENCY is to know yourself, your heritage, and the health/HEALTH and illness/ILLNESS beliefs and practices derived from your heritage—ethnic, religious, or both. It was pointed out in Chapters 5 and 6 that many daily HEALTH practices have their origins in one's heritage, yet may not be thought of in this context.

The following interview procedure is useful for making you aware of the overall history and health/HEALTH belief and practice-related folklore and ethnocultural knowledge of your family. Because the ethnocultural history of each family is unique, you may want to discover more than health/HEALTH beliefs and practices with this interview. Ask your parents or grandparents questions about your family surname, traditional first names, family stories, the history of family "characters" or notorious family members, how historical events affected your family in past generations, and so forth. Next, ask the person you are interviewing the questions in the Heritage Assessment, found in Appendix E. Then, in interviewing your grandmothers, great-aunts, and mother, obtain answers to the following questions:

1. What did they do to maintain health/HEALTH? What did their mothers do?
2. What did they do to protect health/HEALTH? What did their mothers do?
3. Do they wear, carry, or hang in their home objects that protect their HEALTH and home?
4. Do they follow a particular dietary regimen or refrain from eating restricted foods?

Physical, mental, and spiritual aspects are implicit in each of the next 3 questions:

1. What home remedies do they use to restore health/HEALTH? What did their mothers use?
2. What are their traditional beliefs regarding pregnancy and childbirth?
3. What are their traditional beliefs regarding dying and death?

There are 2 reasons for exploring your familial heritage. First, it draws your attention to your ethnocultural and religious heritage and HEALTH-related belief system. Many of your daily habits relate to early socialization practices that are passed on by parents or additional significant others. Many behaviors are both subconscious and habitual, and much of what you believe and practice is passed on in this manner. By digging into the past, remote and recent, you can recall some of the rituals you observed either your parents or your grandparents perform. You are then better able to realize their origin and significance. There are many beliefs and practices that are ethnically similar, and socialization patterns may tend to be similar among ethnic groups as well. Religion also plays a role in the perception of, interpretation of, and behavior in health/HEALTH and illness/ILLNESS.

The maternal side is ideal for your interview because, in today's society of interethnic, interracial, and interreligious marriages and complex family structures, it is assumed that the ethnic beliefs and practices related to health/HEALTH and illness/ILLNESS of the family may be more in tune with the mother's family than with the father's. By and large, family nurturance and health/HEALTH maintenance, protection, and/or restoration have been the domain of women in most cultures and societies. The mother tends to be the gate-keeper—the person within a family who cares for family members when illness/ILLNESS occurs. She also tends to be the prime mover in protecting health/HEALTH and seeking health/HEALTH care. It is the mother who tells the child what and how much to eat and drink, when to go to bed, and how to dress in inclement weather. She shares her knowledge and experience with her offspring, but usually the daughter is singled out for such experiential sharing. However, this is not a "universal" circumstance, and in many family heritages it is the father who is the family caregiver. If that is true for your family, it is your paternal family whom you must interview. Given the complex familial changes and social changes related to family life, it behooves you to question both your maternal and your paternal relatives.

The second reason for this examination of familial health/HEALTH practices is to sensitize you to the role your ethnocultural and religious heritage has played. You must reanalyze the concepts of health/HEALTH and illness/ILLNESS and view your own definitions from another perspective. If your familial background is presented in a class or another group setting, the peer group is able to see the people in a different light. A group observes similarities and differences among its members. You discover peer beliefs and practices that you originally had no idea existed. You may then be able to identify the "why" behind many daily health/HEALTH habits, practices, and beliefs in your family.

You may be amazed to discover the origins of the health/HEALTH practices. The "mysterious" behavior of a roommate or friend may be explained by reflecting on its origin. It is interesting to discover cross-ethnic practices within one's own group, as some people believe that a given practice is an "original," done only by their family. Many religious customs, such as the blessing of the throat, are now conceptualized in terms of health/HEALTH behavior. Table 7–1

Table 7–1   Family Health Histories Obtained from Students of Various Ethnic Backgrounds and Religions

Austrian (United States), Jewish

HEALTH Maintenance

Bake own bread
Eat wholesome foods, homegrown fruits, and vegetables

HEALTH Protection

Camphor around the neck (in the winter) in a small cloth bag to prevent measles and scarlet fever

HEALTH Restoration

Boils: Fry chopped onions, make a compress, and apply to the infections
Sore throat: Go to the village store, find a salted herring, wrap it in a towel, put it around the neck, and let it stay there overnight; gargle with salt water

Black and Native American, Baptist

HEALTH Maintenance

Dress right for the weather
Eat balanced meals 3 times a day

HEALTH Protection

Blackstrap molasses
Keep everything clean and sterile
Regular checkups
Stay away from people who are sick

HEALTH Restoration

Bloody nose: Place keys on a chain around neck to stop
Sore throat: Suck yolks out of eggshell; honey and lemon; baking soda, salt, and warm water and lemon; onions around the neck; and/or salt water to gargle

Black African (Ethiopia), Orthodox Christian

HEALTH Maintenance

Keep the area clean
Pray every morning when getting up from bed

HEALTH Protection

Eat hot food, such as pepper, fresh garlic, and lemon

Table 7–1 *continued*

HEALTH Restoration

Eat hot and sour foods, such as lemons, fresh garlic, hot mustard, and/or red pepper
Make a kind of medicine from leaves and roots of plants mixed together
Colds: hot boiled milk with honey
Evil eye: They put some kind of plant root on fire and make the man who has the evil eye
  smile and the man talks about his illness

Canadian, Catholic

HEALTH Maintenance

Cleanliness
Food: People should eat well (fat people used to be considered healthy)
Prayer: HEALTH was always mentioned in prayer

HEALTH Protection

Elixirs containing herbs and brewed, given as a vitamin tonic
Lots of good food
Sleep
Wear camphor around the neck to ward off any evil spirit; use Father John's medicine from
  November to May

HEALTH Restoration

Aches and pains: hot Epsom salt baths
Colds: hot lemons
Cough: shot of whiskey
Eye infections: Potatoes are rubbed on them or a gold wedding ring is placed on them and
  the sign of the cross is made 3 times
Fever: Lots of blankets and heat make you sweat out a fever
Headache: Lie down and rest in complete darkness
Infected wounds: raw onions placed on wounds
Kidney problems: herbal teas
Sinuses: camphor placed in a pouch and pinned to the shirt

Eastern Europe (United States), Jewish

HEALTH Maintenance

Doctor only when pregnant (grandmother)
Go to doctor when sick (mother)
Health care for others, not self (mother)
Health for self not a priority (grandmother)
Physician twice a year (mother)
Reluctantly sought medical help (grandmother)

HEALTH Protection

Not much to prevent illness—very ill today with chronic diseases (grandmother)
Observe precautions, such as dressing warmly, not going out with wet hair, getting enough
  rest, staying in bed if not feeling well (mother)
Vitamins and water pills

(continued)

Table 7-1 *continued*

HEALTH Restoration

Colds: fluids, aspirin, rest
Insomnia: glass of wine
Muscle aches: Massage with alcohol
Sore throat: Gargle with salt water; tea with lemon and honey
Stomach upset: Eat light and bland foods
Chicken soup used by mother and grandmother

English, Baptist

HEALTH Maintenance

Daily walks
Eat well
Keep warm
Read

HEALTH Restoration

Cold: Heat glass and put on back
Earache: honey and tea; warm cod-liver oil in ear; stay in bed

English, Catholic

HEALTH Maintenance

Bedroom window open at night
Good housekeeping
Immediate cleanup after meals; wash pan before meals
Lots of exercise; proper sleep; lots of walking; no drinking or smoking; hard work
Never wear dirty clothing
Rest
Take baths

HEALTH Protection

Keep kitchen at 90°F in winter and house will be warm
Maintain a good diet: fresh vegetables, vitamins, little meat, lots of fish, no fried foods; lots of sleep
Strict enforcement of lifestyle

HEALTH Restoration

Colds: chicken soup; herb tea made from roots; alcohol concoctions; Vicks and hot towels
   on chest; lots of fluids, rest; Vicks, sulfur, and molasses
Cuts: wet tobacco
Rashes: burned linen and cornstarch
Sore throat: 4 onions and sugar steeped to heal and soothe the throat

English, Episcopal

HEALTH Maintenance

Cod-liver oil
Enough sleep
Thorough diet, vitamins

Table 7-1 *continued*

HEALTH Restoration

Colds and sore throats: camphor on chest and red scarves around chest

French (France), Catholic

HEALTH Maintenance

Proper food; rest; proper clothing; cod-liver oil daily

HEALTH Protection

Every spring give sulfur and molasses for 3 days as a laxative to get rid of worms

HEALTH Restoration

Colds: Rub chest with Vicks; honey

French Canadian, Catholic

HEALTH Maintenance

Wear rubbers in the rain and dress warmly; take part in sports; active body; lots of sleep

HEALTH Protection

Cod-liver oil in orange juice
No "junk foods"; play outside; walk; daily use of Geritol; camphor on clothes; balanced
  meals
Sulfur and molasses in spring to clear the system

HEALTH Restoration

Back pain: mustard packs
Colds: brandy with warm milk; honey and lemon juice; hot poultice on the chest; tea,
  whiskey, and lemon
Rashes: oatmeal baths
Sore throat: Wrap raw potatoes in sack and tie around neck; soap and water enemas
Warts: rub potato on wart, run outside, and throw it over left shoulder

German (United States), Catholic

HEALTH Maintenance

Good diet
Take aspirin
Take shots
Wash before meals; change clothes often
Wear rubbers; never go barefoot; long underwear and stockings

HEALTH Protection

Cod-liver oil
Drink glass of water at meals
Exercise
No sweets at meals
Plenty of milk
Spring tonic; sulfured molasses

(continued)

Table 7–1 *continued*

HEALTH Restoration

Coughs: honey and lemon; hot water and Vicks; boiled onion water, honey and vinegar
Constipation: Ivory soap suppositories
Cramps: ginger tea
Earache: few drops of warm milk in the ear; laxatives when needed
Fever: Mix whiskey, water, and lemon juice and drink before bed—causes person to perspire and break fever
Headache: Boil a beef bone and break up toast in the broth and drink
Recovery diet: boil milk and shredded wheat and add a dropped egg—first thing eaten after an illness
Sore back: hot mustard plaster
Sore throat: saltwater gargle
Stye: cold tea-leaf compress
Swollen glands or mumps: Put pepper on salt pork and tie around the neck

Iran (United States), Islam

HEALTH Maintenance

Cleanliness
Diet

HEALTH Protection

Dress properly for the season and weather; keep feet from getting wet in the rain
Inoculations

HEALTH Restoration

Cough: honey and lemon
Indigestion: baking soda and water
Rashes: Apply cornstarch
Sore throat: Gargle with vinegar and water
Sore muscles: alcohol and water

Irish (Catholic)

HEALTH Maintenance

Attitudes important: "good living habits and good thinking"; "eat breakfast—if late for school, eat a good breakfast and be a little late"; "don't be afraid to spend on groceries—you won't spend on the doctor later"
Avoid "fast foods"
Be clean, wear clean clothes
Blessing of the throat
Brush teeth; if out of toothpaste use table salt, or Ivory soap, or Dr. Lyon's Tooth Powder
Dress warmly
Early to bed ("rest is the best medicine")
Good food, balanced diet
Keep clean
Keep feet warm and dry

Table 7-1 *continued*

Outdoor exercise, enjoy fresh air and sunshine
Plenty of rest
Vitamins
Wear holy medals, green scapular

HEALTH Protection

Avoid sick people
Be goal-oriented
Clean out bowels with senna for 8 days
Drink senna tea at every vacation—cleans out the system
During flu season, tie a bag of camphor around the neck
Eat lots of oily foods
Every spring, drink a mixture of sulfur and molasses to clean blood
Maintain a strong family with lots of love
Never go to bed with wet hair
Nurture a strong religious faith
Onions under the bed to keep nasal passages clear
Prevent evil spirits: Don't look in mirror at night and close closet doors
Take Father John's medicine every so often

HEALTH Restoration

Chicken soup for everything from colds to having a baby
See doctor only in emergency
Acne: Apply baby's urine
Backache: Apply hot oatmeal in a sock; place a silver dollar on the sore area, light
  a match to it; while the match is burning, put a glass over the silver dollar and
  then slightly lift the glass, and this causes a suction, which is said to lift the
  pain out
Boils: cooked oatmeal wrapped in a cloth (steaming hot) applied to drain pus; oatmeal
  poultice
Colds: tea and toast; chest rub; vaporizer; hot lemonade and a tablespoon of whiskey;
  mustard plasters; Vicks on chest; whiskey; Vicks in nostrils; hot milk with butter, soups,
  honey, hot toddies, lemon juice, and egg whites; ipecac ("cruel but good medicine");
  whiskey with hot water and sugar; soak feet in hot water and sip hot lemonade; boiled
  wines; coffee with anisette
Colic: warm oil on stomach
Coughs: cough syrup (available on stove all winter) made from honey and whiskey; Vicks on
  chest; mustard plaster on chest; onion-syrup cough medicine; steam treatment; swallow
  Vicks; linseed poultice on chest; flaxseed poultice on back, red flannel cloth soaked in hot
  water and placed on chest all night
Cramps: crème de menthe
Cuts: boric acid
Earache: Heat salt, put in stocking behind the ear
Fever: spirits of niter on a dry sugar cube or mix with water; cold baths; alcohol rubdowns;
  cover with blankets to sweat it out

(continued)

Table 7-1   *continued*

HEALTH Restoration *(continued)*

Headache: Fill a soup bowl with cold water and put some olive oil in a large spoon; hold
  the spoon over the bowl in front of the person with the headache; while doing this, recite
  words in Italian and place index finger in the oil in the spoon; drop 3 drops of oil from the
  finger into the bowl; by the diameter of the circle the oil makes when it spreads in the
  water, the severity of the headache can be determined (larger = more severe); after this
  is done 3 times, the headache is gone; or place a hot poultice on forehead; hot facecloth;
  cold, damp cloth to forehead; in general, stay in bed, get plenty of rest and sleep, a glass of
  juice about once an hour, aspirin, and lots of food to get back strength; kerchief with ice
  in it is wrapped around the head; mint tea
High blood pressure: In Italy for high blood pressure, colonies of blood suckers were kept
  in clay, where they were born; the person with high blood pressure would have a blood
  sucker put on his fanny, where it would suck blood; it was thought that this would lower
  his blood pressure; the blood suckers would then be thrown in ashes and would then
  throw up the blood they had sucked from the person. If the blood sucker died, it alerted
  the person to see a doctor because it sometimes meant that there was something wrong
  with the person's blood
Insect bites: Vaseline or boric acid
Menstrual cramps: hot milk sprinkled with ginger; shot of whiskey, glass of warm wine; warm
  teas; hot-water bottle on stomach
Muscle pain: Heat up carbon leaves (herb) and bundle in a hot cloth to make a pack
  (soothes any discomfort)
Nausea and other stomach ailments: hot teas; castor oil; hot ginger ale; bay leaf; cup of hot
  boiled water; potato for upset stomach; baking soda; gruel
Pimples: to draw contents, apply hot flaxseed
Poison ivy: yellow soap suds
Sore throat: honey; apply Vicks on throat at bedtime and wrap up the throat; paint throat
  with iodine, honey and lemon, Karo syrup; paint with kerosene oil internally with a rag
  and then tie a sock around the neck; paint with iodine or Mercurochrome and gargle with
  salt and water, honey, melted Vicks
Splinters: flaxseed poultice
Sprains: beat egg whites, apply to part, and wrap part
Stomachache: camilla and maloa (herbs) added to boiled water
Stye: hot tea bag to area
Sucking thumb: Apply hot pepper to thumb
Sunburn: Apply vinegar; put milk on cloth and apply to burn; a cold, wet tea bag on small
  areas such as eyelids
To build up blood: eggnog with brandy; marsala wine and milk
Toothache: whiskey applied topically
Upset stomach: herb tea made with herbs sent from Italy

Italian (United States), Catholic

HEALTH Maintenance

Eat (solved emotional and physical problems); fruit at end of meal cleans teeth; early to bed
  and early to rise
Hearty and varied nutritional intake; lots of fruit, pasta, wine (even for children), cheese,
  home grown vegetables, and salads; exercise in form of physical labor; molasses on a piece
  of bread, or oil and sugar on bread; hard bread (good for the teeth)

Table 7–1 *continued*

Pregnancy:
Two weeks early: girl
Two weeks late: boy
Heartburn: baby with lots of hair

HEALTH Protection

Eat properly
Garlic cloves strung on a piece of string around the neck of infants and children to prevent
  colds and "evil" stares from other people, which they believed could cause headaches and
  a pain or stiffness in the back or neck (a piece of red ribbon or cloth on an infant served
  the same purpose)
If infants got their nights and days mixed up, they were tied upside down and turned all the
  way around
Keep feet warm
Keep warm in cold weather
Never wash hair before going outdoors or at night
Never wash hair or bathe during period
Stay out of drafts
To prevent bowlegs and keep ankles straight, up to the age of 6 to 8 months a bandage was
  wrapped around the baby from the waist to the feet
To prevent "evil" in the newborn, a scissor was kept open under the mattress of the crib

Norwegian (Norway), Lutheran

HEALTH Maintenance

Cleanliness
Cod-liver oil
Rest

HEALTH Protection

Immunizations

HEALTH Restoration

Colds and sore throat: hot peppermint drink and Vicks

Nova Scotian, Catholic

HEALTH Maintenance

Sleep; proper foods

HEALTH Protection

Cut up some onions and put them on back of stove to cook; feed them to all

HEALTH Restoration

Cold: Boil carrots until jellied, add honey; as expectorant boil onions, add honey
Cold in the back: Alcohol was put in a small metal container, a piece of cotton on a stick
  was placed in the alcohol, ignited, and put in a *banky* (a type of glass resembling a whiskey
  glass); this was put on the back where the cold was and left for half an hour and a hickey-
  like rash would develop; it was believed that the rash would drain the cold

(continued)

Table 7–1 *continued*

HEALTH Restoration *(continued)*

Earache: Put few drops of heated camphorated oil in ear; melt chicken fat and sugar, put in ear
Earache with infection: To drain the infection, cut a piece of salt pork about 2 inches long and 3/4 inch thick and insert it into the infected ear and leave for a few days
Psoriasis: Hang a piece of lead around the neck
Skin ulcer and infection: A sharp blade was sterilized and used to make a small incision in the skin, and live blood suckers were placed in the opening, they would drain the infection out; when the blood sucker was full, it would fall to a piece of paper, be bled, placed in alcohol, and reused
Sore throat: Coat a tablespoon of molasses with black pepper

Polish (United States), Catholic

HEALTH Maintenance

Cod-liver oil
Eating good, nutritious foods
Plenty of rest
Use of physician

HEALTH Protection

Eat fresh, homegrown foods
Exercise
Good diet
Good personal hygiene
Work

HEALTH Restoration

Colds: Drink hot liquids, chicken soup, honey
Headache: Take aspirin, hot liquids
Sore muscles: heating pads and hot compresses

Swedish (United States), Protestant

HEALTH Maintenance

A lot of walking
Cod-liver oil
Eat well-balanced meals
Routine medical examinations

HEALTH Protection

Blessing of the throat on St. Blaise Day
Dress appropriately for weather
Eat an apple a day
Eat sorghum molasses for general, all around good health
"I don't do a blooming thing"; eat well

HEALTH Restoration

Anemia: cod-liver oil
Bee stings: poultice
Black eye: leeches

Table 7-1 *continued*

Congestion: steamy bathroom
Cough: warm milk and butter
Earache: warm oil
Fever: blankets to sweat it out
Lumbago: Drink a yeast mixture
Rundown and tired: Eat a whole head of lettuce
Sick: lots of juices and decarbonated ginger ale; lots of rest
Sore throat: gargle with salt and take honey in milk; herringbone wrapped in flannel around the neck
Upset stomach: baking soda

---

lists a sample of responses to the questions that students obtained from members of the maternal side of their families regarding the maintenance, protection, and restoration of health/HEALTH. Table 7–2 describes selected answers to questions regarding birth and death beliefs and practices. These methods, beliefs, and practices are examples to trigger your questions and help you to probe the memories of the person you are questioning.

■ Consciousness Raising

The experience of sharing one's familial HEALTH practices raises one's consciousness in several ways, helps participants see themselves and others in a different context, and facilitates the understanding of patients' practices.

Recognizing Similarities

In my experience, as discussion continues, people realize that many personal beliefs and practices do, in fact, differ from what they are being taught in nursing or medical education to accept as the right way of doing things. Participants begin to admit that they do not seek medical care when the first symptoms of illness appear. On the contrary, they usually delay seeking care and often elect to self-treat at home. They also recognize that there are many preventive and health maintenance acts learned in school with which they choose not to observe. Sometimes, they discover that they are following self-imposed regimen for health-related problems and are not seeking any outside intervention.

Another facet of a group discussion is the participants' exposure to the similarities that exist among them in terms of HEALTH maintenance and protection. To their surprise and delight, they find that many of their daily acts— routines they take for granted—directly relate to methods of maintaining and protecting HEALTH.

As is common in most large groups, students seem to be shy at the beginning of this exploration. As more and more members of the group are willing to share their experiences, however, other students feel more comfortable and share more readily. A classroom tactic I have used to break the ice is to reveal an experience I had on the birth of my first child. My mother-in-law, an immigrant from Eastern Europe, drew a circle around the child's crib with her

Table 7-2 Examples of Selected Familial Ethnocultural and Religious Beliefs and Practices Related to Birth and Death

Nation of Origin and Religion	Birth Beliefs	Death Beliefs
Cape Verde—Catholic	Baptism	Death is a part of life
England—Christian	Baptism Natural event	Body dying Everlasting life with Christ Funeral and prayer Person goes to heaven
Germany—Lutheran	Birth is sacred	Body dies when we die— souls go to heaven and enjoy ever-lasting life
	Do not take baby out until it is baptized	Celebrate person's life and the promise of eternal life
	Mother does not go to the baptism	God's will
Greece—Orthodox	After 40 days mother and newborn go to church—baby is blessed and prayers are said to keep away the evil spirits	After a death, light a candle that burns all night
	Baptized at 2	Bones are unburied after 3 years, are put into a holy box, and are placed in the church or are reburied in the family grave
	Gifts given to the baby to protect it from the evil eye— charms of white and blue beads are worn on the wrist	In mourning, women wear black for the rest of their lives and men grow facial hair
	If the baby cries excessively, exorcism may be performed	Hold a special service on the 40th day
	Wrap the baby in blankets and pin to sheets to relax	Some older people believe in ghosts
		The good go to paradise; the bad go to hell
		Visit grave daily
Ireland—Catholic	Baby shower before birth but never set up the crib until after birth	After death, the body is washed and prepared for the wake at home by a neighbor and then the wake and mass
	Men not present at birth	Blessing with oils and receive the Eucharist for the last time
	Tell of pregnancy after 3 months	Dying person wears a Rosary around the neck to keep evil spirits away and God closer

Table 7-2 *continued*

		Dying: Pray the Rosary aloud as it is a stepping stone to the Virgin Mary, asking her to watch over this person and guide him or her to everlasting peace Final separation of the soul from the body—soul lives on and is transported to God Mourning: keening—a ritual of professional criers coming to the home and crying for hours over the death of a family member Wake—"a party with one less person"
Italy—Catholic	Life begins at conception	Closed casket Cremation
Japan—Shinto	Umbilical cord saved—a lasting bond between mother and child 100-day-old child taken to the Shrine	Cremation
Lithuania—Catholic	Baptism	Pray for the dead Visit graves
Portugal—Catholic	Throw a party for the birth of a boy (relates to the time when males were needed to work on the farms) Women during pregnancy get less pretty with a girl because the baby is taking her mother's looks	A party comforts the loved ones but if one dies in a painful way there is no celebration Celebrate a painless death—means the person has been good and is now with Jesus Widow must forever wear black—this serves as a warning to other men that she has suffered a loss and is not attractive to prevent shame from being brought to her
Sicily—Catholic	Baptism Gift from God	Close all shades and never go out during daylight The day you were born, it was known the day you were to die Women mourn for years, wearing only black and seldom going outside

fingers and spat on the baby 3 times to prevent the evil spirits from harming him. Once such an anecdote is shared, other participants have less difficulty in remembering similar events that took place in their own homes.

Students have a variety of feelings about the self-care practices of their families. One feeling discussed by many students is shame. A number of students express conflict in their attitudes: They cannot decide whether to believe the old ways when they have continued to be practiced or to drop them and adopt the more modern ones they are learning in school. For example, a young man from Ethiopia revealed that he experienced angst when he had an upper respiratory infection and his mother offered him herbs from their homeland. (This is an example of cognitive dissonance.) Many admit that this is the first time they have disclosed these HEALTH beliefs and practices in public, and they are relieved and amazed to discover similarities with other students. Frequently, there is a logical explanation as to why a given practice is successful. The acts may have different names or be performed in a slightly different manner, but the uniting thread among them is to prevent ILLNESS and to maintain and/or restore HEALTH.

Transference to Patients and Others

The effects of such a verbal catharsis are long remembered and often quoted or referred to throughout the remainder of a course. The awareness we gain helps us understand the behavior and beliefs of patients and, for that matter, other people better. Given this understanding, we are comfortable enough to ask patients how they interpret a symptom and how they think it ought to be treated. We begin to be more sensitive to people who delay in seeking health care or fail to comply with preventive measures and treatment regimens. We come to recognize that we do the same thing. The increased familiarity with home health/HEALTH practices and remedies helps us project this awareness and understanding to the patients who are served.

Analyzed from a "scientific" perspective, the majority of these practices have a sound basis. In the area of health/HEALTH maintenance (see Table 7–1), one notes an almost universal adherence to activities that include rest, balanced diet, and exercise.

In the area of health/HEALTH protection, various differences arise, ranging from visiting a physician to wearing a clove of garlic around the neck. Although the purpose of wearing garlic around the neck is "to keep the evil spirit away," the act also forces people to stay away: What better way to cut down exposure to wintertime colds than to avoid close contact with people?

One person remembered that during her childhood her mother forced her to wear garlic around her neck. Like most children, she did not like to be different from the rest of her schoolmates. As time went on, she began to have frequent colds, and her mother could not understand why this was happening. The mother followed her child to school some weeks later and discovered that she removed the garlic on her way to school, hiding it under a rock and then replacing it on the way home. There was quite a battle between the mother and daughter! The youngster did not like this method of protection because her peers mocked her.

A discussion of home remedies is of further interest when each of the methods presented is analyzed for its possible "medical" analogy and for its prevalence among various religious and ethnic groups. Many of the practices and remedies, to the surprise and relief of students, tend to run throughout groups but have different names or contain different ingredients.

In this day of computers and sophisticated medicine, including transplants, cloning, and intricate surgery, the most prevalent need expressed by people who practice traditional medicine is to protect people and prevent "evil" from harming them or to remove the "evil" that may be the cause of their HEALTH problem. As students, we analyze and discuss a problem and its traditional treatments and we begin to see how evil continues to be considered the cause of ILLNESS and how often the treatment is then designed to remove it.

Each person testifies to the efficacy of a given remedy. Many state that, when their grandmothers and mothers shared these remedies with them, they experienced great feelings of nostalgia for the good old days, when things seemed so simple. Some people may express a desire to return to these practices of yesteryear, whereas others openly confess that they continue to use such measures—sometimes in addition to what a health care provider tells them to use or often without even bothering to consult a provider.

The goal of this kind of consciousness-raising session is to reawaken the participant to the types of health/HEALTH practices within her or his own family. The other purpose of the sharing is to make known the similarities and differences that exist as part of a cross-ethnocultural and religious phenomenon. We are intrigued to discover the wide range of beliefs that exists among our peers' families. We had assumed that people thought and believed as we did. For the first time, we individually and collectively realize that we all practice a certain amount of traditional medicine, that we all have ethnocultural-specific ways of treating ILLNESS, and that we, too, often delay in seeking professional health care. We learn that most people prefer to treat themselves at home and that they have their own ways of treating a particular set of symptoms—with or without a prescribed medical regimen. The previously held notion that "everybody does it this way" is shattered. The greatest challenge in this activity is to encourage students and others to think of HEALTH, rather than simply health. This exercise brings you to the window on the glass door pictured in the introduction.

Explore MediaLink

Go to the Student Resource Site at nursing.pearsonhighered.com for chapter-related review questions, case studies, and activities. Contents of the CULTURALCARE Guide and CULTURALCARE Museum can also be found on the Student Resource Site. Click on Chapter 7 to select the activities for this chapter.

Box 7–1: Keeping Up

FOLKLIFE CENTERS
The following is a listing of selected folklife centers in the United States. From these centers, and others readily discovered on the World Wide Web, one may obtain films and literature related to folklife and medicine.

Alabama
The Alabama Folklife Program and The Alabama Folklife Association
410 N. Hull Street
Montgomery, AL 36104
334-242-3601
334-269-9098 Fax
http://www.arts.state.al.us/folklife/folklife.htm

Arizona
Southern Arizona Folklife Center
University of Arizona
Tucson, AZ 85721
520-621-2211
http://www.library.arizona.edu/images/folkarts/folkhome.html

California
Center for Study of Comparative Folklore and Mythology
University of California, Los Angeles
Los Angeles, CA 90024
http://www.folkmed.ucla.edu

Kentucky
Appalshop
P.O. Box 743A
Whitesburg, KY 41858
http://www.appalshop.org

Missouri
Missouri Folk Arts Program
157 McReynolds Hall
University of Missouri–Columbia
Columbia, MO 65211
573-882-6296
573-882-0360 Fax
http://museum.research.missouri.edu/mfap/

New England
Folk Arts Center of New England
42 West Foster Street
Melrose, MA 02176
http://facone.org/

Utah
The Utah Arts Council
617 East South Temple
Salt Lake City, UT 84102-1177
801-236-7555 Voice
800-346-4128 TDD
801-236-7556 Fax
http://arts.utah.gov/

Washington, DC
Within the federal government, resources for folklore and folklife endeavors in Washington, DC, are concentrated in 4 agencies:

1. The Library of Congress: http://www.loc.gov
2. The Smithsonian Institution: http://www.si.edu
3. National Endowment for the Arts: http://arts.endow.gov/
4. National Endowment of the Humanities: http://www.neh.gov/

American Folklife Center
The Library of Congress
Washington, DC 20540
202-287-6590
Folkline 202-287-2000: a telephone information service, http://www.loc.gov
Folklife Sourcebook: a resource guide to relevant organizations
This center was created by Congress in 1976 to "preserve and present" American folklife. It is an educational and research program.

Archive of Folk Culture
The Library of Congress
Washington, DC 20540
202-287-5510
http://www.loc.gov/folklife/cg.html
This is the public reference and archival arm of the American Folklife Center.

The American Folklore Society
1703 New Hampshire Avenue, NW
Washington, DC 20009
Membership in this society, founded in 1888, is open to all persons interested in folklore. It serves as a forum for the preservation of folklore.

■ References

Kennet, F. (1976). *Folk medicine—Fact and fiction: Age-old cures, alternative medicine, natural remedies.* New York: Crescent Books.

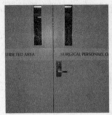 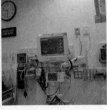 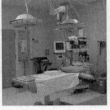 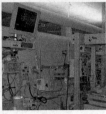

Figure 8-1   Figure 8-2   Figure 8-3   Figure 8-4

Chapter 8

Health and Illness in Modern Health Care

■ Objectives

1. Discuss the professional socialization of nurses, physicians, and other members of the health care delivery system.
2. Describe the "culture" of the health care providers.
3. Compare the growth of the gross domestic product and national health care expenditures over time.
4. Compare the expenditures for health care in the United States with those of other nations.
5. Itemize how the "dollar" spent for health care is allocated.
6. Recognize the interrelationships and trends of sociocultural, public health, and medical events that have produced the crises in today's modern health care system.
7. Break down the complex web of factors that impedes a person's passage through the health care system.
8. Chart the "Amazing Maze of Health Care" and give examples of your personal and professional experience.
9. Describe barriers to health care.
10. Identify the factors that determine medicine to be an institution of social control.
11. Compare and contrast modern medical care and CULTURALCARE.

The opening images for this chapter depict the inner depths of the modern health care system's culture. Figure 8–1 is an example of the doors to an emergency room or a surgical suite. These doors are closed to all except those sanctioned to enter. Few people outside of this closed system understand the intricacies of the cultures of health care and the meanings of the culture's knowledge and rituals, beliefs, and practices. Figure 8–2 is a well-equipped modern emergency room. Figure 8–3 is an operating room, and Figure 8–4 is a neo-natal intensive care unit. Each of the last 3 images illustrates the amount of high-technological equipment that is found in today's hospital. The knowledge and training necessary to use these items are extensive and costly. The equipment is extremely expensive, and many institutions have many units equipped such as these. The personnel responsible for delivering care in these technical settings are highly skilled. These 3 images suggest one of the reasons for the extraordinary costs of health care to be discussed in this chapter. In fact, as will be discussed in this chapter, it has been frequently demonstrated that the high cost of health care is not proof of high quality (Abelson, 2007, p. A-1) What are the unique symbols of your profession within the overall culture of modern health care? What settings or objects would you choose to represent your experiences of modern health care delivery?

The health care system of this nation has been in crisis, and the visionary words and observations of Dr. John Knowles in 1970 ring true today:

> American medicine, the pride of the nation for many years, stands on the brink of chaos. Our medical practitioners have their great moments of drama and triumph. But, much of U.S. medical care, particularly the everyday business of preventing and treating illness, is inferior in quality, wastefully dispensed, and inequitably financed.

What is it about our health care system and the people who practice within it that generated and continue to generate these comments? This chapter presents an overview of the issues inherent in the acculturation of health care providers and the health care delivery system in the United States. It begins by discussing the norms of the health care provider "cultures" and then examines many of the salient issues regarding the health care system in general.

■ The Health Care Provider's Culture

The providers of health care—nurses; physicians; social workers; dietitians; physical, occupational, respiratory, and speech therapists; and laboratory and departmental professionals—are socialized into the culture of their profession. Professional socialization teaches the student a set of beliefs, practices, habits, likes, dislikes, norms, and rituals. Each of the professional disciplines has its own language and objects, rituals, garments, and myths, which become an inherent part of the scope of students' education, socialization, and practice. The providers view time in their own ways, and they believe that their view of a health and illness situation and subsequent interventions are the only possible answers to the complex questions surrounding a health-related event. This newly learned information regarding health and illness differs in varying degrees from that of the individual's heritage. As students become more and more immersed and knowledgeable in the scientific and technological domains, they usually move further and further from their past belief systems and, indeed, further from the population at large in terms of its understanding and beliefs regarding health/HEALTH and illness/ILLNESS. Just as it is not unusual to hear providers say, "Etoh, bid, tid, im, iv," and so forth, it is not uncommon to hear patients say things such as "I have no idea what the nurses and doctors are saying!" "They speak a foreign language!" "What they are doing is so strange to me." In addition, there exists an underlying cultural norm among health care providers that "all must be done to save a patient, regardless of the patient's and family's wishes" and regardless of the financial consequences to the patient and family, to the health care system, or to society in general. A consequence of this philosophy has been the rise of iatrogenic health problems and the escalation of out-of-control health care costs.

As a result, health care providers can be viewed as an alien or foreign culture or ethnic group. They have a social and cultural system; they experience "ethnicity" in the way they perceive themselves in relation to the health care consumer and often each other. Even if they deny the reality of the situation, health care providers must understand that they are ethnocentric. Not only are they ethnocentric, but also many of them are xenophobic. To appreciate this critical issue, consider the following. A principal reason for the difficulty experienced between the health care provider and the consumer is that health care providers, in general, adhere rigidly to the modern allopathic, or Western, system of health care delivery. (These terms may be used interchangeably to describe health care.) With few exceptions, they do not publicly sanction any methods of protection or healing other than scientifically proved ones. They ordinarily fail to recognize or use any sources of medication other than those that have been deemed effective by scientific means. The only types of healers that are sanctioned are those that have been educated, licensed, and certified according to the requirements of this culture.

What happens, then, when people of one belief system encounter people who have other beliefs regarding health and illness (either in protection or in treatment)? Is the provider able to meet the needs as perceived and defined by the patient? More often than not, a wall of misunderstanding arises between the two. At this point, a breakdown in communications occurs, and the consumer ends up at a disadvantage.

Providers think that they comprehend all facets of health and illness and may frequently take a xenophobic view to HEALTH and ILLNESS and traditional HEALERS. Although in training and education health care providers have a significant advantage over the consumer-patient, it is entirely appropriate for them to explore other ideas regarding health/HEALTH and illness/ILLNESS and to adjust their approach to coincide with the needs of the specific patient. Health care providers have tried to force Western medicine on one and all, regardless of results.

The following list outlines the more obvious aspects of the health care provider's culture. In connection with later chapters, it can be referred to as a framework for comparing various other ethnic and cultural beliefs and practices.

1. Beliefs
   a. Standardized dualistic definitions of *health* and *illness*
   b. The omnipotence of technology
2. Practices
   a. The maintenance of health and the protection of health or prevention of disease through such mechanisms as the avoidance of stress, the use of immunizations, and the high use of costly medications
   b. Annual physical examinations and diagnostic procedures, such as Pap smears, mammographies, and colonoscopies.
3. Habits
   a. Charting
   b. The constant use of jargon
   c. The use of a systematic approach and problem-solving methodology
   d. Observing and depending on electronic monitors and other devices
4. Likes
   a. Promptness
   b. Neatness and organization
   c. Compliance
5. Dislikes
   a. Tardiness
   b. Disorderliness and disorganization
6. Customs
   a. Professional deference and adherence to the pecking order found in autocratic and bureaucratic systems
   b. Hand washing
   c. The use of certain procedures attending birth and death
7. The expectation of recovery no matter the cost or consequences of therapy

As noted, inherent in the socialization into the health care professions, nursing, medicine, social work, and the various therapies, there are countless cultural traits that are passed on both verbally and nonverbally. Remember, the doors in Figure 8–1 illustrate the closed aspects of the entire health care system.

Today, the problems of health care delivery have grown exponentially, and solutions are more elusive than ever. Doctors in the United States administer the world's most expensive medical (illness) care system. The costs of U.S. health care soared from $4 billion in 1940 to $27.5 billion in 1960, to the staggering 2008 figure of $2.3 trillion (U.S. Department of Health and Human Services, 2010, p. 366). Health care is an enterprise that exceeds all the goods and services produced by half the states in the country. Health has become this country's biggest business, and it accounts for 16.2% of our gross domestic

**Table 8-1   Gross Domestic Product, National Health Expenditures,
and Per Capita Expenditures, Selected Years: 1960–2008**

	Gross Domestic Product (GDP) in Billions of Dollars	National Health Expenditures in Billions of Dollars	National Health Expenditures Per Capita ($)
1960	526	27.5	148
1980	2,788	253.4	1,100
2000	13,399	1,352.9	4,789
2008	14,441	2,338	7,681

Source: U.S. Department of Health and Human Services. (2010). National Center for Health Statistics. Health, United States, 2010: With Special Feature on Death and Dying. Hyattsville, MD. 2011: Author. Retrieved from www.cdc.gov/nchs/data/hus/hus10.pdf 2011, December 18, 2011, p. 366.

Table 8-2   Per Capita Health Expenditures, Selected Years: 1960–2008

	National Health Expenditures ($)	Private Health Expenditures ($)	Public Health Expenditures ($)
1960	148	1,100	36
1980	1,100	638	462
2000	4,790	4,789	2,111
2008	7,681	4,046	3,635

Source: U.S. Department of Health and Human Services. (2010). National Center for Health Statistics. Health, United States, 2010: With Special feature on Death and Dying. Hyattsville, MD. 2011: Author. Retrieved from www.cdc.gov/nchs/data/hus/hus10.pdf 2011, December 18, 2011, p. 366.

product, as shown in Table 8–1. In fact, $7,681 was spent in 2008 per capita on health care for every man, woman, child, and fetus (U.S. Department of Health and Human Services, 2010, p. 366). Table 8–2 displays the per capita health expenditures and breaks down the figures as to the amount of money coming from private and public funds. The increment of expenditures from 1960 to 2008 is staggering.

Four questions then present themselves:

1. *What are the costs of health care?*
2. *How do we pay for health care?*
3. *Is health care in America better than in any other place on Earth?*
4. *Why is health care so expensive?*

■ Health Care Costs

What Are the Costs of Health Care?

This question is critical, and there are countless ways to answer it. However, it is certainly at the root of the problems we now face. The American health care system is both a source of national pride—if one has an expensive and adequate health insurance package or the money, it certainly is possible to get the finest medical/technological care in the world—and a source of deep embarrassment—those who are poor or uninsured may be wanting for care as people with a low family income, do not have consistent health insurance. According to Kinney, "the elephant in the room when it comes to healthcare is its cost." She explains that

> the inflation in healthcare costs in the United States are due to:
> (1) the advances in medical science and associated technology and pharmaceutical products; and
> (2) the advent of widespread health insurance coverage. (2010, p. 406)

The advances in technology contribute to overall health care costs and expenditures.

In Table 8–3 you can examine the growth in national health expenditures from 1960–2008.

Table 8-3 National Health Expenditures: United States, Selected Years: 1960–2008

	(Amount in Billions)			
	1960	1980	2000	2008
National health expenditures	$27.5	$253.4	$1,352.9	$2,338.7
Health services and supplies	24.9	233.5	1,264.1	2,181.3
Personal health care	23.3	214.8	1,139.2	1,952.3
Hospital care	9.2	101.0	416.9	718.4
Professional services	8.3	67.3	426.8	731.2
Physicians and clinical services	5.4	47.1	288.6	496.2
Other professional services	0.4	3.6	39.1	65.7
Dental services	2.0	13.3	62.0	101.2
Other personal health care services	0.6	3.3	37.1	68.1
Nursing home and home health	0.9	20.9	125.8	203.1
Home health care	0.1	2.4	30.5	64.7
Nursing home care	0.8	18.5	95.3	138.4
Retail outlet sales of medical products	4.9	25.7	169.8	299.6
Prescription drugs	2.7	12.0	120.6	234.1
Other medical products	2.3	13.6	49.2	65.5
Government administration and net cost of private health insurance	1.2	12.2	81.8	159.6
Government public health activities	0.4	6.4	43.0	69.4
Investment	**2.6**	**19.9**	**88.8**	**157.5**
Research	0.7	5.4	25.6	43.6
Structures and equipment	1.9	14.5	63.2	113.9

Source: U.S. Department of Health and Human Services. (2010). National Center for Health Statistics. Health, United States, 2010: With Special feature on Death and Dying. Hyattsville, MD. 2011: Author. Retrieved from www.cdc.gov/nchs/data/hus/hus10.pdf 2011, December 18, 2011, p. 369.

Table 8-4   Costs for Hospitalizations with Procedures: 1999 and 2006

	Amount in Millions (2006 dollars)	
Procedure	1999	2006
Respiratory intubation and mechanical ventilation	10,687	15,729
Percutaneous transluminal coronary angioplasty (PTCA)	6,407	13,327
Cardiac pacemaker, cardioverter, or defibrillator	3,518	8,693
Coronary artery bypass graft (CABG)	8,344	8,085
Knee arthroplasty (knee replacement)	3,573	7,920
Spinal fusion	2,651	7,670

Source: U.S. Department of Health and Human Services. (2009). National Center for Health Statistics. Health, United States, 2009: With Special Feature on Medical Technology. Hyattsville, MD. 2010: Author. Retrieved from www.cdc.gov/nchs/data/hus/hus09.pdf 2011, December 18, 2011, pp. 102–104.

Table 8–4 compares the costs for hospitalizations with procedures from 1999 with those of 2006. In addition, personal health care expenditures also soared between 1998–2008. They nearly doubled from $1.0 trillion to nearly $2.0 trillion.

When I was studying nursing in 1960:

- National health expenditures were $27.6 billion; in 2008, they were $2,338.7 trillion.
- Hospital care expenditures were $9.2 billion; in 2008, they were $1,952.3 billion.
- Physician and clinical services expenditures were $5.4 billion; in 2008, they were $496.2 billion.
- Nursing home expenditures were $0.8 billion; in 2008, they were $138.4 billion.
- Research funding was $0.7 billion; in 2008, it was $43.6 billion (Table 8–5 depicts the ways the health care dollar was spent from 1960 to 2008).

Table 8–4 also displays the costs of the most costly procedures in 1999 and 2006. The 6 most expensive principal procedures were selected based on aggregate national hospital costs in 2006. The costs were for the entire hospital stay, including the cost of performing the principal procedure.

How Do We Pay for Health Care?

The sources for paying for care in 1960 were primarily personal, out of pocket or private insurance; Medicare and Medicaid did not yet exist until 1965. It is obvious that they now make over 50% of health care expenditures possible— coverage shifted from the private sector to the public sector and is presently shifting back to the private sector. Technology has exploded, the costs of health care have soared, and many of the health care-related programs are seen as "entitlements." The costs of services are blindly covered and quite often it is impossible for a patient to get an itemized bill, yet, when people get them, they are astonished at the costs but state, "My insurance covers it and it costs me nothing." However, for more and more people the costs of heath care have become so high that their health insurance companies either disallow desired procedures or stop payments after a certain amount is reached. Families are left bankrupt in many instances or finding it necessary to choose between care or financial insolvency.

Affordable Health Care

On March 23, 2010, President Obama signed the Affordable Care Act. The law put in place comprehensive health insurance reforms that will roll out over 4 years and beyond, with most changes taking place by 2014. At this writing, the law has been in effect for over 1 year and the following changes have occurred:

1. Providing small business health insurance tax credits,
2. Relief for 4 million seniors who hit the Medicare prescription drug "donut hole,"
3. Providing access to insurance for uninsured Americans with pre-existing conditions,
4. Providing free preventive care,
5. Establishing consumer assistance programs in the states,
6. Free preventive care for seniors, and
7. Improving health care quality and efficiency.

It does not matter whether a person or family gets health benefits through work, buys insurance themselves, has a small business and desire to provide health coverage to their employees, are on Medicare, or don't currently have insurance, the Affordable Care Act gives a better control of decisions about health coverage. It is designed to make health care insurance affordable by providing small businesses with a tax credit to provide coverage, and in 2014 it will provide tax credits to those who need help in buying insurance. This facet represents the largest middle-class tax cut for health care in history. The Affordable Care Act is projected to reduce premium costs for millions of families and small business owners who are priced out of coverage today (2011). This could help as many as 32 million Americans who have no health care receive coverage.

Is Health Care in America Better Than in Any Other Place on Earth?

Table 8–5 compares, over time, the amount of money paid per capita in the United States and several other nations for health care. In 2007, the amount of money paid per capita in the United States was more than double the amount spent in Denmark. Yet, despite the high expenditures for

Table 8-5   Per Capita Health Expenditures Adjusted to U.S. Dollars in Selected Countries and Selected Years: 1960–2007

	1960	1980	2000	2007
United States	149	1,091	4,704	7,290
Switzerland	166	1,017	3,217	4,417
Norway	49	668	3,039	4,763
Germany	___	971	2,671	3,588
Canada	125	780	2,516	3,895
Denmark	___	896	2,378	3,512
Spain	16	393	1,536	2,671
Japan	30	585	1,967	2,581 (in 2006)
Mexico	___	___	508	823

Source: U.S. Department of Health and Human Services. (2010). National Center for Health Statistics. Health, United States, 2010: With Special feature on Death and Dying. Hyattsville, MD. 2011: Author. Retrieved from www.cdc.gov/nchs/data/hus/hus10.pdf 2011, December 19, 2011, p. 365.

health care, we were *not* healthier in 2006 than people from other nations. The infant mortality rate is the figure used as a standard for measuring the overall health of a nation. Infant mortality rates in the United States have been steadily declining since 1960 and the national average stood at 6.7 deaths in 2006, the most recent year that data is available from per 1,000 births; yet, some southern states are experiencing a rise in their infant mortality rates. In fact, 26 other nations had lower infant mortality rates than the United States. Table 8–6 illustrates infant mortality rates from selected countries, 1960 and 2006 and the estimates for 2012 (U.S. Department of Health and Human Services, 2010, p. 131). In addition, the World Factbook, published by the Central Intelligence Agency in 2009 includes estimated infant mortality rates for 2012. The entry gives the number of deaths of infants under 1 year old in a given year per 1,000 live births and ranks each country from highest to lowest number of deaths. Afghanistan, with 121.63 deaths ranks first; Monaco, with 1.80 deaths ranks 222 last; and, the United States ranks 174 with 5.98 deaths (The World Factbook, 2009). The infant mortality estimated rates for other nations are included in Table 8–6.

How did we get to this costly and critical situation? What factors converged to bring us to this dramatic breaking point? Because of the unprecedented growth of biomedical technology, we have witnessed the tremendous advancement in medical science and in the ability to perform an astounding variety of lifesaving procedures; now, not only can we no longer afford to finance these long-dreamed-of miracles, but the dream has become a nightmare.

The last question—"Why is it that health care is so expensive?"—may be answered by exploring the trends in the development of the health care system, but factored into this analysis is also the increase in the population; the desire

Table 8-6 **Infant Mortality Rates for Selected Countries in the Organization for Economic Co-operation and Cuba: 1960, 2006, and 2007, and 2012 estimates**

Nation	Number of Infant Deaths/1,000 Live Births: 1960	Number of Infant Deaths/1,000 Live Births: 2006	Number of Infant Deaths/1,000 Live Births: 2012 (est.)
Cuba	37.3	5.3	4.83
Czech Republic	20.0	3.3	3.70
Finland	21.0	2.8	3.40
France	27.7	3.8	3.37
Japan	30.7	2.6	2.21
Luxembourg	31.5	2.5	4.39
Norway	18.9	3.2	3.50
Portugal	77.5	3.3	4.60
Spain	43.7	3.8	3.37
Sweden	16.6	2.8	2.74
United States	26.0	6.7	5.98

Source: U.S. Department of Health and Human Services. (2010). National Center for Health Statistics. Health, United States, 2010: With Special feature on Death and Dying. Hyattsville, MD. 2011: Author. Retrieved from www.cdc.gov/nchs/data/hus/hus10.pdf 2011; U.S. Department of Health and Human Services. (2009). National Center for Health Statistics. Health, United States, 2009: With Special Feature on Medical Technology. Hyattsville, MD. 2011: Author. Retrieved from www.cdc.gov/nchs/data/hus/hus09.pdf 2011, p. 104; and Central Intelligence Agency. (2012). The World Factbook. Retrieved from https://www.cia.gov/library/publications/the-world-factbook/rankorder/2091rank.html, March 9, 2012.

by health care providers, researchers, and vendors to cure all diseases; and the public's expectation that all illnesses can be cured. Each event has contributed to this situation, and the results are the ongoing issues we are confronting today.

■ Trends in Development of the Health Care System

During the days of the early colonists, our health care system was a system of superstition and faith. It has evolved into a system predicated on a strong belief in science; the epidemiological model of disease; highly developed technology; and strong values of individuality, competition, and free enterprise. Two major forces—free enterprise and sciences—have largely shaped the problems we now face. Health problems have evolved from the epidemics of 1850 to the chronic diseases of today, notwithstanding the resurgence of tuberculosis and the AIDS epidemic. In 1850, health care technology was virtually nonexistent; today, it dominates the delivery of health care. We now take for granted such dramatic procedures as kidney, heart, and liver transplants. New technologies and biomedical milestones are materializing daily (Torrens, 1988, pp. 3–31). However, the consequences of these events are also rising daily in terms of extraordinary costs and countless practice issues and errors, discussed earlier.

Social organizations and peer review bodies to control the use of technology did not exist in 1850; today they proliferate, and the federal government is expected to play a dominant role. The belief that health care is a right for all Americans is still a prominent philosophy, yet the fulfillment of that right is still in question. The trends, begun in the 1980s and early 1990s, such as the cutbacks in federal funding for health services and the attempt to turn the clock back on social programs have led to a diminished and denigrated role for the government in people's health. On the other hand, the events of September 11, 2001, have pointed out the consequences of these cuts and the enormous and compelling need to boost public health and national security efforts.

There is growing and grave concern about the realization of this basic human right of health and health care. Mounting social problems, such as toxic waste, homelessness, and millions of people without health insurance, confound the situation. These factors all affect the delivery of health care. The problems of acquiring and using the health care system are legendary and ongoing.

The year 1960 is the benchmark being used to compare health care costs and significant events. A brief overview of these landmark events follows. These events have contributed to what we see today as the health care "nightmare." We are in a situation where health care delivery has become less and less personal and more and more technological in many health care settings. The barriers to health care are increasing and, as evidenced earlier, more and more people are unable to obtain health care, in spite of having health insurance. The events depicted that have occurred in the health care system, whether within the public health or medical sector, have happened within the context of the longer societal framework. The public sector events include those related to the collective responsibility for the health of large populations in many dimensions—prevention, surveillance, disease control, and so forth—and those events, positive and negative, that affect large population cohorts. The medical events are those that include the development of diagnostic and/or therapeutic methods that are problem-specific and affect limited numbers of people. The public health events include government laws and policies that were designed initially to increase the scope of the health care system and later to control medical costs.

This information is further embedded in the key health system issues of the century and the start of this decade, the key health problems, and the selected key health strategies of the time. The key issues are professionalization, infrastructure building, improved access, cost control, market forces, and the reinvention of government. The key health problems are reemerging infectious diseases, chronic diseases, and the modern care changes. Key health strategies include maternal and infant health, antibiotics, screen and treat, and managed care.

At the turn of the 20th century, 1900–1930, efforts were underway to identify medicine as a profession and to eradicate all philosophies of care that were not under the umbrella of the Flexner definition of a profession. Agents such as quinine for malaria and the diphtheria antitoxin for immunization were discovered, and the use of radium to treat cancer began.

Infectious diseases, including pneumonia and influenza, were pandemic. The main health strategy was maternal and child health, given the large numbers of new immigrants. In 1929, third-party payment for health care began with the creation of Blue Cross and Blue Shield.

Between 1930 and 1960, the health care system issue was infrastructure building. The passage of the Hill-Burton Act in 1946 provided funding for the building of hospitals and other health care resources. The system was on a roll—the development of today's extraordinarily costly tests and treatments began, and the settings for their use were built. The development of vaccines and antibiotics paved the way to a decrease in the occurrence of communicable disease, and a false sense of freedom from illness began to develop. At the same time, it began to become obvious that, for many, access to health care was becoming more and more difficult.

In 1965, President Lyndon B. Johnson's War on Poverty became the focal point of social and health policy and, among other laws, Medicare and Medicaid came into being. The Health Professionals Education Assistance Act was passed, which led to the proliferation of medical nursing and other allied health programs. In 1967, the first heart transplant was performed by Dr. Christiaan Barnard in South Africa, and a whole new focus on science and technology was born. Today, transplants have become nearly ordinary events, and an entitlement philosophy is applied to receiving them.

The 1960s were an explosive time—there were too many assassinations, too many riots—yet strides were made in the struggle for civil rights. The war in Vietnam was a nightly television event until the truce in 1975. The 1970s, 1980s, and 1990s all had their share of strife and progress. Progress in health care was accompanied by the escalation of costs and the limiting of comprehensive care. The cases of HIV/AIDS continue to increase, and the threat of anthrax and other forms of bioterrorism are present in the minds of most people. In addition, the 1960s were a decade of profound change in the delivery of health care, public health, and available methods of treating health problems and funding new resources. Selected highlights include the:

- Development of the vaccines for polio and rubella (1961 and 1963)
- Development of the methods for external cardiac pacing (1961)
- Development of liver transplant method (1963) and first human heart transplanted (1967)
- Surgeon General's Report on Smoking (1964)
- War on Poverty, Medicare/Medicaid passed (1965)

The 1970s brought even greater strides in medical technology and public health:

- Professional Standards Review Organization established, Clean Water Act passed, and the Tuskegee experiment[1] ended (1972)
- Comprehensive Health Planning; "Certificate of Need" (1974)
- HBV—the hepatitis vaccine was developed (1978)

[1]The Tuskegee syphilis experiment began in 1932.

- First test tube baby born (1978)
- Biotechnical Explosion (1979)
- Cyclosporine developed (1979)

At the end of the 1970s, efforts were developed to "control" the costs of health care, yet the seductiveness of the "advances" in technology actually began the out-of-control escalation of the rise of health care costs. The following are examples of events in the 1980s that further fed the rising costs of health care and the emerging expectation of people to be entitled to better and better levels of technological diagnosis and illness care that would provide longer life expectancies:

- Nuclear magnetic resonance introduced (1980)
- The beginning of the HIV/AIDS epidemic and the HIV virus isolated at the Institute Pasteur, Paris (1981)
- Monoclonal antibodies (1984)
- Retroviral oncogenes (1985)

The 1990s to the present time have presented even greater challenges to the availability and affordability of health care. In 1993 and 1994, President and Mrs. Clinton made an extraordinary effort to study our complex health care system and sought ways to reform it. That effort did not materialize, and the present political energy has shifted from health care reform to welfare reform and the saving of Social Security and Medicare. The nation's 76 million baby boomers will soon be able to retire, which will necessitate large payouts from Social Security and Medicare, but it is unknown how many workers will there be to contribute to the system. The size of the shortfall depends on the changes in longevity, the birth rate, and immigration rates (Zitner, 1999). Efforts such as managed care (Saltus, 1999) and the discounting of payments for medications for the elderly were short-term and controversial approaches to managing funds. These efforts, too, have not succeeded.

Meanwhile, the costs of health care continue to soar, causing some hospitals to downsize their nursing staff in an effort to reduce costs. Ultimately, it was believed that the Clinton plan would create a few giant insurers, and health maintenance organizations (HMOs) would dominate the market; most people would be forced into low-cost plans, doctors would be employed by the insurers or HMOs, hospitals would be controlled by insurers and HMOs, care would be multitiered, the bureaucracy would increase, costs would not be contained, and financing would be regressive. The overall goal of health care reform was to make health care accessible, comprehensive, and affordable—a right and not a privilege of all residents of the United States. However, technology is advancing and our use of it is increasing, and we continue to spend vast sums on the care of patients in the last year of life while delivering less and less preventive care. In addition, the costs of for-profit care continue to explode, and the dominant force in managed care is the for-profit HMO.

The following are examples of health care events in the 1990s and 2012:

- Human Genome Project (1992)
- Assisted suicide; Dr. J. Kevorkian (1996)
- Hantavirus pulmonary syndrome (1993)
- Septuplets born and survive (1997)
- Octuplets born; 7 survive (1998)
- Stem cell cloning (1998)
- Biologics and follow-on biologics (2004)
- Affordable Care Act (2010)
- The Supreme Court upheld the Affordable Care Act (June 28, 2012)

With the catastrophe of September 11, 2001, the need to immunize people for smallpox and countless other public health issues emerged, as did the need for emergency preparedness.

Biologics are complex medicines that are manufactured with the use of living organisms. The increasing use of biologics and new follow-on biologics are the cutting edge of pharmaceutical therapies. The biogeneric market is about $2 billion. The Biotechnology Industry Organization has stated that "the safety and effectiveness of a chemical drug can be established by the specification of its active ingredient, but the safety and effectiveness of a biotech product is determined by the manner in which it is made" (Samalonis, 2004). In other words, the consequences of this pioneering medicine will be expensive iatrogenic problems.

Grave concern is being expressed regarding the high costs of health care, and that the costs of durable medical supplies and medications continue to rise, and so on. On one hand, we are seeking to ever expand therapeutic miracles; on the other hand, there is shock and dismay at the ever-increasing costs of health care. It is apparent when one realizes that the costs of health care for a family of 4 has more than doubled in 9 years (2002–2011) from $9,235 to $19,393 (Strachen, 2011).

■ Common Problems in Health Care Delivery

Many problems exist within today's health care delivery system. Some of these problems affect all of us, and others are specific to the poor and to emerging majority populations. It has been suggested that the health care delivery system fosters and maintains a childlike dependence and depersonalized condition for the consumer. The following sections describe problems experienced by most consumers of health care, as categorized by Ehrenreich and Ehrenreich (1971, pp. 4–12). It is interesting to note that this historical framework was developed in 1971, yet it holds as a framework today.

Finding Where the Appropriate Care Is Offered at a Reasonable Price

It may be difficult for even a knowledgeable consumer to receive adequate care. One summer, I was on vacation with my 11-year-old daughter. She complained of a sore throat for 2 days, and, when she did not improve on the third day, I decided to take her to a pediatrician and have a throat culture taken. She was running a low-grade fever, and I suspected a strep infection. I phoned the emergency room of a local teaching hospital for the name of a pediatrician, but I was instructed to "bring her in." I questioned the practicality of using an emergency room, but the friendly voice on the other end of the line assured me: "If you have health insurance and the child has a sore throat, this is the best place to come." After a rather long wait, we were seen by an intern who was beginning his first day in pediatrics. To my dismay and chagrin, the young man appeared to have no idea of how to proceed. The resident entered and patiently demonstrated to the fledgling intern—using my daughter—how to go about doing a physical examination on a child. Since I had brought the child to the emergency room merely for a throat culture, I felt that what they were doing was unnecessary and said so. After much delay, the throat culture was taken; we were told we could leave and should call back in 48 hours for the report. As we left the cubicle, we had to pass another cubicle with an open curtain—where a woman was vomiting all over herself, the bed, and the equipment while another intern was attempting to insert a gastric tube. Needless to say, my daughter was distressed by the sight, which she could not help but witness. The reward for this trial was an inflated bill.

Two days later, I called back for the report. It could not be located. When it was finally "found," the result was negative. I took issue with this because it took 30 minutes for them to find the report. Perhaps this sounds a bit over-stated; however, I had the feeling that they told me it was negative just to get me off the phone.

I related this personal experience to bring out two major points. First, it is not easy to obtain what I, as a health care provider, consider to be a rather minor procedure. Second—and perhaps more important—it was expensive!

The average health care consumer in such a circumstance may very well have no idea of what is really going on. When health care is sought, one should have access to professionally performed examinations and treatment. When one is seeking the results of a laboratory test, the results should be available immediately at the agreed-on time and place instead of being lost in a jungle of bureaucracy.

Finding One's Way Amidst the Many Available Types of Medical Care

A friend's experience illustrates how hard it may be to find appropriate medical care. She had minor gastric problems from time to time and initially sought help from a family physician. He was unable to treat the problem adequately;

therefore, she decided to go elsewhere. However, for many reasons—including anger, embarrassment, and fear of reprisal—she chose not to tell the family physician that she was dissatisfied with his care, nor did she request a referral. She was essentially on her own in terms of securing an appointment with either a gastroenterologist or a surgeon. She very quickly discovered that no physician who was a specialist in gastroenterology would see her on a self-referral. In order to get an appointment, she had to ask her own general practitioner for a referral or else seek initial help from another general practitioner or internist. Since she had little money to spend on a variety of physicians, she decided to wait to see what would happen. In this instance, she was fortunate and has had few further problems.

As a teaching and learning experience, I ask students to describe how they go about selecting a physician and where they go for health care. The younger students in the class generally seek the services of their families' physicians. The older or married students often have doctors other than those with whom they "grew up." These latter students generally are quite willing to share the trials and tribulations they have experienced. When given the freedom to express their actions and reactions, most admit to having a great deal of difficulty in getting what they perceive to be good health care. A number of the older students state that they select a physician on the staff of the institution where they are employed. They have had an opportunity to see him or her at work and can judge, firsthand, whether he or she is "good" or "bad." One mother stated that she worked in pediatrics during her pregnancy solely to discover who was the best pediatrician. A newly married student stated that she planned to work in the delivery room to see which obstetrician delivered a baby with the greatest amount of concern for both the mother and the child.

That is an ideal situation for members of the nursing profession, but what about the average layperson who does not have access to this resource? This question alerts the students to the specialness of their personal situations and exposes them to the immensity of the problem that the average person experiences. After individual experiences are shared, the class can move on to work through a case study such as the following.

Ms. B. is a new resident in this city. She discovers a lump in her breast and does not know where to turn. How does she go about finding a doctor? Where does she go?

One initial course of action is to call the American Cancer Society for advice. From there, she is instructed to call the County Medical Society, since the American Cancer Society is not allowed to give out physicians' names. During a phone call to the County Medical Society, she is given the names of 3 physicians in her part of the city. From there, she is on her own in attempting to get an appointment with one of them. It is not uncommon for a stranger to call a physician's office and be told (1) "The doctor is no longer accepting new patients," (2) "There is a 6-month wait," or (3) "He or she sees no one without a proper referral."

The woman, of course, has another choice: She can go to an emergency room or a clinic, but then she discovers that the wait in the emergency room is intolerable for her. She may rationalize that because a "lump" is not really an "emergency," she should choose another route. She may then try to secure a clinic appointment, and once again she may experience a great deal of difficulty in getting an appointment at a convenient time. She may finally get one and then discover that the wait in the clinic is unduly long, which may cause her to miss a day of work.

Figuring Out What the Physician Is Doing

It is not always easy for members of the health professions to understand what is happening to them when they are ill. What must it be like for the average person who has little or no knowledge of health care routines and practices?

Pretend that you are a layperson who has just been relieved of all your clothes and given a paper dress to put on. You are lying on a table with strange eyes peering down at you. A sheet is thrown over you, and you are given terse directions—"breathe," "cough," "don't breathe," "turn," "lift your legs." You may feel without warning a cold disk on your chest or a cold hand on your back. As the physical examination process continues, you may feel a few taps on the ribs, see a bright light shining in your eye, feel a cold tube in your ear, and gag on a stick probing the inside of your mouth. What is going on? The jargon you hear is unfamiliar. You are being poked, pushed, prodded, peered at and into, and jabbed, and you do not know why. If you are female and going for your first pelvic examination, you may have no idea what to expect. Perhaps you have heard only hushed whisperings, and your level of fear and discomfort is high. Insult is added to injury when you experience the penetration of a cold, unyielding speculum: "What is the doctor doing now and why?"

These hypothetical situations are typical of the usual physical examinations that you may encounter routinely in a clinic or a private physician's office. Suppose you have a more complex problem, such as a neurological condition, for which the diagnostic procedures may indeed be painful and complicated. Have you ever had a CT scan? A magnetic resonance image (MRI)? An angioplasty? Quite often, those who deliver care have neither experienced nor witnessed the vast number of procedures that are performed in diagnostic workups and in treatment. They have little awareness of what the patient is thinking, feeling, and experiencing. Similarly, because the names and the purposes of the procedures are familiar to health care workers—don't forget, this is their culture—they may take their own understanding of the procedures for granted and have difficulty appreciating why the patient cannot understand what is happening.

Finding Out What Went Wrong

What did you do the last time a patient asked to read the chart? Traditionally, you uttered an authoritative "tsk," turned abruptly on white-heeled shoes, and walked briskly away. Who ever heard of such nerve? A patient asking to read a chart! Today, there is the "patient's bill of rights." One of its mandates is that the patient has the right to read his or her own medical record. Experience, however, demonstrates that this right is still not always granted; and in certain situations 2 records are kept. Suppose one enters the hospital for what is deemed to be a simple medical or surgical problem. All is well if everything goes according to routine. However, what happens when complications develop? The more determined the patient is to discover what the problem is or why there are complications, the more he or she believes that the health care providers are trying to hide something. The cycle perpetuates itself, and a tremendous schism develops between provider and consumer. Quite often, "the conspiracy of silence" tends to grow as more questions are asked. This unpleasant situation may continue until the patient is locked inside his or her subjective world. It is rare for a person to truly understand unforeseen complications. Nurses all too often enter into this collusion and play the role of a silent partner with the physician and the institution.

Overcoming the Built-in Racism and Male Chauvinism of Doctors and Hospitals

Students tend to have little difficulty in describing many incidents of racism and male chauvinism: that they are mostly women suffices and that they are nurses adds meaning to the problem. Classroom discussion helps identify subtle incidents of racism. For example, students may realize that Black patients may be the last to receive morning or evening care, meal trays, and so forth. If this is a normal occurrence on a floor, it is an indictment in itself. Racism may take another tack. Is it an accident that the Black person is the last patient to receive routine care, or has he or she consciously been made to wait? Does the fact that the Black person may have to wait longest for water or a pill demonstrate racism on a conscious level, or is it subliminal?

Nurses recognize the subtle patronization of both themselves and female patients. Once the situation is probed and spelled out, the students adopt a much more realistic attitude toward the insensitivity of those who choose a racist or chauvinistic style of giving care. Students have noted that, when they are aware of what is happening, they are better able to take steps to block future occurrences. Some have written letters to me after they have begun or returned to the practice of nursing, stating that knowing the phenomenon is common helps them project a stronger image in their determination to work for change.

■ Pathways to Health Services

When a health problem occurs, there is an established system whereby health care services are obtained. The classical theoretical work that was developed in the mid-1960s and the 1970s continues to establish a viable framework for describing sources of patient problems. Suchman (1965) contends that the family is usually the first resource. It is in the domain of the family that the person seeks validation that what he or she is experiencing is indeed an illness. Once the belief is validated, health care outside of the home is sought. It is not unusual for a family to be receiving care from many different providers, with limited or no communication among the attending caregivers. Problems and complications erupt when a provider is not aware that other providers are caring for a patient. Let us not forget that, in rural and remote areas, comprehensive health care is difficult to obtain. For patients who are forced to use the clinics of a hospital, there is certainly no continuity of care because intern and resident physicians come and go each year. This is known as the level of first contact, or the entrance into the health care system.

The second level of care, if needed, is found at the specialist's level: in clinics, private practice, or hospitals. Obstetricians, gynecologists, surgeons, neurologists, and other specialists make up a large percentage of those who practice medicine. Recently, hospitalists have been added.

The third level of care is delivered within hospitals that provide inpatient care and services. Care is determined by need, whether long term (as in a psychiatric setting or rehabilitation institute) or short term (as in the acute care setting and community hospitals).

An in-depth discussion of the different kinds of hospitals—voluntary or profit-making and nonprofit institutions—is more appropriate to a book dealing solely with the delivery of health care. In our present context, the issue is "what does the patient know about such settings, and what kind of care can he or she expect to receive?"

To many students, the health care delivery problems of a given hospital unit are far removed from the scope of practice they know from nursing school and from what they ordinarily see in a work setting (unless they choose to work in a city or county public hospital). Many students assume that the care they observe and deliver in a suburban or community private hospital is the universal norm. This is a fundamental error in experience and understanding, which can be corrected if students are assigned to visit first the emergency room of a city hospital and then the emergency room of a suburban hospital in order to compare the two milieus. Unless students visit each setting, they fail to gain an appreciation of the major differences—how vastly such facilities differ in the scope of patients' treatment. Students typically report that, in the suburban emergency room, the patients are called by name, their families wait with them, and every effort is made to hasten their visit. The contrast with people in urban emergency rooms—who have waited for extended periods of time, are sometimes not addressed by name, and are not allowed to have family members come with them while they are examined—is astounding. The noise and confusion are also factors that confront and dismay students when they are exposed to big-city emergency rooms.

Figure 8–5 illustrates the maze of health care and the variety of obstacles a patient must deal with in attempting to navigate this complex system. Indeed, the patient not only needs to navigate an internal system of a given hospital but also needs to understand all the types of care available. Just to complicate matters more deeply, many people are given information that contradicts itself—as with the diagnosis and treatment of breast cancer or the use of estrogen replacement therapy—and then the patient is asked to make the choices.

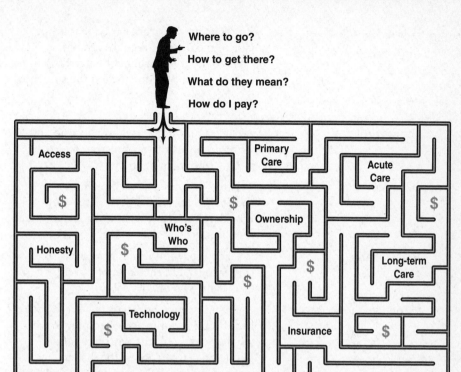

Where to go?

How to get there?

What do they mean?

How do I pay?

Figure 8-5 Navigating the Amazing Maze of Health Care.

■ Barriers to Health Care

There are countless factors, or barriers, in addition to financial that thwart a person's or family's ability to use the health care system to its greatest potential. The following are some examples:

Access	A person is unable to enter into the system because he or she lacks money, health insurance, or the ability to get to a center where health care is delivered. Another access factor is that primary care physicians are leaving their practices, either to retire or to limit the scope of their practices to "concierge" services.
Age	The person is too young or too old to enter into the system and is unaware of ways to overcome this.

(continued)

Class	A person may be from a class that is not part of the dominant culture, limiting their ability to determine the need for health care and to understand the subtleties involved in making health care system choices.
Education	A person may not know how to read and write English and may not read and write in his or her native tongue.
Gender	Existing services may be limited to a specific gender or the person may be unwilling or unable to access a system that does not deliver gender-specific care.
Geography	A person may not reside near a health care facility, and the costs of traveling to a facility may be unaffordable.
Homelessness	A person may be homeless in a place where health care is not provided to people who are homeless, and the person does not know the ways to access the system.
Insurance	A person may not have health insurance, or it may be inadequate to cover the scope of the person's needs.
Language	A person may not speak or understand English and adequate interpreter services may not be available.
Manners	A person's manners or expectations of the provider's manners may not be congruent.
Philosophy	The philosophy of an institution may not be congruent with a person's religious or personal philosophy.
Prejudice	The person seeking health care may sense the prejudice that the providers and institution exhibit.
Race	There may be residuals of racial prejudice as part of the institution's philosophy.
Racism	The institution may have specific barriers in place to not treat people from other races than the race of the owners of the facility.

Religion	A patient may not desire to be treated in an institution that is not derived from his or her religious background, and there may be manifest prejudice on both sides—patient and institution. A given religion's teachings regarding HEALTH and ILLNESS may contradict modern health care practices.
SES (socioeconomic status)	The 2 extremes of socioeconomic status are poverty or great wealth; poverty can limit access to care; wealth may prevent people from seeking care in institutions where they prefer to not go because of the patient population served there.
Technology	A person may not be able to afford or want the plethora of diagnostic tests and therapies offered to him or her.
Transportation	There may be no public transportation available from where the patient resides to the institution.

■ Medicine as an Institution of Social Control

The people of today's youth-oriented, cure-expecting, death-denying society have unusually high expectations of the healers of our time. We expect a cure (or if not a cure, then the prolongation of life) as the normal outcome of illness. The technology of modern health care dominates our expectations of treatment, and our primary focus is on the curative aspects of medicine, not on prevention.

As control over the behavior of a person has shifted from the family and church to a physician, "be good" has shifted to "take your medicine." The role that physicians play within society in terms of social control is ever-growing, so that conflict frequently arises between medicine and the law over definitions of accepted codes of behavior and the relative status of the 2 professions in governing American life. Zola (1966, 1972) uses the following examples to illustrate the "medicalization" of society.

Through the Expansion of What in Life Is Deemed Relevant to the Good Practice of Medicine

This factor is exemplified by the change from a specific etiological model of disease to a multicausal one. The "partners" in this new model include greater acceptance of comprehensive medicine, the use of the computer, and the practice of preventive medicine. In preventive medicine, however, the medical person must get to the layperson before the disease occurs: Clients must be sought out. Thus, forms of social control emerge in an attempt to prevent disease: eating a low-cholesterol diet, avoiding stress, stopping smoking, and getting proper and adequate exercise.

Through the Retention of Absolute Control over Certain Technical Procedures

This step is, in essence, the right to perform surgery and the right to prescribe drugs. In the life span of human beings, modern medicine can often determine life or death from the time of conception to old age through genetic counseling; abortion; surgery; and technological devices, such as computers, respirators, and life-support systems. Medicine has at its command drugs that can cure or kill—from antibiotics to the chemotherapeutic agents used to combat cancer. There are drugs to cause sleep or wakefulness, to increase or decrease the appetite, and to increase or decrease levels of energy. There are drugs to relieve depression and stimulate interest. (In the United States, those mood-altering drugs are consumed at a rate higher than the medications prescribed and used to treat specific diseases.) In addition, medicine can control what medications are available for legal consumption.

Through the Expansion of What in Medicine Is Deemed Relevant to the Good Practice of Life

This expansion is illustrated by the use of medical jargon to describe a state of being—such as the *health* of the nation or the *health* of the economy. Any political or economic proposal or objective that enhances the "health" of those concerned wins approval.

There are numerous areas in which medicine, religion, and law overlap. For example, public health practice, law, and medicine overlap in the creation of laws that establish quarantine and the need for immunization. As another example, a child is unable to enter school without proof of having received certain inoculations. Medicine and law also merge in areas of sanitation and rodent and insect control. A legal-medical dispute can arise over the guilt or innocence of a criminal as determined by his or her "mental state" at the time of a crime.

Some diseases carry a social stigma: One must be screened for tuberculosis before employment, a history of typhoid fever permanently prevents a person from commercially handling food, venereal disease must be reported and treated, and even the ancient disease of leprosy continues to carry a stigma.

Abortion represents an area replete with conflict that involves politics, law, religion, and medicine. Those in favor of abortion rights believe that it is a woman's right to have an abortion and that the matter is confidential between the patient and her physician. Opponents argue on religious and moral grounds that abortion is murder. At present, the law sanctions abortion. In many states, however, Medicaid will no longer pay for an abortion unless the mother's life is in danger, a policy that makes it increasingly difficult for the poor to obtain these services.

Another highly charged area of conflict involves the practice of euthanasia. With the burgeoning of technological improvements, the definition of *death* has changed in recent years. It sometimes takes a major court battle to "pull the plug," such as in the Nancy Cruzan case. The battles with the late Dr. Jack Kevorkian have stretched these issues even further.

Finally, although many daily practical activities are undertaken in the name of health—taking vitamins, practicing hygiene, using birth control, engaging in dietary or exercise programs—the "diseases of the rich" (cancer, heart disease, and stroke) tend to capture more public attention and funding than the diseases of the poor (malnutrition, high maternal and infant death rates, sickle-cell anemia, and lead poisoning).

In this chapter, we have explored, in a very limited way, the culture and characteristics inherent in the socialization into the health care professions; many of the issues surrounding the American health care delivery system by examining the history and trends that led to its present character; the experiences a person may have in attempting to obtain care; and how medicine is now an institution of social control. Table 8–7 brings closure to this chapter by comparing medical care and CULTURALCARE.

Table 8-7   Comparison: Medical Care and CULTURALCARE

	Medical Care	CULTURALCARE
Definition	"The art and science of the diagnosis and treatment of disease and the maintenance of health"	Professional health care that is culturally sensitive, culturally appropriate, and culturally competent
Goals	Prevention of disease and injury and promotion and maintenance of health Relief of pain and suffering caused by maladies Care and CURE of those with a malady and care of those who cannot be cured Avoidance of premature death and pursuit of a peaceful death	Provision of care that is *culturally sensitive*—the provider possesses some basic knowledge of and constructive attitudes toward the health traditions observed among the diverse cultural groups found in the setting in which he or she is practicing *Culturally appropriate*—the provider applies the underlying background knowledge that must be possessed to provide a patient with the best possible health care *Culturally competent*—within the delivered care, the provider understands and attends to the total context of the patient's situation and it is a complex combination of knowledge, attitudes, and skills Assistance to patient/family in pursuit of HEALTH and HEALING

(continued)

Table 8–7   *continued*

Philosophy	Allopathic—body and mind "With enough money, energy, and scientific zeal, there are no diseases or maladies that it cannot cure or remedy"	Holistic care predicated on HEALTH traditions and patient/family/community articulated needs and situation
Challenges	Should life support be used far beyond the natural trajectory of a given episode? Should disease and death ever be accepted? Should such controversial issues such as physician-assisted suicide and euthanasia be accepted as part of medical practice? Ever-rising costs and iatrogenic problems	Disparagement and nonacceptance of HEALTH, ILLNESS, and HEALING traditions
Sources of Stress	Former success Rise in chronic illness	Nonrecognition by modern providers of the meanings of HEALTH, ILLNESS, and HEALING traditions
Scientific and Technological Developments	Sophisticated, costly technology Experimental treatments Follow-on biologics	Steeped in ethnocultural HEALTH-related traditions
Cultural Pressures	"Scientific progress" High quality = best available in diagnosis and treatment Assumption = better to come	Antithetical at times to allopathic practice Patient may be seen as "noncomplier" or to not appreciate provider efforts
Medicalization of Life	Apply medical model and technologies to problems historically not thought of as medical in nature	Apply knowledge to entire sociocultural and HEALTH context of patients
Medicine and Society	Fed by large amounts of money—public and private; influenced by social mores, values, and economics; and a substrate of dominant culture	Many traditions neither recognized nor known within the dominant culture Many beliefs and practices hidden
Define health/ HEALTH	*Health* = "the experience of well-being and integrity of mind and body"	HEALTH = "the balance of the person, both within one's being—physical, mental, and spiritual—and in the outside world—natural, communal, and metaphysical, is a complex, interrelated phenomenon"

Table 8-7   *continued*

Define illness/ *ILLNESS*	Malady, disease, illness, and sickness—loss of freedom or opportunity, or the loss of pleasure	ILLNESS = "the imbalance of one's beings—physical, mental, and spiritual—and in the outside world—natural, communal, and metaphysical"
Causes of illness/ *ILLNESS*	Viruses, bacteria, stress, etc.	Evil eye, or spirits; God's punishment; internal imbalance; jealousy; envy?
Maintain Health	Health promotion—activities to stay well	Daily health practices, such as following dietary taboos, special clothing, and prayer
Protect Health	Immunization	Protective items worn, carried, or hung in the home
Restore Health	Technology Human experimentation Radical measures "Hope" at all costs	Traditional remedies—herbs, prayer, pilgrimages to shrines— both religious and secular
Birth Practices	Medicalization Hospitalization In vitro fertilization	Use of midwife when possible Traditional rituals Prayer
Death Practices	"Everything done to prevent" Long-term use of life support Experimental therapies	Prayer, vigils, acceptance
Attitudes Toward Other Health Care Systems	Skeptical and sometimes contemptuous of "alternative medicine" Seen as a danger	May see modern medicine as an alternative to ethnocultural or religious traditions

Source: Adapted from: Hanson, M. J., & Callahan, D. (Eds.). (1999). *The goals of medicine.* Washington, DC: Georgetown Press.

The struggles continue as we attempt to find a balance between the high technology of the 21st century and primary preventive care and a strong public health care system. There must also be a balance between the forces of modern medical care and CULTURALCARE.

Explore 🌐 MediaLink

Go to the Student Resource Site at nursing.pearsonhighered.com for chapter-related review questions, case studies, and activities. Contents of the CULTURALCARE Guide and CULTURALCARE Museum can also be found on the Student Resource Site. Click on Chapter 8 to select the activities for this chapter.

Box 8–1: Keeping Up

It goes without saying that much of the data presented in this chapter will be out of date when you read this text. However, at this final stage of writing, it is the most recent information available. The following resources will be most helpful in keeping you abreast of the frequent changes in health care events, costs, and policies:

1. The National Center for Health Statistics publishes *Health, United States*, an annual report on trends in health statistics. It can be retrieved from http://www.cdc.gov/nchs/hus.htm. *Health, United States, 11* is not available and *Health, United States, 12* will be published in May, 2012.
2. Health related data and other statistics are available at http://www.cdc.gov/DataStatistics/.
3. Information regarding the Affordable Care Act can be found at www.healthcare.gov.
4. Information regarding selected health statistics and other relevant information in a global context can be found at https://www.cia.gov/library/publications/the-world-factbook/index.html.

■ Internet Sources

Samalonis, L. B. (2004). Follow-on biologics: The next frontier. Retrived from http://www.drugtopics.com/drugtopics/article/articleDetail.jsp?id=115886, June 27, 2007.

Strachen. (2011). U.S. Health care costs per family more than doubled in nine years, report finds. Huff Post Business. Retrieved from http://www.huffingtonpost.com/2011/05/16/us-healthcare-costs-double-report_n_862677.html, March 8, 2012.

The World Factbook. (2009). Washington, DC: Central Intelligence Agency. Retrieved from https://www.cia.gov/library/publications/the-world-factbook/index.html, March 9, 2012.

U.S. Department of Health and Human Services. (2009). National Center for Health Statistics. Health, United States, 2009: With Special Feature on Medical Technology. Hyattsville, MD. 2010: Author. Retrieved from www.cdc.gov/nchs/data/hus/hus09.pdf 2011, p. 104.

U.S. Department of Health and Human Services. (2010). National Center for Health Statistics. Health, United States, 2010: With Special feature on Death and Dying. Hyattsville, MD. 2011: Author. Retrieved from www.cdc.gov/nchs/data/hus/hus10.pdf 2011.

U.S. Department of Health and Human Services. (2010). Retrieved from HealthCare.gov http://www.healthcare.gov/index.html, July, 2011.

■ References

Abelson, R. (2007, June 14). In health care, cost isn't proof of high quality. *New York Times*, p. A-1.

Ehrenreich, B., & Ehrenreich, J. (1971). *The American health empire: Power, profits, and politics.* New York: Random House, Vintage Books. (The headings that follow this reference in the text are quoted from this book.)

Kinney, E. D. (2010). For profit Enterprise in Health care: Can it contribute to health reform? *American Journal of Law and Medicine, 36,* 405–435.

Knowles, J. (1970, January). "It's time to operate." *Fortune,* 79.

Saltus, R. (1999, February 18). Managed, yes, but couple wonders, is care? *Boston Globe.* P. A-1.

Suchman, E. A. (1965). Stages of Illness and Medical Care. *Journal of Health and Human Behavior, 6(3),* 114–128.

Torrens, P. R. (1988). Historical evolution and overview of health services in the United States. In S. J. Williams & P. R. Torrens (Eds.), *Introduction to health services* (3rd ed.). New York: John Wiley & Sons.

Zitner, A. (1999, March 14). Demographers caught looking on US trends. *Boston Sunday Globe.* Web References.

Zola, I. K. (1996, October). Culture and symptoms: An analysis of patients presenting complaints. *American Sociological Review, 31,* 615–630.

Zola, I. K. (1972, November). Medicine as an institution of social control. *Sociological Review, 20(4),* 487–504. (The headings that follow this reference in the text are quoted from this article.)

Unit

III

HEALTH
and ILLNESS
Panoramas

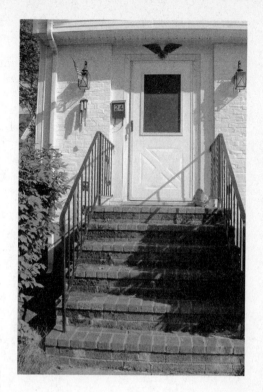

Thus far, this book has discussed 4 of the 6 steps to CULTURALCOMPETENCY. The first 7 chapters presented the underlying theoretical rationale that is the foundation for CULTURALCOMPETENCY and brought you to the transparent door depicted in the introduction, to "observe" the various "bricks" philosophies, concepts, and situations involved in the theoretical development of CULTURALCOMPETENCY.

- Chapter 1 presented the theoretical foundation and rationale for the development of "CULTURALCOMPETENCY."
- Chapter 2 set the theoretical foundation of what was the first step, *know your personal heritage*, as it reviewed the sociological components of heritage.
- Chapter 3 developed the background necessary to understand the role that the changing demographics of the larger communities have had in society in general and specifically in the delivery of health care—this is the second step.
- Chapters 4, 5, and 6 explored the dynamics involved in health/HEALTH, illness/ILLNESS, and curing/HEALING—the third step.
- Chapter 7 provided the opportunity to look intensely inside this door from your personal experience and presented information regarding the exciting and challenging intricacies of exploring *your* heritage and

207

your family's health/HEALTH and illness/ILLNESS beliefs and practices. As stated, this completes the first and most important step in becoming CULTURALLY COMPETENT.

■ Chapter 8 examined the "culture" of health care providers and that of the health care delivery system and introduced arguments relevant to the trends in the development of the health care system, common problems in the delivery of health care, pathways to health services, and medicine as an institution of social control and compared modern and traditional philosophies of health care delivery.

The first 5 chapters in this unit embrace the fifth step—traditional HEALTH care—and will provide a framework for learning about the communities you may be practicing in. It presents examples of the *traditional* HEALTH, ILLNESS, and HEALING beliefs and practices of selected populations. Each chapter introduces the

■ background of the population,
■ *traditional* definitions of *HEALTH/ILLNESS/HEALING*,
■ *traditional* methods of HEALTH maintenance and protection,
■ *traditional* methods of HEALTH restoration,
■ current health problems, and
■ health disparities in morbidity and mortality rates and manpower.

These are areas that can be applied in researching information regarding the populations you are caring for and working with. The World Wide Web is extremely helpful in gathering the demographic and modern health-related data applicable to a given population. Chapter 14 illustrates the journey on the Road to CULTURALCOMPETENCY and how this knowledge is vital to a person's development in this discipline.

My experiences have taught me that people are thirsty for knowledge regarding tradition, be it their own or the traditions of others. The need for historical, pertinent, and compelling information was recently driven home when I was discussing New Year's Day with a cohort of fifteen 21-year-old college senior students. The students did not know that New Year's Day—January 1—is a religious holiday; they believed it was a secular holiday. The conversation that resulted from this incident revealed a "thirst" for knowledge regarding *tradition*. They were eager to learn about traditions and the HEALTH traditions and other cultural events from their own ethnocultural heritage, the heritages of peers, and the heritages of other people. Thus, an effort has been exerted to maintain the integrity of older references and the primary data that have been gathered regarding HEALTH beliefs and practices over the 37 years I have developed this text. In the race to modernity, science, technology, and "scholarly" endeavors, the HEALTH traditions of family and others may well be lost—as the saying goes, the baby was "thrown away with the bath water," to this generation.

The first 5 chapters in Unit III will present an overview of relevant historical and contemporary theoretical content that will help you:

1. Develop a level of awareness of the background and health/HEALTH problems of both the emerging majority and White ethnic populations.
2. Understand and describe selected *traditional* HEALTH beliefs and practices.
3. Understand the *traditional* pathways to HEALTH care and the relationship between these pathways and the American health care system.
4. Understand certain manpower problems of each of the communities discussed.
5. Be more familiar with the available literature regarding each of the communities.

The following exercises are inherent in Chapter 14 and are appropriate to all chapters in Unit III:

1. Familiarize yourself with some literature of the given community—that is, read literature, poetry, or a biography of a member of each of the communities.
2. Familiarize yourself with the history and sociopolitical background of each of the communities.

The questions that follow should be thoughtfully considered:

1. What are the traditional definitions of *HEALTH* and *ILLNESS* in each of the communities? Are they alike or different?
2. What are the traditional methods of maintaining HEALTH?
3. What are the traditional ways of protecting HEALTH?
4. What are the traditional ways of restoring HEALTH?
5. Who are the traditional HEALERS? What functions do they perform?

This is an extraordinary way to build connections between communities and to see how much different ethnocultural and religious communities have in common. Since HEALTH is the metaphor for this text, it brings to the forefront a way to analyze and understand some of the variability in health care.

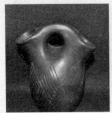 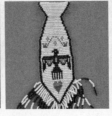 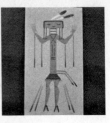

Figure 9-1   **Figure 9-2**   **Figure 9-3**   **Figure 9-4**

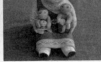

Chapter 9

HEALTH and ILLNESS in the American Indian and Alaska Native Population

To "make medicine" is to engage upon a special period of fasting, thanksgiving, prayer, and self denial, even self-torture.

—*Wooden Leg (late 19th century) Cheyenne*

■ Objectives

1. Discuss the background of the American Indian and Alaska Native population.
2. Discuss the demographic profile of the American Indian and Alaska Native population.
3. Describe the traditional definitions of HEALTH and ILLNESS of the American Indian and Alaska Native population.
4. Describe the traditional methods of HEALING of the American Indian and Alaska Native population.
5. Describe the practice of a traditional healer.
6. Describe current health care problems of the American Indian and Alaska Native population.
7. Describe the services rendered by the Indian Health Service.

8. Describe demographic disparity as it is seen in health manpower distribution of the American Indian and Alaska Native population as represented in the health care delivery system.

The opening images for this chapter depict objects related to traditional American Indian HEALTH beliefs and practices. Figure 9–1 is Cherokee pottery, a wedding vase that symbolizes the union of 2 lives to become one—a HEALTHY beginning for a family. The couple drinks from each side of the vessel. Figure 9–2 is a woman holding children symbolizing the grandmother relating stories to her children or grandchildren. This is a way to pass on the cultural heritage of the family. It is an example of Acoma Pueblo pottery from Sky City, New Mexico. Figure 9–3 is a woven beaded thunderbird tie. The thunderbird has many meanings for American Indian people, such as their ability to control rainfall. Some people believe they are protective of HEALTH because of their strength. Beadwork is a traditional art for many people and is a spiritual undertaking. This tie was a gift from a traditional Micmac man in Boston, Massachusetts. Figure 9–4 is a sand painting. The Navajo medicine man creates the sand paintings during the diagnostic phase of a healing ceremony.

■ Background

The descendants of the original inhabitants of the North American continent and Alaska numbered 2.9 million people, or 0.9% of the total population of the United States in Census 2010. This number reported American Indian and Alaska Native alone and represented a growth from 2.5 million people in 2000 (Humes, Nicholas, & Jones, 2011, p. 4). When compared to "U.S. all races," the American Indian/Alaska Native (AI/AN) population lags behind in several areas, including lower educational levels and higher unemployment rates. The AI/AN population is a young population. The median age of the population is 28.0 years, compared with 35.3 years for all races in the United States. The population has larger families, less health insurance (the number of AI/ANs without health insurance is over double that for U.S. all races), and a poverty level nearly twice that of the rest of the population. The American Indian population served by the Indian Health Service is living longer than it did 30 or even 20 years ago. In fact, statistics on age at death show that during 1972–1974, life expectancy at birth for the American Indian population was about 63.6 years and has now increased to 72.6 years, but it is still 5.2 years less than the U.S. all races life expectancy of 77.8 years (2003–2005 rates) (U.S. Department of Health and Human Services, 2012). Diseases of the heart, malignant neoplasm, unintentional injuries, diabetes mellitus, and chronic liver diseases and cirrhosis are the 5 leading causes of Indian deaths in 2007 (U.S. Department of Health and Human Services, 2011).

The first time that American Indians were counted as a separate group was in the 1860 census, and the 1890 census was the first to count American Indians throughout the country. The counting of American Indians before 1890 was limited to those living in the general population of the various states; the American Indians residing in American Indian territory and on American Indian reservations were not included. Alaska Natives, in Alaska, have been counted since 1880, but until 1940 they were generally reported in the "American Indian" racial category. The people were enumerated separately (as Eskimo and Aleut) in 1940 in Alaska. It was not until the 1970 census that separate response categories were used to collect data on the Eskimo and Aleut population, and then only in Alaska.

The American Indian nations that were the largest populations include the Cherokee, Navajo, Latin American Indian, Choctaw, Sioux, and Chippewa. The largest Alaska Native group was Eskimo.

To realize the plight of today's American Indians, it is necessary to journey back in time to the years when Whites settled in this land. Before the arrival of Europeans, this country had no name but was inhabited by groups of people who called themselves nations. The people were strong both in their knowledge of the land and in their might as warriors. The Vikings reached the shores of this country about A.D. 1010. They were unable to settle on the land and left after a decade of frustration. Much later, another group of settlers, since termed the "Lost Colonies," were repulsed. More people came to these shores, however, and the land was taken over by Europeans.

As the settlers expanded westward, they signed "treaties of peace" or "treaties of land cession" with the American Indians. These treaties were similar to those struck between nations, although in this case the agreement was imposed by the "big" nation onto the "small" nation. One reason for treaties was to legitimize the takeover of the land that the Europeans had "discovered." Once the land was "discovered," it was divided among the Europeans, who set out to create a "legal" claim to it. The American Indians signed the resultant treaties, ceding small amounts of their land to the settlers and keeping the rest for themselves. As time passed, the number of Whites rapidly grew, and the number of Indians diminished because of wars and disease. As these events occurred, the treaties began to lose their meaning; the Europeans disregarded them. They decided that these "natives" had no real claim to the land and shifted them around like cargo from one reservation to another. Although the American Indians tried to seek just settlements through the American court system, they failed to win back the land that had been taken from them through misrepresentation. For example, in 1831, the Cherokees were fighting in the courts to keep their nation in Georgia. They lost their legal battle, however, and, like other American Indian nations after the time of the early European settlers, were forced to move westward. During this forced westward movement, many died, and all suffered. Today, many nations are seeking to reclaim their land through the courts (Brown, 1970; Deloria 1969, 1974; Fortney, 1977). Several claims, such as those of the Penobscot and Passamaquoddy tribes in Maine, have been successful. The number of federally recognized tribes has increased from just over 100 as recently ago as the 1980s to the present (2012) 564 (United States Department of the Interior, Bureau of Indian Affairs, 2010).

As the American Indians migrated westward, they carried with them the fragments of their culture. Their lives were disrupted, their land was lost, and many of their leaders and teachers perished, yet much of their history and culture somehow remained. Today, more and more American Indians are seeking to know their history. The story of the colonization and settlement of the United States is being retold with a different emphasis.

American Indian people have sought ways to rebuild Indian communities and to maintain an Indian future in America. The American Indian Movement (AIM) was born in Minnesota in 1968. Today, it is apparent that the movement has transformed policy making into programs and organizations that have served Indian people in many communities. The policies were consistently made in consultation with spiritual leaders and elders. In fact, the movement was founded to turn the attention of Indian people toward a renewal of spirituality and at the heart of AIM is deep spirituality and a belief in the connectedness of all Indian people (Waterman & Salinas, 2006).

American Indians live predominantly in 26 states (including Alaska), with most residing in the western part of the country as a result of the forced westward migration. Although many American Indians remain on reservations and in rural areas, just as many people live in cities, especially on the West Coast. Oklahoma, Arizona, California, New Mexico, and Alaska have the largest numbers of American Indians (IHS, 2007). Today, more and more people are claiming to have American Indian roots.

■ Traditional Definitions of HEALTH and ILLNESS

Although each American Indian Nation or tribe had its own history and belief system regarding HEALTH and ILLNESS and the traditional treatment of ILLNESS, some general beliefs and practices underlie the more specific tribal ideas. The terms HEALTH and ILLNESS are used to indicate that, among traditional people, the connotations are holistic, as defined and discussed in Chapters 5 and 6. The data—collected through an ongoing review of the literature and from interviews granted by members of the groups—come from the Navajo Nation, Hopis, Cherokees, Shoshones, and New England Indians with whom I have worked closely.

The traditional American Indian belief about HEALTH is that it reflects living in "total harmony with nature and having the ability to survive under exceedingly difficult circumstances" (Zuckoff, 1995). Humankind has an intimate relationship with nature (Boyd, 1974). The Earth is considered to be a living organism—the body of a higher individual, with a will and a desire to be well. The Earth is periodically HEALTHY and less HEALTHY, just as human beings are. According to the American Indian belief system, a person should treat his or her body with respect, just as the Earth should be treated with respect. When the Earth is harmed, humankind is itself harmed and, conversely, when humans harm themselves, they harm the Earth. The Earth gives food, shelter, and medicine to humankind; for this reason, all things of the Earth belong to human beings and nature. "The land belongs to life, life belongs to the land, and the land belongs to itself." In order to maintain

HEALTH, Indians must maintain their relationship with nature. "Mother Earth" is the friend of the American Indian, and the land belongs to the American Indian (Boyd, 1974).

According to American Indian belief, as explained by a medicine man, Rolling Thunder, the human body is divided into 2 halves, which are seen as plus and minus (yet another version of the concept that every whole is made of 2 opposite halves). There are also—in every whole—2 energy poles: positive and negative. The energy of the body can be controlled by spiritual means. It is further believed that every being has a purpose and an identity. Every being has the power to control him- or herself and, from this force and the belief in its potency, the spiritual power of a person is kindled (Boyd, 1974).

In all American Indian cultures, disease is associated with the religious aspect of society as supernatural powers are associated with the causing and curing of disease. Disease is conceived of in a wide variety of ways. It is believed to occur due to a lack of prevention, which is given by wearing or using charms; the presence of some material object that has intruded into the body via sorcery; or the absence of the free soul from the body (Lyon, 1996, pp. 60–61). One example of an amulet is *Duklij*, turquoise or green malachite that is believed to contain supernatural qualities that ward off the evil spirits and bring rain (Lyon, 1996, p. 68).

Many American Indians with traditional orientations believe there is a reason for every sickness or pain. They believe that ILLNESS is the price to be paid either for something that happened in the past or for something that will happen in the future. In spite of this conviction, a sick person must still be cared for. Everything is seen as being the result of something else, and this cause-and-effect relationship creates an eternal chain. American Indians do not generally subscribe to the germ theory of modern medicine. ILLNESS is something that must be. Even the person who is experiencing the ILLNESS may not realize the reason for its occurrence, but it may, in fact, be the best possible price to pay for the past or future event(s) (Boyd, 1974).

The Hopi Indians associate ILLNESS with evil spirits. The evil spirit responsible for an ILLNESS is identified by the medicine man, and the remedy for the malady resides in the treatment of the evil spirit (Leek, 1975, p. 16).

According to legend, the Navajo people originally emerged from the depths of the Earth—fully formed as human beings. Before the beginning of time, they existed with holy people, supernatural beings with supernatural powers, in a series of 12 underworlds. The creation of all elements took place in these underworlds, and there all things were made to interact in constant harmony. A number of ceremonies and rituals were created at this time for "maintaining, renewing, and mending this state of harmony" (Bilagody, 1969, p. 21).

When the Navajo people emerged from the underworlds, 1 female was missing. She was subsequently found by a search party in the same hole from which they had initially emerged. She told the people that she had chosen to remain there and wait for their return. She became known as death, sickness, and witchcraft. Because her hair was unraveled and her body was covered with dry red ochre, the Navajos today continue to unravel the hair of their dead and to cover their bodies with red ochre. Members of the Navajo nation believe that "witchcraft exists and that certain humans, known as witches, are able to interact with the evil spirits. These people can bring sickness and other unhappiness to the people who annoy them" (Bilagody, 1969, p. 36).

Traditionally, the Navajos see ILLNESS, disharmony, and sadness as the result of one or more combinations of the following actions: "(1) displeasing the holy people; (2) annoying the elements; (3) disturbing animal and plant life; (4) neglecting the celestial bodies; (5) misuse of a sacred Indian ceremony; or (6) tampering with witches and witchcraft" (Bilagody, 1969, p. 57). If disharmony exists, disease can occur. The Navajos distinguish between 2 types of diseases: (1) contagious diseases, such as measles, smallpox, diphtheria, syphilis, and gonorrhea and (2) more generalized ILLNESSES, such as "body fever" and "body ache." The notion that ILLNESS is caused by a microbe or another physiological agent is alien to the Navajos. The cause of disease, of injury to people or to their property, or of continued misfortune of any kind must be traced back to an action that should not have been performed. Examples of such infractions are breaking a taboo and contacting a ghost or witch. To the Navajos, the treatment of an ILLNESS, therefore, must be concerned with the external causative factor(s), not with the ILLNESS or injury itself (Kluckhohn & Leighton, 1962, pp. 192–193).

■ Traditional Methods of HEALING

Traditional HEALERS

The traditional HEALER of Native America is the medicine man or woman, and American Indians, by and large, have maintained their faith in him or her over the ages. The medicine men and women are wise in the ways of the land and of nature. They know well the interrelationships of human beings, the Earth, and the universe. They know the ways of the plants and animals, the sun, the moon, and the stars. Medicine men and women take time to determine first the cause of an ILLNESS and then the proper treatment. To determine the cause and treatment of an ILLNESS, they perform special ceremonies, which may take up to several days.

A medicine man or woman is also known among many people as a *Kusiut*, a "learned one." The acquisition of full shamanic powers takes many years, often as many as 30 years of training before one has the ability to cure illness. The shaman's power is accumulated through solitary vision quests and fasts repeated over the years. The purification rituals include scrubbing oneself in freezing cold water and ingesting emetics (Lyon, 1996, p. 141).

As a specific example, Boyd describes the medicine man, Rolling Thunder—the spiritual leader, philosopher, and acknowledged spokesman of the Cherokee and Shoshone tribes—as being able to determine the cause of ILLNESS when the ILL person does not know it. The "diagnostic" phase of the treatment may take as long as 3 days. There are numerous causes of ILLNESS and a great number of reasons—good or bad—for having become ILL.

These causes are of a spiritual nature. When modern physicians see a sick person, they recognize and diagnose only the physical illness. Medicine men and women, in contrast, look for the spiritual cause of the problem. To the American Indian, "every physical thing in nature has a spiritual nature because the whole is viewed as being essentially spiritual in nature." The agents of nature, herbs, are seen as spiritual helpers, and the characteristics of plants must be known and understood. Rolling Thunder states that "we are born with a purpose in life and we have to fulfill that purpose" (Boyd, 1974, pp. 124, 263). The purpose of the medicine man or woman is to cure, and their power is not dying out.

The medicine man or woman of the Hopis uses meditation in determining the cause of an ILLNESS and sometimes even uses a crystal ball as the focal point for meditation. At other times, the medicine man or woman chews on the root of jimsonweed, a powerful herb that produces a trance. The Hopis claim that this herb gives the medicine man or woman a vision of the evil that has caused a sickness. Once the meditation is concluded, the medicine man or woman is able to prescribe the proper herbal treatment. For example, fever is cured by a plant that smells like lightning; the Hopi phrase for fever is "lightning sickness" (Leek, 1975, p. 16).

The Navajo Indians consider disease to be the result of breaking a taboo or the attack of a witch. The exact cause is diagnosed by divination, as is the ritual of treatment. There are 3 types of divination: motion in the hand (the most common form and often practiced by women), stargazing, and listening. The function of the diagnostician is first to determine the cause of the ILLNESS and then to recommend the treatment—that is, the type of chant that will be effective and the medicine man or woman who can best do it. A medicine man or woman may be called on to treat obvious symptoms, whereas the diagnostician is called on to ascertain the cause of the ILLNESS. (A person is considered wise if the diagnostician is called first.) Often, the same medicine man or woman can practice both divination (diagnosis) and the singing (treatment). When any form of divination is used in making the diagnosis, the diagnostician meets with the family, discusses the patient's condition, and determines the fee.

The practice of motion in the hand includes the following rituals. Pollen or sand is sprinkled around the sick person, during which time the diagnostician sits with closed eyes and face turned from the patient. The HEALER's hand begins to move during a song. While the hand is moving, the diagnostician thinks of various diseases and various causes. When the arm begins to move in a certain way, the diagnostician knows that the right disease and its cause have been discovered. He or she is then able to prescribe the proper treatment (Wyman, 1966, pp. 8–14). The ceremony of motion in the hand also may incorporate the use of sand paintings. (These paintings are a well-known form of art.) Four basic colors are used—white, blue, yellow, and black—and each color has a symbolic meaning. Chanting is performed as the painting is produced, and the shape of the painting determines the cause and treatment of the ILLNESS. The chants may continue for an extended time (Kluckhohn & Leighton, 1962, p. 230), depending on the family's ability to pay and the capabilities of the singer. The process of motion in the hand can be neither inherited nor learned. It comes to a person suddenly, as a gift. It is said that people able to diagnose their own ILLNESSES are able to practice motion in the hand (Wyman, 1966, p. 14).

Unlike motion in the hand, stargazing can and must be learned. Sand paintings are often but not always made during stargazing. If they are not made, it is either because the sick person cannot afford to have one done or because there is not enough time to make one. The stargazer prays the star prayer to the star spirit, asking it to show the cause of the ILLNESS. During stargazing, singing begins and the star throws a ray of light that determines the cause of the patient's ILLNESS. If the ray of light is white or yellow, the patient will recover; if it is red, the illness is serious. If a white light falls on the patient's home, the person will recover; if the home is dark, the patient will die (Wyman, 1966, p. 15).

Listening, the third type of divination, is somewhat similar to stargazing, except that something is heard rather than seen. In this instance, the cause of the ILLNESS is determined by the sound that is heard. If someone is heard to be crying, the patient will die (Wyman, 1966, p. 16).

The traditional Navajos continue to use medicine men and women when an ILLNESS occurs. They use this service because, in many instances, the treatment they receive from the traditional HEALERS is better than the treatment they receive from the health care establishment. Treatments used by singers include massage and heat treatment, the sweatbath, and use of the yucca root—approaches similar to those common in physiotherapy (Kluckhohn & Leighton, 1962, p. 230).

The main effects of the singer are psychological. During the chant, the patient feels cared for in a deeply personal way as the center of the singer's attention, since the patient's problem is the reason for the singer's presence. When the singer tells the patient recovery will occur and the reason for the ILLNESS, the patient has faith in what is heard. The singer is regarded as a distinguished authority and as a person of eminence with the gift of learning from the holy people. He or she is considered to be more than a mere mortal. The ceremony—surrounded by such high levels of prestige, mysticism, and power—takes the sick person into its circle, ultimately becoming one with the holy people by participating in the sing that is held on the patient's behalf. The patient once again comes into harmony with the universe and subsequently becomes free of all ILLS and evil (Kluckhohn & Leighton, 1962, p. 232).

The religion of the Navajos is one of good hope when they are sick or suffer other misfortunes. Their system of beliefs and practices helps them through the crises of life and death. The stories that are told during ceremonies give the people a glimpse of a world that has gone by, which promotes a feeling of security because they see that they are links in the unbroken chain of countless generations (Kluckhohn & Leighton, 1962, p. 233).

Many Navajos believe in witchcraft, and, when it is considered to be the cause of an ILLNESS, special ceremonies are employed to rid the individual of the evil caused by witches. Numerous methods are used to manipulate the supernatural. Although many of these activities may meet with strong social disapproval,

Navajos recognize the usefulness of blaming witches for ILLNESS and misfortune. Tales abound concerning witchcraft and how the witches work. Not all Navajos believe in witchcraft but, for those who do, it provides a mechanism for laying blame for the overwhelming hardships and anxieties of life.

Such events as going into a trance can be ascribed to the work of witches. The way to cure a "witched" person is through the use of complicated prayer ceremonies that are attended by friends and relatives, who lend help and express sympathy. The victim of a witch is in no way responsible for being sick and is, therefore, free of any punitive action by the community if the ILLNESS causes the victim to behave in strange ways. However, if an incurably "witched" person is affected so that alterations in the person's established role severely disrupt the community, the victim may be abandoned (Kluckhohn & Leighton, 1962, p. 244). Box 9–1 presents selected beliefs of a traditional Cherokee medicine man.

Box 9–1

Hawk Littlejohn, 1941–2000

I had the privilege of working with Hawk Littlejohn, a traditional medicine man, in 1979 at the Boston (Massachusetts) Indian Council. Thomas Crowe wrote in his obituary that Hawk Littlejohn "embraced tradition in the modern world. He was a native of Western North Carolina and a member of the Eastern Band of the Cherokee nation. He was unique both in his skills in the traditional methods of natural and psychological healing and in his sensitivity and concern for his fellow man." I interviewed him in June 1979. Here are several of his thoughts in his own words:

- A medicine man sees himself in my tribe as a person who is many, many things. Not just as a HEALER or not just as a priest. We like to see ourselves like the fingers on a hand. They are separated and work independently of the hand if requested to, but they're still part of the whole. And each one of these fingers can do different things. It's like when I go to visit a home and there is a child there who is suffering from malnutrition but in our medicine we're more interested in the cause not the symptom. So, I've left my role as a HEALER and a priest to a role that might turn out to be social or political to find out why the child is hungry, why this child is feeling this way. And that might be dealing with the tribal government or some kind of social situation. We elect to see ourselves as representatives of our people's needs.
- The medicine man or HEALER in my tribe is considered to be chosen by the Great Spirit. For a couple of years the medicine men check all children for unusual marks, it is not any particular mark on the body but something they consider very unusual as a sign. The unusual marks that were on me were Simian Creases, the line that goes across my hand. I'm told it is unusual to have one of these but to have two, one on each hand, is very unusual. I was perhaps two or three years old when I was chosen.
- As a child I was taught that there are three parts of us and the most obvious part is the physical aspect, then the second part is the intellectual part,

(continued)

and the third part is the spiritual aspect of a person. The physical is the tangible, the one we can see and touch and be with all the time. We go through acceptance of our physical being. This is what I have to walk the path of life with and I accept it for what it is. The intellectual aspect is the part that interprets things for you—dreams, visions, feelings, and what the spirit is saying to you. The spiritual aspect of a person of is the slowest and the last in most cases to mature. The spiritual aspect is kept in harmony and in balance by the awareness that it is part of everything else. We believe that all life forms have a spirit and the relationship of man to all other beings that are alive is a spiritual one. When all three aspects are working together it is called balance and harmony, or the center of the earth.

- Let's say a student, for example, puts a lot of emphasis on the intellect and neglects the physical and the spiritual aspect of him, we believe that there are natural forces which always try to seek a balance. For instance, if you get a cut, you heal because it is natural to try to seek balance. We believe that there are many subtle things the Great Spirit made and very obvious things that the Great Spirit made like creatures like elephants, whales, and the obvious. And then much more subtle creatures like what you call germs and viruses and when we believe that when the Great Spirit created life, he created laws to govern life, that the wolf wouldn't eat the deer in one day, that there would be laws to govern these kinds of things. One of the laws was what we call a "*skilly*." It is a being or a creature and it has no good or bad. When a person neglects the spiritual and physical part for the intellect, and does not seek balance, the *skilly* comes in and one of the effects of the *skilly* is sickness and disease.

- One of the ways to treat people is indirectly. When I go to see people we talk about their corn and their lives and they talk about my corn and my life and then we get down to the reason why I am there. They don't tell me their physical symptoms. One of the things we've realized is that sickness isolates people from other people and the sickness has separated the person from the community and from his family. So we automatically try to make him or bring him back out of that isolation and one of the ways we do that is to include the family and friends in the HEALING process.

- In my tribe we have knowledge of about 500 different plants and use about 350 of them on a pretty regular basis. We see the plants as other life forms, but the commonality between all life forms is this spiritual aspect. We believe that each thing that is alive has a spirit and its spirit has a personality, so I use the spirit of the plant to cure another spirit—when the spirit of the sickness is not compatible with the spirit of the plant, the disease dissipates. We call the plants, plant people. My people's medicine started off as a trial and error, like most medicine did, using the plants. If you had a sickness that reminded them of a rabbit, for example, a plant that reminded them of a fox would be used to treat it.

- I think the solution to Indian problems is for Indian people to start identifying themselves. I see as a traditional person that one of the steps on this long journey is to gain pride and dignity in oneself. Naturally, I believe it is in traditionalism. Traditionalism is a philosophy, a way of life and living, a holistic sort of thing that we're a part of.

Source: Crowe, T. (2001). "Hawk Littlejohn embraced the old ways in the modern world. SMN Archives/Regional News, 1/17/01. Retrieved from http://www.smokymountainnews.com/issues/1_01/1_17_01/front_littlejohn.shtml, April 16, 2012.

Traditional Remedies

American Indians practice an act of purification in order to maintain their harmony with nature and to cleanse the body and spirit. This is done by total immersion in water in addition to the use of sweatlodges, herbal medicines, and special rituals. Purification is seen as the first step in the control of consciousness, a ritual that awakens the body and the senses and prepares a person for meditation. The participants view it as a new beginning (Boyd, 1974, pp. 97–100).

The basis of therapy lies in nature, hence the use of herbal remedies. Specific rituals are to be followed when herbs are gathered. Each plant is picked to be dried for later use. No plant is picked unless it is the proper one, and only enough plants are picked to meet the needs of the gatherers. Timing is crucial, and the procedures are followed meticulously. So deep is their belief in the harmony of human beings and nature that the herb gatherers exercise great care not to disturb any of the other plants and animals in the environment (Boyd, 1974, pp. 101–136).

One plant of interest, the common dandelion, contains a milky juice in its stem and is said to increase the flow of milk from the breasts of nursing mothers. Another plant, the thistle, is said to contain a substance that relieves the prickling sensation in the throats of people who live in the desert. The medicine used to hasten the birth of a baby is called *weasel medicine* because the weasel is clever at digging through and out of difficult territory (Leek, 1975, p. 17).

The following is a list of common ailments and herbal treatments used by the Hopi Indians (Leek, 1975, pp. 17–26):

1. Cuts and wounds are treated with globe mallow. The root of this plant is chewed to help mend broken bones.
2. To keep air from cuts, piñon gum is applied to the wound. It is used also in an amulet to protect a person from witchcraft.
3. Cliff rose is used to wash wounds.
4. Boils are brought to a head with the use of sand sagebrush.
5. Spider bites are treated with sunflower. The person bathes in water in which the flowers have been soaked.
6. Snakebites are treated with the bladder pod. The bitter root of this plant is chewed and then placed on the bite.
7. Lichens are used to treat the gums. They are ground to a powder and then rubbed on the affected areas.
8. Fleabane is used to treat headaches. The entire herb is either bound to the head or infused and drunk as a tea.
9. Digestive disorders are treated with blue gillia. The leaves are boiled in water and drunk to relieve indigestion.

10. The stem of the yucca plant is used as a laxative. The purple flower of the thistle is used to expel worms.

11. Blanket flower is the diuretic used to provide relief from painful urination.

12. A tea is made from painted cup and drunk to relieve the pain of menstruation.

13. Winter fat provides a tea from the leaves and roots and is drunk if the uterus fails to contract properly during labor.

The use of American Indian cures and herbal remedies continues to be popular. Among the Oneida Indians, the following remedies are used (Knox & Adams, 1988):

Illness	Remedy
Colds	Witch hazel, sweet flag
Sore throat	Comfrey
Diarrhea	Elderberry flowers
Headache	Tansy and sage
Ear infection	Skunk oil
Mouth sores	Dried raspberry leaves

Among the Micmac Indians of Canada, the following remedies have been reported to be used (Basque & Young, 1984):

Illness	Remedy
Warts	Juice from milkweed plant
Obesity	Spruce bark and water
Rheumatism	Juniper berries
Diabetes	Combination of blueberries and huckleberries
Insomnia	A head of lettuce a day
Diarrhea	Tea from wild strawberry

Drums are another source of treatment. HEALING ceremonies are accompanied by drumming, rattles, and singing. The noise consists of sounds that interfere with the negative work of the spirits of the disease. The rhythm of the drumming plays a role in altering human consciousness (Lyon, 1996, p. 67). "Drumming is essential in helping the shaman make the transition from an ordinary state of consciousness to the shamanistic state of consciousness" (p. 68). Quiet HEALING ceremonies are unheard of.

Table 9–1 summarizes the cultural phenomena affecting American Indians, Aleuts, and Eskimos.

Table 9-1 **Examples of Cultural Phenomena Affecting Health Care Among the American Indian and Alaska Native Population**

Nations of Origin	Five hundred sixty-one American Indian nations indigenous to North America; Aleuts and Eskimos in Alaska
Environmental Control	Traditional HEALTH and ILLNESS beliefs may continue to be observed by "traditional" people Natural and magico-religious folk medicine tradition Traditional HEALER—medicine man or woman
Biological Variations	Accidents Heart disease Cirrhosis of the liver Diabetes mellitus
Social Organization	Extremely family-oriented to both biological and extended families Children taught to respect traditions Community social organizations
Communication	Tribal languages Use of silence and body language
Space	Space is very important and has no boundaries
Time Orientation	Present

Source: Spector, R. (1992). Culture, ethnicity, and nursing. In P. Potter & A. Perry (Eds.), *Fundamentals of Nursing* (3rd ed.). St. Louis, MO: Mosby-Year Book. Reprinted with permission. This material was published in Potter & Perry's Fundamentals of Nursing, Jackie Crisp and Catherine Taylor (Eds), Copyright Elsevier (2009)."

■ Current Health Care Problems

Today, American Indians are faced with a number of health-related problems and health disparities. Many of the old ways of diagnosing and treating illness have not survived the migrations and changing ways of life of the people. Because these skills often have been lost and because modern health care facilities are not always available, American Indian people are frequently caught in limbo when it comes to obtaining adequate health care. Many of the illnesses that are familiar among White patients may manifest themselves differently in American Indian patients. Native peoples experience higher disease rates and lower life expectancy than any other racial or ethnic group in the country. The rates of diabetes, mental disorders, cardiovascular disease, pneumonia, influenza, and injuries of Indians are exponentially higher, the infant mortality rate is 150% greater for Indians than that of White infants. As alluded to at the beginning of this chapter, suicide rates among the young are high—a rate that is more than 3 times that of the general population (Nieves, 2007, p. A-9) and life expectancy is 5 years less than the rest of the U.S. population. The impact of this is felt throughout the community. In addition, at least one third of American Indians exist in a state of abject poverty. With this destitution come poor living conditions and attendant problems, as well as diseases of the poor—including malnutrition, tuberculosis, and high maternal and infant death rates. Poverty and isolated living serve as further barriers that keep American Indians from using limited health care facilities even when they are available (National Congress for American Indians, 2010).

The traumas that the American Indians in the Plains states experienced over the past 175 years, such as the massacre at Wounded Knee, are part of the problem, as is the decimation of the land and culture.

Morbidity and Mortality

The American Indian and Alaska Native people have long experienced lower health status when compared with other Americans. Lower life expectancy and the disproportionate disease burden exist perhaps because of inadequate education, disproportionate poverty, discrimination in the delivery of health services, and cultural differences. These are broad quality-of-life issues rooted in economic adversity and poor social conditions.

American Indians and Alaska Natives born today have a life expectancy that is 2.4 years less than the U.S. population of all races (74.5 to 76.9 years, respectively). American Indian and Alaska Native infants die at a rate of nearly 10 per every 1,000 live births, as compared to 7 per 1,000 for the U.S. population (2001–2003 rates). Given the higher health status enjoyed by most Americans, the lingering health disparities of American Indians and Alaska Natives are troubling. In trying to account for the disparities, health care experts, policymakers, and tribal leaders are looking at many factors that impact the health of Indian people, including the adequacy of funding for the American Indian health care delivery system (U.S. Department of Health and Human Services, IHS, 2011).

The American Indian and Alaska Native population has several characteristics different from the U.S. population that would impact assessing the cost for providing similar health services enjoyed by most Americans. The American Indian population is younger, because of higher mortality, than all other U.S. races. The Indian Health Service (IHS) population is predominately rural, which should suggest lower costs; however, the disproportionate incidence of disease and medical conditions experienced by the American Indian population raises the costs, which almost obliterates the lower cost offsets. Table 9–2 compares selected health status indicators for all races and American Indians. As can be seen in Table 9–2, the crude birth rate among American Indians/Alaska Natives is higher than that of the general population; the infant mortality rate is higher; and the male suicide and homicide rates in 2004 are higher than in the general population. The incidence of both breast cancer and prostate cancer is lower.

The bold entries in Table 9–3 illustrate the greatest areas of disparity between American Indians and all other races in the United States. Diabetes, homicide, infant deaths, and so forth are notably higher. Another way to realize the gravity of the disparities is to examine Table 9–3 that presents the ratios between the total U.S. population and the American Indian/Alaska Native populations.

Table 9-2   Comparison of Selected Health Status Indicators—All Races and American Indians and Alaska Natives: 2007

Health Indicator	All Races	American Indians and Alaska Natives
Crude birth rate per 1,000 population by race of mother, 2007	14.3	**15.3**
Percentage of live births of women receiving prenatal care first trimester, 2007	67.5	53.2
Percentage of live births of women receiving third-trimester or no prenatal care, 2007	8.4	14.0
Percentage of live births to teenage childbearing women—under 18, 2007	3.4	6.1
Percentage of low birth weight per live births >2,500 grams, 2007	8.22	7.46
Infant mortality per 1,000 live births, 2006	6.7	**8.3**
Cancer—all sites per 100,000 population, 2007	446.7	332.0
Lung cancer incidence per 100,000 population, 2007	Men: 65.4 Women: 47.4	Men: — Women: —
Breast cancer incidence per 100,000, 2007	122.5	83.4
Prostate cancer incidence per 100,000, 2007	158.3	77.9
Male death rates from suicide, all ages, age adjusted per 100,000 resident population, 2007	11.3	**18.1**
Male death rates from homicide, all ages, age adjusted per 100,000 resident population, 1999/2003	9.6	**9.2**

Source: National Center for Health Statistics. Health, United States (2010). With Special Feature on Death and Dying. Hyattsville, MD. 2011: Author, pp. 102, 106, 107, 110, 124, 137, and 204.

Mental Illness

The family in this population is often a nuclear family, with strong biological and large extended family networks. Children are taught to respect traditions, and community organizations are growing in strength and numbers. Many American Indians tend to use traditional medicines and HEALERS and are knowledgeable about these resources. People may frequently be treated by a traditional medicine man or woman. The sweat lodge and herbs are frequently used to treat mental symptoms. Several diagnostic techniques include the use of divination, conjuring, and stargazing.

"Ghost sickness" is a culture bound syndrome that affects some American Indians. This mental health problem involves a preoccupation with death, an intense fear of ghosts and the deceased and is associated with witchcraft. It is thought to be caused by the touch of a ghost. The ghosts of the recently departed may cause illness or even death among the living. Symptoms include bad dreams, weakness, feelings of danger, loss of appetite, and confusion (Admin., 2011).

Methamphetamine (meth) abuse and suicide are 2 top concerns in Indian country. Methamphetamine is a low-cost, highly addictive stimulant drug. Its

Table 9-3 Mortality Disparities Rates Between American Indians and Alaska Natives (AI/AN) in the IHS Service Area 2004–2006 Age-Adjusted Rates per 100,000 Population

	AI/AN Rate 2004–2006	U.S. All Races Rate—2005	Ratio: AI/AN to U.S. All Races
All Causes	980.0	798.8	1.2
Alcohol-Induced	43.0	7.0	6.1
Breast Cancer	21.0	24.1	0.9
Cerebrovascular	46.6	46-6	1.0
Cervical Cancer	3.3	2.4	1.4
Diabetes	68.1	24.6	2.8
Heart Disease	206.2	211.1	1.0
HIV Infection	3.0	4.2	0.7
Homicide (Assault)	11.7	6.1	1.9
Infant Deaths[a]	8.0	6.9	1.2
Malignant Neoplasm	176.2	183.8	1.0
Maternal Deaths	16.9	15.1	1.1
Pneumonia/Influenza	27.1	20.3	1.3
Suicide	19.8	10.9	1.8
Tuberculosis	1.2	0.2	6.0

Source: U.S. Department of Health and Human Services, Indian Health Service. (2011). *Facts on health disparities.* Retrieved from http://info.ihs.gov/.

[a]Infant deaths per 1,000 live births.

Note: Rates are adjusted to compensate for misreporting of American Indian and Alaska Native race on state death certificates. American Indian and Alaska Native death rate columns present data for the 3-year period specified. U.S. all races columns present data for a 1-year period. ICD-10 codes were introduced in 1999; therefore, comparability ratios were applied to deaths for 1996–1998. Rates are based on American Indian and Alaska Native alone; 2000 census with bridged-race categories.

introduction to Indian Country has destabilized and disrupted entire health and social systems. Meth is a synthetic artificial stimulant with a number of effects on the brain and the rest of the body. People who use this chemical may display high levels of aggression and may injure or kill themselves and others. Meth also causes significant physical complications including neurological/organic brain changes. Hand in hand with meth abuse is the high suicide rate. There are a wide range of general risk factors, such as "getting into trouble," that have been shown to contribute to suicide in adolescents. AI/AN young people face, on average, a greater number of these risk factors and/or the risk factors are more severe in nature. Research suggests that factors that protect Native youth and young adults against suicidal behavior are their sense of belonging to their culture, strong tribal spiritual orientation, and cultural continuity (Grenier & Lockjer, 2007).

Alcoholism is a major mental health problem among American Indians. A comparison of the 10 leading causes of death among American Indians/Alaska Natives and the general population reveals that unintentional injuries (#3), chronic liver disease and cirrhosis (#4), and suicide (#6) rank higher as

Table 9–4 Comparison: The 10 Leading Causes of Death for American Indians and Alaska Natives and for All Persons, 2007

American Indians and Alaska Natives	All Persons
1. Diseases of heart	Diseases of heart
2. Malignant neoplasms	Malignant neoplasms
3. Unintentional injuries	Cerebrovascular diseases
4. Chronic liver disease and cirrhosis	Chronic lower respiratory diseases
5. Diabetes mellitus	Unintentional injuries
6. Suicide	Alzheimer's disease
7. Chronic lower respiratory diseases	Diabetes mellitus
8. Cerebrovascular diseases	Influenza and pneumonia
9. Homicide	Nephritis, nephrotic syndrome, and nephrosis
10. Influenza and pneumonia	Septicemia

Source: National Center for Health Statistics. Health, United States, 2010: With Special Feature on Death and Dying. Hyattsville, MD. 2011: Author, pp. 145–146.

causes of death than for the population at large. Each of these causes of death is related to mental health problems, including alcoholism.

Table 9–4 compares the 10 leading causes of death between all persons and American Indians and Alaska Natives. The sixth leading cause of death is suicide and the ninth cause of death is homocide—these 2 causes do not place among the top 10 causes of death in the total population.

Fetal Alcohol Syndrome

"My son will forever travel through a moonless night with only the roar of the wind for company" (Dorris, 1989, p. 264). This quote reflects on the tragedy of fetal alcohol syndrome, an affliction that affects countless American Indian children. A new study from the Substance Abuse and Mental Health Services Administration (SAMHSA) shows that American Indians and Alaska Natives continue to have higher rates of alcohol use and illicit drug use disorders than other racial groups.

The markings of fetal alcohol syndrome include

- abnormal growth in height, weight, and/or head circumference, including microcephaly;
- central nervous system problems such as behavioral and/or mental health problems, including learning disabilities and abnormal sleeping and eating patterns; and
- appearance with a specific pattern of recognizable deformities, such as the three key facial features, a smooth philtrum, a thin vermillion border, and small palpebral fissures. (Bertrand, Floyd, & Weber, 2005, p. 3).

An estimated 70,000 fetal alcohol children are born every year in the United States, many of whom are American Indians. The worldwide numbers vary, with a range of 0.2–1.5 cases per 1,000 live births being most frequently reported (Bertrand et al., 2005, p. 3). Dorris (1989, p. 231) further points out that the son of an alcoholic biological father is 3 times more likely to become an abusive drinker.

This problem has grown over time, and the impact increases with each generation. Mortality and morbidity rates for American Indians are directly affected by alcohol abuse. Alcohol abuse is the most widespread and severe problem in the American Indian community. It is extremely costly to the people and underlies many of their physical, mental, social, and economic problems, and the problem is growing worse. Hawk Littlejohn, the medicine man of the Cherokee nation, Eastern band, attributes this problem, from a traditional point of view, to the fact that American Indians have lost the opportunity to make choices. They can no longer choose how they live or how they practice their medicine and religion. He believes that, once people return to a sense of identification within themselves, they begin to rid themselves of this problem of alcoholism. Whatever the solution may be, the problem is indeed immense (Littlejohn, 1979).

Domestic Violence

Another problem related to alcohol abuse in the American Indian people is domestic violence, sexual abuse, and the battering of women. A battered woman is one who is physically assaulted by her husband, boyfriend, or another significant other. The assault may consist of a push; severe, even permanent injury; sexual abuse; child abuse; or neglect. Once the pattern of abuse is established, subsequent episodes tend to get worse. This abuse is not traditional in American Indian life but has evolved. True American Indian love is based on a tradition of mutual respect and the belief that men and women are part of an ordered universe where the people should live in peace. In the traditional American Indian home, children were raised to respect their parents, and they were not corporally punished. Violence toward women was not practiced. In modern times, however, the sanctions and protections against domestic violence have decreased, and the women are far more vulnerable. Many women are reluctant to admit that they are victims of abuse because they believe that they will be blamed for the assault. Hence, the beatings continue. A number of services are available to women who are victims, such as safe houses and support groups. It is believed that the long-range solution to this problem lies in teaching children to love—to nurture children and give them self-esteem, to teach boys to love and respect women, and to give girls a sense of worth. Amnesty International calls sexual abuse against American Indian women a "maze of injustice." It is "the failure to protect Indigenous women from sexual violence in the USA." The disproportionate impact on American Indian women is derived from disparate communities that vary with respect to law enforcement, jurisdiction, and health care and support services (Grenier & Lockjer, 2007, p. 3).

Domestic violence has a profound effect on the community and on the family. A pattern of abuse is easily established. It begins with tension: The female attempts to keep peace but the male cannot contain himself, a fight erupts, and then the crisis arrives. The couple may make up, only to fight again. Attempts to help must be initiated, or the cycle escalates. The problem is extremely complex. Some of the services available to a household experiencing domestic violence include

1. tribal health: direct services for physical and mental health,
2. law enforcement: police protection may be necessary, and
3. legal assistance: assistance for immediate shelter and emergency food and transportation.

Urban Problems

More than 50% of American Indians live in urban areas; for example, in Seattle, Washington, there are over 15,000 American Indians. Although this population is not particularly dense, its rates of diphtheria, tuberculosis, otitis media with subsequent hearing defects, alcohol abuse, inadequate immunization, iron-deficiency anemia, childhood developmental lags, mental health problems (including depression, anxiety, and coping difficulties), and caries and other dental problems are high. As in all dysfunctional families, problems arise that are related to marital difficulties and financial strain, which usually are brought about by unemployment and the lack of education or knowledge of special skills. The tension often is compounded further by alcoholism.

Between 5,000 and 6,000 American Indians live in Boston, Massachusetts. They experience the same problems as American Indians in other cities, yet there is an additional problem. Few non-Indian residents are even aware that there is an American Indian community in that city or that it is in desperate need of adequate health and social services.

Health Care Provider Services

Some historical differences in health care relate to geographic locations. American Indians living in the eastern part of this country and in most urban areas are not covered by the services of the Indian Health Service, services that are available to American Indians living on reservations in the West. In 1923, tribal government—under the control of the Bureau of Indian Affairs—was begun by the Navajos, who established treaties with the U.S. government, but in the areas of health and education the United States did not honor these treaties. Health services on the reservations were inadequate. Consequently, the people were sent to outside institutions for the treatment of illnesses, such as tuberculosis and mental health problems. As recently as 1930, the vast Navajo lands had only 7 hospitals with 25 beds each. Not until 1955 were American Indians finally offered concentrated services with modern physicians. Only since 1965 have more comprehensive services been available to the Navajos.

■ The Indian Health Service

The IHS is an agency within the U.S. Department of Health and Human Services. It is responsible for providing federal health services to American Indians and Alaska Natives. The provision of health services to members of federally recognized tribes grew out of the special government-to-government relationship between the federal government and Indian tribes. This relationship was established in 1787. It is based on Article I, Section 8, of the Constitution and has been given form and substance by numerous treaties, laws, Supreme Court decisions, and executive orders. The IHS is the principal federal health care provider and health advocate for American Indian people. Its goal is to raise their health status to the highest possible level.

Between 1990 and 2007, the U.S. AI/AN population increased by 65% from 2.0 to 3.3 million people. The IHS service area population comprises approximately 56% of the U.S. Indian population and increases at a rate of approximately 1.9% per year. The Indian health system is challenged to meet even 65% of the health needs of Indian country. The increase in the IHS service population is the result of natural increase (births minus deaths) and the expansion of the IHS service delivery area, as the result of the federal recognition of tribes. It must be noted that 43% of the Indian population resides in rural areas (U.S. Department of Health and Human Services, IHS, 2007). The principal legislation authorizing federal funds for health services to recognized Indian tribes is the Snyder Act of 1921. It authorized funds for "the relief of distress and conservation of health . . . [and] for the employment of . . . physicians . . . for Indian tribes throughout the United States." Congress passed the Indian Self-Determination and Education Assistance Act (Public Law 93-638, as amended) to provide tribes the option of either assuming from the IHS the administration and operation of health services and programs in their communities or remaining within the IHS-administered direct health system. Congress subsequently passed the Indian Health Care Improvement Act (P.L. 94-437), which is a health-specific law that supports the options of P.L. 93-638. The goal of P.L. 94-437 is to provide the quantity and quality of health services necessary to elevate the health status of American Indians and Alaska Natives to the highest possible level and to encourage the maximum participation of tribes in the planning and management of health services.

The IHS provides a comprehensive health services delivery system for American Indians and Alaska Natives with an opportunity for maximum tribal involvement in developing and managing programs to meet health needs. The IHS goal is to ensure that comprehensive, culturally acceptable personal and public health services are available and accessible to all American Indian people.

In order to carry out its mission, attain its goal, and uphold its foundation, the IHS

1. assists tribes in developing their health programs through activities, such as health management training, technical assistance, and human resource development and

2. assists tribes in coordinating health planning, in obtaining and using health resources available through federal, state, and local programs, and in operating comprehensive health care services and health programs.

Preventive measures involving environmental, educational, and outreach activities are combined with therapeutic measures into a single national health system. Within these broad categories are special initiatives in traditional medicine, elder care, women's health, the care of children and adolescents, injury prevention, domestic violence and child abuse, health care financing, state health care, sanitation facilities, and oral health. Most IHS funds are appropriated for American Indians who live on or near reservations. Congress also has authorized programs that provide some access to care for American Indians who live in urban areas.

IHS services are provided directly and through tribally contracted and operated health programs. Health services also include health care purchased from private providers. The federal system consists of 28 hospitals, 58 health centers, 31 health stations, and 5 school centers. There are also 17 tribal hospitals, 235 tribal health centers, 166 Alaska village clinics, 92 tribal health stations, and 28 tribal school health centers. In addition, 34 urban Indian health projects provide a variety of health and referral services. Approximately 600,000 American Indians and Alaska Natives reside in counties served by urban Indian health programs. IHS serves the members of 565 federally recognized tribes and 2 million American Indians and Alaska Natives residing on or near reservations.

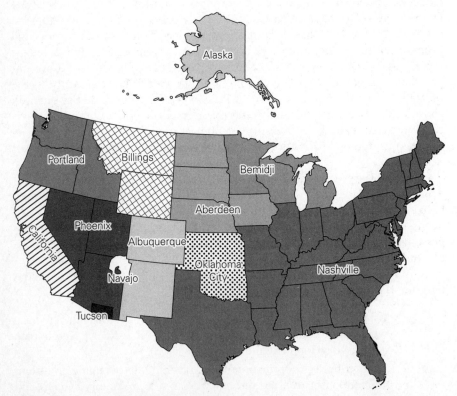

Figure 9–5　Indian Health Service.

The budget for FY 2011 was estimated to be $829 million (U.S. Department of Health and Human Services, Indian Health Service Fact Sheets).

The IHS headquarters is located in Rockville, Maryland. Some headquarters' functions are conducted in IHS offices in Phoenix and Tucson, Arizona, and in Albuquerque, New Mexico. IHS regional administrative units, called *area offices*, are located in the following cities (as shown on the map—Figure 9–5). The map is "live" on the Internet and each area, when tapped, presents pertinent information about the communities it serves. The web page is http://www.ihs.gov/PublicAffairs/IHSBrochure/map.asp.

Aberdeen, South Dakota	605-226-7582
Anchorage, Alaska	907-729-3689
Albuquerque, New Mexico	505-248-4500
Bemidji, Minnesota	218-444-0452
Billings, Montana	406-247-7248
Nashville, Tennessee	615-467-1500
Oklahoma City, Oklahoma	405-951-3820
Phoenix, Arizona	602-364-5039
Portland, Oregon	503-414-5555
Sacramento, California	916-930-3927
Tucson, Arizona	520-295-2405
Window Rock, Arizona	928-871-5811

The ineligibility of American Indians living on the East Coast to secure such services has caused numerous difficulties for needy American Indians. Health care providers generally seem to think that American Indians should receive health services from the IHS and try to send them there. Unfortunately, there simply is no IHS on the East Coast, so American Indians tend to be shifted around among the regional health care resources that are available.

Many providers of health care and social services are not aware that many of the American Indians on the East Coast have dual citizenship as a result of the Jay Treaty of 1794, which allows for international citizenship between the United States and Canada, a fact that raises questions about whether American Indians can freely cross the border between the United States and Canada and whether those who live in the United States are eligible for welfare or Medicaid.

Cultural and Communication Problems

A factor that inhibits the American Indian use of White-dominated health services is a deep, cultural problem: American Indians suffer disease when they come into contact with White health care providers. American Indians feel uneasy because for too many years they have been the victim of haphazard care and disrespectful treatment. All too often, conflict arises between what the American Indians perceive their illness to be and what the physicians diagnose.

American Indians, like most people, do not enjoy long waits in clinics; separation from their families; the unfamiliar, regimented environment of the hospital; or the unfamiliar behavior of the nurses and physicians, who often display demeaning and demanding attitudes. Their response to this treatment varies. Sometimes, they remain silent; other times, they leave and do not return. Many American Indians request that, if the ailment is not an emergency, they be allowed to see the medicine man or woman first and then receive treatment from a physician. Often, when a sick person is afraid of receiving the care of a physician, the medicine man or woman encourages the person to go to the hospital.

Health care providers must be aware of several factors when they communicate with American Indians. One is recognition of the importance of nonverbal communication. Often, American Indians observe providers and say very little. A patient may expect a provider to deduce the problem through instinct rather than by the extensive use of questions during history taking. In part, this derives from the belief that direct quoting is intrusive on individual privacy. When examining an American Indian with an obvious cough, a provider might be well advised to use a declarative statement—"You have a cough that keeps you awake at night"—and then allow time for the patient to respond to the statement.

It is American Indian practice to converse in a very low tone of voice. It is expected that the listener will pay attention and listen carefully in order to hear what is being said. It is considered impolite to say, "Huh?" or "I beg your pardon" or to give any indication that the communication was not heard. Therefore, an effort should be made to speak with patients in a quiet setting, where they will be heard more easily.

Note taking is taboo. Indian history has been passed through generations by means of verbal storytelling. American Indians are sensitive about note taking while they are speaking. When one is taking a history or interviewing, it may be preferable to use memory skills rather than to record notes. This more conversational approach may encourage greater openness between the patient and the provider.

Another factor to be considered is differing perceptions of time between the American Indian patient and the provider. Life on the reservation is not governed by the clock but by the dictates of need. When an American Indian moves from the reservation to an urban area, this cultural conflict concerning time often exhibits itself as lateness for appointments. One solution is the use of walk-in clinics.

American Indian Health Care Manpower

The percentage of American Indians enrolled in most health programs in selected health professions is low; when compared to the population percentages in Census 2010, demographic disparity is found in each of the professions. Table 9–5 gives the percentage of American Indians compared with total program percentages of enrollment and non-Hispanic White enrollment.

Table 9–5   **Percentage of American Indians Enrolled in Selected Health Profession Schools, Compared with Non-Hispanic Whites: 2004–2005**

	Number Enrolled	Non-Hispanic White (%)	American Indian (%)
Dentistry	19,342	60.6	0.6
Allopathic Medicine	74,518	62.4	0.9
Osteopathic Medicine	15,634	70.5	0.7
Optometry	5,556	60.3	0.3
Pharmacy	50,691	59.5	0.5
Podiatry	2,095	62.2	0.5
Public Health	22,604	59.3	0.7

Source: National Center for Health Statistics. (2007). Health, United States, 2010: With Special Feature on Death and Dying. Hyattsville, MD: Author, p. 352.

Recent nursing data are missing from the overall health professions enrollment data in Table 9–5. However, the National Sample Survey of Registered Nurses 2008 prepared by the Bureau of Health Professions of the Health Resources Administration provides relevant information regarding the demographic profile of American Registered Nurses. It estimates that the registered nurse population in the United States in 2008 was 3,063,162, with 2,596,599 registered nurses employed in nursing. Of this number, 83.2% were White non-Hispanic and 0.3% were AI/AN (non-Hispanic) (United States Department of Health and Human Services, Health Resources and Services, 2010). Given that in 2010 the White population was 63% of the total population and AI/AN (non-Hispanic) people comprised 0.9% of the resident population; this is a clear indication that there is not demographic parity in the percentage of AI/AN (non-Hispanic) people in nursing. This demographic picture and the percentages in the tables demonstrate a situation that is an ongoing concern. Somnath and Shipman, who reviewed a total of 55 studies, found that minority patients tend to receive better interpersonal care from practitioners of their own race or ethnicity, particularly in primary care and mental health settings, and that non–English speaking patients experience better interpersonal care, greater medical comprehension, and greater likelihood of keeping follow-up appointments when they see a language-concordant practitioner.

They concluded their study by stating that "the findings indicated greater health professions diversity will likely lead to improved public health by increasing access to care for underserved populations, and by increasing opportunities for minority patients to see practitioners with whom they share a common race, ethnicity or language." They also stated that "race, ethnicity, and language concordance, which is associated with better patient-practitioner relationships and communication, may increase patients' likelihood of receiving and accepting appropriate medical care" (Somnath & Shipman, 2006, p. 17). The Research on Culture box illustrates an example of research conducted in American Indian communities.

RESEARCH ON CULTURE

A large amount of research has been conducted among members of the American Indian and Alaska Native population. The following study is one example:

> Strickland, C. J., & Cooper, M. (2011) . Getting into trouble: perspectives on stress and suicide prevention among Pacific Northwest Indian youth. *Journal of Transcultural Nursing, 22*(3), 240–247.

This descriptive, ethnographic study in a Pacific Northwest tribe seeks to gain an understanding of the life experiences of the youth in the studied community. Focus groups and observations were conducted with 30 Indian youth between the ages of 14 to 19 years. The youths were asked to discuss their stressors, sense of family and community, and hopes for the future.

The youths reported major stress and noted that friends and family were both a support and also a source of stress. The stressors included "getting into trouble." This was doing something in home, community, or society that would result in sanctions or discipline. The coping skills were found to be "speaking up for oneself" often resulting in more trouble. It was further discovered that the youth desired to "stay on track." They want to strengthen their cultural values, experience economic development, and future opportunity. The findings provide insight about the suicide risk among Indian youth.

Explore 🌐 MediaLink

Go to the Student Resource Site at nursing.pearsonhighered.com for chapter-related review questions, case studies, and activities. Contents of the CULTURALCARE Guide and CULTURALCARE Museum can also be found on the Student Resource Site. Click on Chapter 9 to select the activities for this chapter.

Box 9–3: Keeping Up

It goes without saying that much of the data presented in this chapter will be out of date when you read this text. However, at this final stage of writing, it is the most recent information available. The following resources will be most helpful in keeping you abreast of the frequent changes in HEALTH and ILLNESS in the American Indian and Alaska Native communities:

1. The National Center for Health Statistics publishes *Health, United States*, an annual report on trends in health statistics. It can be retrieved from http://www.cdc.gov/nchs/hus.htm. *Health, United States, 11* is not available and *Health, United States, 12* will be published in May, 2012.

2. Health related data and other statistics are available at http://www. cdc.gov/DataStatistics/.
3. National Congress of American Indians. (2012). Health. Retrieved from http://www.ncai.org/Health.48.0.html.
4. United States Department of Health and Human Services, Indian Health Service Fact Sheets, 2011 IHS Year Profile. Retrieved from http://www.ihs.gov/PublicAffairs/IHSBrochure/Profile2010.asp.
5. United States Department of the Interior, Bureau of Indian Affairs. Retrieved from http://www.artnatam.com/tribes.html.

■ Internet Sources

Admin. (2011). Culture-bound syndromes: Ghost sickness. Multicultural Psychology. Retrieved from http://www.learnmax.in/Multicultural-Psychology/351.html, June 22, 2011.

Crowe, T. (2001). Hawk Littlejohn embraced the traditional ways in the modern world. Smokey Mountain News. Retrieved from http://www. smokymountainnews.com/issues/1_01/1_17_01/front_littlejohn.shtml, April 16, 2012.

Grenier, D., & Lockjer, R. (2007). Domestic violence. IHS Fact Sheet, Behavioral Health. 2011. Retrieved from http://www.ihs.gov/MedicalPrograms/MCH/M/obgyn0607_Feat.cfm#dv, March 11, 2012.

Indian Health Service, 2011. Fact Sheet, author. Retrieved from http://www.ihs.gov, July, 2007.

National Congress of American Indians. (2012). Health. Retrieved from http://www.ncai.org/Health.48.0.html, March 11, 2012.

National Museum of the American Indian. (2008). Home Page. Washington, DC: Smithsonian. Retrieved from http://www.nmai.si.edu/, June 22, 2011.

Somnath, S., & Shipman, S. (2006). The Rationale for Diversity in the Health Professions: A Review of the Evidence. Washington, DC: U.S. Department of Health and Human Services, Health Resources and Services Administration Bureau of Health Professions. Retrieved from http://www.hrsa.gov/, March 11, 2012.

United States Department of Commerce, U.S. Census Bureau. (2011). Census 2010. Retrieved from http://www.census.gov/, June 22, 2011.

United States Department of Health and Human Services. Indian Health Service Fact Sheets. (2011). IHS Year Profile. Retrieved from http://www.ihs.gov/PublicAffairs/IHSBrochure/Profile2010.asp, June 25, 2011.

United States Department of Health and Human Services, Health Resources and Services. (2004). The National Survey of Registered Nurses 2008 Documentation for the General Public Use File, 2006, Bureau of Health Professions Health Resources and Services Administration. HRSA/BHPr and the National Sample Survey of Registered Nurses. Retrieved from http://www.hrsa.gov/.

United States Department of Health and Human Services. (2011). National Center for Health Statistics. (2011). Health, United States, 2010: With Special Feature on Death and Dying. Hyattsville, MD: Author. Retrieved from www.cdc.gov/nchs/data/hus/hus10.pdf 2011, March 11, 2012.

United States Department of Health and Human Services, Indian Health Service, IHS. (2011). Fact Sheets Indian Population Trends, Indian Health Service Trends. Retrieved from http://info.ihs.gov/, June 2011.

United States Department of Health and Human Services, Indian Health Service. (2007). Indian Population Trends, 2007. Retrieved from http://info.ihs.gov/, February 24, 2008. p. 1.

United States Department of Health and Human Services, Health Resources and Services. (2010). The National Survey of Registered Nurses 2008 Documentation for the General Public Use File, 2006, Bureau of Health Professions Health Resources and Services Administration. HRSA/BHPr and the National Sample Survey of Registered Nurses. Retrieved from http://www.hrsa.gov/data-statistics/index.html, June 28, 2011.

United States Department of the Interior, Bureau of Indian Affairs. (2010). Federal Register: October 1, 2010 V. 75, No. 190, Federally Recognzed Indian Tribes. Retrieved from http://www.artnatam.com/tribes.html, December 1, 2011. pp. 60810–60814.

Waterman, L., & Salinas, E. J. (2006). A Brief History of the American Indian Movement. Retrieved from http://www.aimovement.org/ggc/history.html, March 11, 2012.

■ References

Basque, E., & Young, P. (1984). Personal Interviews, Boston Indian Council.

Bertrand, J., Floyd, R. L., & Weber, M. K. (2005). Guidelines for identifying and referring persons with fetal alcohol syndrome. *MMWR.* V.54/RR-11.

Bilagody, H. (1969). An American Indian looks at health care. In R. Feldman & D. Buch (Eds.), *The ninth annual training institute for psychiatrist-teachers of practicing physicians.* Boulder, CO: WICHE, No. 3A30.

Boyd, D. (1974). *Rolling thunder.* New York: Random House.

Brown, D. (1970). *Bury my heart at Wounded Knee.* New York: Holt.

Deloria, V., Jr. (1969). *Custer died for your sins.* New York: Avon Books.

Deloria, V., Jr. (1974). *Behind the trail of broken treaties.* New York: Delacorte.

Dorris, M. (1989). *The broken cord.* New York: Harper & Row.

Fortney, A. J. (1977, January 23). Has White man's lease expired? *Boston Sunday Globe,* pp. 8–30.

Humes, K. R., Jones, N. A. and Ramirez, R. R. (2011). Overview of Race and Hispanic Origin: 2010. Census Briefs, p. 4. Retrieved from http://2010.census.gov/2010census/data/, June 26, 2011.

Kluckhohn, C., & Leighton, D. (1962). *The Navaho* (Rev. ed.). Garden City, NY: Doubleday.

Knox, M. E., & Adams, L. (1988). *Traditional health practices of the Oneida Indian.* Oshkosh: University of Wisconsin, College of Nursing.

Leek, S. (1975). *Herbs: Medicine and mysticism.* Chicago: Henry Regnery.

Littlejohn, Hawk. (1979). Personal interview. Boston, MA.

Lyon, W. S. (1996). *Encyclopedia of Native American healing.* New York: Norton.

Nieves, E. (2007, June 9). Indian reservation reeling in weave of youth suicides and attempts. *New York Times,* p. A-9.

Spector, R. (1992). Culture, ethnicity, and nursing. In P. Potter & A. Perry (Eds.), *Fundamentals of nursing* (3rd ed.). St. Louis: Mosby-Year Book.

Strickland, C. J., & Cooper, M. (2011). Getting into trouble: perspectives on stress and suicide prevention among Pacific Northwest Indian youth. *Journal of Transcultural Nursing. 22*(3), 240–247.

Wyman, L. C. (1966). Navaho diagnosticians. In W. R. Scott & E. H. Volkhart (Eds.), *Medical care.* New York: John Wiley & Sons.

Zuckoff, M. (1995, April 18). More and more claiming American Indian heritage. *Boston Globe,* A8.

■ Additional Readings

Bear, S., & Bear, W. (1996). *The medicine wheel.* New York: Fireside.

Catlin, G. (1993). *North American Indian portfolio.* Washington, DC: Library of Congress.

Neihardt, J. G. (1991—original 1951). *When the tree flowered.* Lincoln: University of Nebraska Press.

Neihardt, N. (1993). *The sacred hoop.* Tekamah, NE: Neihardt.

Neihardt, J. G. (1998—original 1961). *Black Elk speaks.* Lincoln: University of Nebraska Press.

Noble, M. (1997). *Sweet Grass: Lives of contemporary Native women of the Northeast.* Mashpee, MA: C. J. Mills.

Peltier, L. (1999). *Prison writings: My life is my sun dance.* New York: St Martin's Press.

Senier, S. (2001). *Voices of American Indian assimilation and resistance.* Norman: University of Oklahoma Press.

Wiebe, R., & Johnson, Y. (1998). *Stolen life—The journey of a Cree woman.* Athens: Ohio University Press.

Wolfson, E. (1993). *From the Earth to the sky.* Boston: Houghton Mifflin.

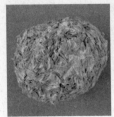 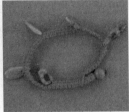 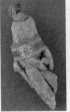 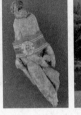

Figure 10–1 **Figure 10–2** **Figure 10–3 Figure 10–4**

Chapter 10

HEALTH and ILLNESS
in the Asian Populations

But when she arrived in the new country, the immigration officials pulled her swan away from her leaving the woman fluttering her arms and with only one swan feather for a memory.

—*Amy Tan*

■ Objectives

1. Discuss the background of the selected communities of the Asian populations.
2. Discuss the demographic profile of selected communities of the Asian populations.
3. Describe the traditional definitions of HEALTH and ILLNESS of selected communities of the Asian populations.
4. Describe the traditional methods of HEALTH maintenance and protection of selected communities of the Asian populations.
5. Describe the traditional methods of HEALING within selected communities of the Asian populations.
6. Describe the practice of a traditional healer.
7. Describe current health care problems of members of selected communities of the Asian populations.

The opening images for this chapter depict objects symbolic of items used to maintain, protect, and restore HEALTH and a traditional place for HEALING that people in the Asian American communities may adhere to. Figure 10–1 is a "1,000-year egg" that is imported from China. The eggs are brought to the United States in large vats and sold in many Asian grocery stores and pharmacies. They are wrapped either in straw or in a carbon-like substance and are solidified over time. The eggs are eaten daily in rice, seen as a source of vitamins and minerals, and are a part of a HEALTH maintenance practice. Figure 10–2 is a small bracelet with jade charms and is placed on a baby for HEALTH protection. Figure 10–3 is a ginseng root. This root is known to be a HEALTH restorative and used to treat countless maladies. Figure 10–4 is the Byodo-In Temple in Kahaluu, Hawaii that was built in the 1960s to commemorate the 100th anniversary of the arrival of the first Japanese immigrant workers in Hawaii who came to work in the sugar plantation fields. It is a replica of the 1,000-year-old Byodo-In Temple located in Uji, Japan on the southern outskirts of Kyoto. It is a non-denominational Buddhist temple located in the Valley of the Temples cemetery and is a place for meditation and prayer and to seek solace.

■ Background

More than 14.7 million people constitute the Asian communities and are the United States' third largest emerging majority group (Humes, Nicholas, & Ramirez, 2011). This number represents 4.8% of the total population, one that has grown 43.3% since the 2000 census—from 10.2 million to 14.6 million people. The term *Asian* refers to people having origins in any of the original peoples of the Far East, Southeast Asia, or the Indian subcontinent (for example, Cambodia, China, India, Japan, Korea, Malaysia, Pakistan, the Philippine Islands, Thailand, and Vietnam). The Asian groups are not limited to nationalities but are characterized by their diversity: More than 30 different languages are spoken and there is a similar number of cultures (Martin, 1995) and many different religions, including, but not limited to, Buddhism, Confucianism, Hinduism, Islam, and Taoism. Over half of all people who reported Asian lived in just 3 states: Hawaii, California, and Washington. The cities with the largest Asian populations are New York, Los Angeles, San Jose, San Francisco, and Honolulu (Barnes & Bennett, 2002, pp. 1–3, 7).

In 2010, there were a total of 1,042,635 Legal Permanent Residents (LPR) in the United States, 46% of whom were new arrivals. People from Asia comprised 40.5% of this population. The nations that the Asian LPRs were from included the People's Republic of China (6.8%), India (6.6%), the Philippines (5.6%), Vietnam (2.9%), and South Korea (2.1%). California, New York, Florida, and Texas had the largest populations of LPRs (Homeland Security, 2011a). There were 619,913 people who naturalized—became citizens of the United States in 2010. Of this number, 40.6% were born in Asia, 9.9% were from

India, 5.7% from the Philippines, 5.5% from the People's Republic of China, and 3.1% from Vietnam. Close to half of the nation's naturalized Asian citizens lived in the metropolitan areas of New York, Los Angeles, or Miami. The median number of years that the people were LPRs was 5 (Homeland Security, 2011b).

This chapter focuses on the traditional HEALTH and ILLNESS beliefs and practices of the Chinese and Indian Americans because the HEALTH and ILLNESS beliefs and practices of many of the other Asians and Pacific Islanders are derived in part from the Chinese and Ayurvedic HEALTH traditions.

Chinese immigration to the United States began over 150 years ago. In 1850, there were only 1,000 Chinese inhabitants in this country; in 1880, there were well over 100,000. This rapid increase occurred in part because of the discovery of gold in California and in part because of the need for cheap labor to build the transcontinental railroads. The immigrants were laborers who met the needs of the dominant society. Like many early immigrant groups, they came here intending only to stay as temporary workers. Most of the immigrants were men, and they clung closely to their customs and beliefs and stayed together in their own communities. The hopes that many had for a better life when they came to the United States did not materialize. Subsequently, many of the workers and their kin returned to China before 1930. Part of the disharmony and disenchantment occurred because these immigrants were not White and did not have the same culture and habits as Whites. For these reasons, they were not welcomed, and many jobs were not open to them. For example, Chinese immigrant workers were excluded from many mining, construction, and other hard-labor jobs, even though the transcontinental railroad was constructed mainly by Chinese laborers. Between 1880 and 1930, the Chinese population declined by nearly 20%. One factor that helped perpetuate this decline in population was a series of exclusion acts halting further immigration. The people who remained behind were relegated to menial jobs, such as cooking and dishwashing. The Chinese workers first took these jobs in the West and later moved eastward throughout the United States. They tended to move to cities where they were allowed to let their entrepreneurial talents surface—their main pursuits included running small laundries, food shops, and restaurants.

The people settled in tightly knit groups in urban neighborhoods that took the name "Chinatown." Here they were able to maintain the ancient traditions of their homeland. They were hard workers and, in spite of the dull, menial jobs usually available to them, they were able to survive.

Both U.S. immigration laws and political problems in China have had an effect on the nature of today's Chinese population. When the exclusion acts were passed, many men were left alone in this country without the possibility that their families would join them. For this reason, a great majority of the men spent many years alone. In addition, the political oppression experienced by the Chinese in the United States was compounded—at a time when immigration laws were relaxed here after World War II, people were unable to return to or leave China because of that country's restrictive new regulations.

By 1965, however, a large number of refugees who had relatives here were able to come to this country. They settled in the Chinatowns of America, causing the population of these areas to swell. The rate of increase since 1965 has been 10% per year.

■ Traditional Definitions of *HEALTH* and *ILLNESS*

Chinese medicine teaches that HEALTH is a state of spiritual and physical harmony with nature. In ancient China, the task of the physician was to prevent ILLNESS. A first-class physician not only cured an ILLNESS but could also prevent disease from occurring. A second-class physician had to wait for patients to become ill before they could be treated. The physician was paid by the patient while the patient was healthy. When illness occurred, payments stopped. Indeed, not only was the physician not paid for services when the patient became ill, but the physician also had to provide and pay for the needed medicine (Mann, 1972, p. 222).

To understand the Chinese philosophy of HEALTH and ILLNESS, it is necessary to look back at the age-old philosophies from which more current ideas have evolved. The foundation rests in the religion and philosophy of Taoism. Taoism originated with a man named Lao-Tzu, who is believed to have been born about 604 B.C. The word *Tao* has several meanings: way, path, or discourse. On the spiritual level, it is the way of ultimate reality. It is the way of all nature, the primeval law that regulates all heavenly and earthly matters. To live according to the Tao, one must adapt oneself to the order of nature. Chinese medical works revere the ancient sages who knew the way and "led their lives in Tao" (Smith, 1958, pp. 175–192).

The Chinese view the universe as a vast, indivisible entity, and each being has a definite function within it. No one thing can exist without the existence of the others. Each is linked in a chain that consists of concepts related to each other in harmonious balance. Violating this harmony is like hurling chaos, wars, and catastrophes on humankind—the end result of which is ILLNESS. Individuals must adjust themselves wholly within the environment. Five elements—wood, fire, earth, metal, and water—constitute the guiding principles of humankind's surroundings. These elements can both create and destroy each other. For example, "wood creates fire," "two pieces of wood rubbed together produce a spark," "wood destroys earth," "the tree sucks strength from the earth." The guiding principles arise from this "correspondences" theory of the cosmos (Wallnöfer & von Rottauscher, 1972, pp. 12–16, 19–21). Tables 10–1 and 10–2 highlight common elements of Asian/Pacific Island religions and give examples of phenomena affecting health care.

For a person to remain HEALTHY, his or her actions must conform to the mobile cycle of the correspondences. The exact directions for achieving this were written in such works as the *Lu Chih Ch'un Ch'iu* (*Spring and Autumn Annals*) written by Lu Pu Wei, who died circa 230 B.C.

Table 10-1 Highlights of Common Elements of Asian Eastern Religions

The teachings of Asian religions, including Confucianism and Buddhism, are complementary and have played a major role in the shaping of the cultural values in Asia.

Buddhism teaches

- Harmony/nonconfrontation (silence as a virtue)
- Respect for life
- Moderation in behavior, self-discipline, patience, humility, modesty, friendliness, selflessness, dedication, and loyalty to others
- Individualism devalued

Confucianism teaches

- Achievement of harmony through observing the 5 basic relationships of society
    1. Ruler and ruled
    2. Father and son
    3. Husband and wife
    4. Older and younger brother
    5. Between friends
- Hierarchical roles, social class system, clearly defined behavioral code
- Importance of family
- Filial piety and respect for elders
- High regard for education and learning

Taoism teaches

- Harmony between humans and nature
- Nature is benign because *yin* (evil) and *yang* (good) are in balance and harmony
- Happiness and a long life
- Charity, simplicity, patience, avoidance of confrontation, and an indirect approach to problems

Shamanism teaches

- Emphasis on nature
- Everything in nature is endowed with a spirit

Hinduism teaches

- "You can have what you want"
    1. Pleasure—through marriage and family
    2. Success—through vocation
    3. Duty—through civic participation
- The community is greater than ourselves
- The stages of life—student, householder, retirement, and *sannyasin*—"one who neither hates nor loves anything"
- Many paths to the same summit

Source: Adapted from material in Romo, R. G. (1995, May 3). Hispanic health traditions and issues. Presented at the Minnesota Health Educators Conference. *Health education expanding our horizons.* Reprinted with permission; and Smith, H. (1998). *The world's religions.* New York: HarperCollins.

Table 10-2 Examples of Cultural Phenomena Affecting Health Care Among Americans of Asian/Pacific Islander Heritage

Nations of Origin	China, Japan, Hawaii, the Philippines, Vietnam, Asian India, Bangladesh, and Pakistan, Korea, Samoa, Guam, and the remaining Asian/Pacific islands
Environmental Control	Traditional HEALTH and ILLNESS beliefs may continue to be observed by "traditional" people
Biological Variations	Hypertension
	Liver cancer
	Stomach cancer
	Coccidioidomycosis
	Lactose intolerance
	Thalassemia
Social Organization	Family—hierarchical structure, loyalty
	Large, extended family networks
	Devotion to tradition
	Many religions, including Taoism, Buddhism, Islam, and Hinduism
	Community social organizations
Communication	National language preference
	Dialects, written characters
	Use of silence
	Nonverbal and contextual cueing
Space	Noncontact people
Time Orientation	Present

Adapted from Spector, R. (1992). Culture ethnicity, and nursing. In P. Potter & A. Perry (Eds.), *Fundamentals of Nursing* (p. 101). St. Louis, MO: Mosby-Year Book. Reprinted with permission. This material was published in Potter & Perry's Fundamentals of Nursing, Jackie Crisp and Catherine Taylor (Eds), Copyright Elsevier (2009).

The holistic concept, as explained by Dr. P. K. Chan (1988), is an important idea of traditional Chinese medicine in preventing and treating diseases. It has 2 main components:

1. A human body is regarded as an integral organism, with special emphasis on the harmonic and integral interrelationship between the viscera and the superficial structures in these close physiological connections, as well as their mutual pathological connection. In Chinese medicine, the local pathological changes always are considered in conjunction with other tissues and organs of the entire body, instead of considered alone.

2. Special attention is paid to the integration of the human body with the external environment. The onset, evolution, and change of disease are considered in conjunction with the geographic, social, and other environmental factors.

Four thousand years before the English physician William Harvey described the circulatory system in 1628, *Huang-ti Nei Ching* (*Yellow Emperor's Book of Internal Medicine*) was written. This is the first known volume that describes the circulation of blood. It described the oxygen-carrying powers of blood and defined the 2 basic world principles: *yin* and *yang*, powers that regulate the universe. *Yang* represents the male, positive energy that produces light, warmth, and fullness. *Yin* represents the female, negative energy—the force of darkness, cold, and emptiness. *Yin* and *yang* exert power not only over the universe but also over human beings.

Yin and *yang* were further explained by Dr. Chan as having been originally a philosophical theory in ancient China. Later, the theory was incorporated into Chinese medicine. The theory holds that "everything in the Universe contains two aspects—*yin* and *yang*, which are in opposition and also in unison. Hence, matters are impelled to develop and change." In traditional Chinese medicine, the phenomena are further explained as follows:

- Matters that are dynamic, external, upward, ascending, and brilliant belong to *yang*.
- Those that are static, internal, downward, descending, dull, regressive, and hypoactive are *yin*.
- *Yin* flourishing and *yang* vivified steadily is the state of health. *Yin* and *yang* regulate themselves in the basic principle to promote the normal activities of life.
- Illness is the disharmony of *yin* and *yang*, a disharmony that leads to pathological changes, with excesses of one and deficiencies of the other, disturbances of vital energy and blood, malfunctioning of the viscera, and so forth (Chan, 1988).

The various parts of the human body correspond to the dualistic principles of *yin* and *yang*. The inside of the body is *yin*; the surface of the body is *yang*. The front part of the body is *yin*; the back is *yang*. The 5 *ts'ang* viscera—liver, heart, spleen, lungs, and kidney—are *yang*; the 6 *fu* structures—gallbladder, stomach, large intestine, small intestine, bladder, and "warmer"—are *yin*. (The "warmer" is now believed to be the lymph system.) The diseases of winter and spring are *yin*; those of summer and fall are *yang*. The pulses are controlled by *yin* and *yang*. If *yin* is too strong, the person is nervous and apprehensive and catches colds easily. If the individual does not balance *yin* and *yang* properly, his or her life will be short. Half of the *yin* forces are depleted by age 40; at 40 the body is sluggish, and at 60 the *yin* is totally depleted, at which time the body deteriorates. *Yin* stores the vital strength of life. *Yang* protects the body from outside forces, and it, too, must be carefully maintained. If *yang* is not cared for, the viscera are thrown into disorder, and circulation ceases. *Yin* and *yang* cannot be injured by evil influences. When *yin* and *yang* are sound, the person lives in peaceful interaction with mind and body in proper order (Wallnöfer & von Rottauscher, 1972).

Chinese medicine has a long history. The Emperor Shen Nung, who died in 2697 B.C., was known as the patron god of agriculture. He was given this title because of the 70 experiments he performed on himself by swallowing a different plant every day and studying the effects. During this period of self-experimentation, Nung discovered many poisonous herbs and rendered them harmless by the use of antidotes, which he also discovered. His patron element was fire, for which he was known as the Red Emperor. The Emperor Shen Nung was followed by Huang-ti, whose patron element was earth. Huang-ti was known as the Yellow Emperor and ruled from 2697 B.C. to 2595 B.C. The greater part of his life was devoted to the study of medicine. Many people ascribe to him the recording of the *Nei Ching*, the book that embraces the entire realm of Chinese medical knowledge. The treatments described in the *Nei Ching*—which became characteristic of Chinese medical practices—are almost totally aimed at reestablishing balances that are lost within the body when ILLNESS occurs. Disrupted harmonies are regarded as the sole cause of disease. Surgery was rarely resorted to; when it was, it was used primarily to remove malignant tumors. The *Nei Ching* is a dialogue between Huang-ti and his minister, Ch'i Po. It begins with the concept of the Tao and the cosmological patterns of the universe and goes on to describe the powers of the *yin* and *yang*. This learned treatise discusses in great detail the therapy of the pulses and how a diagnosis can be made on the basis of alterations in the pulse beat. It also describes various kinds of fevers and the use of acupuncture (Wallnöfer & von Rottauscher, 1972, pp. 26–28).

The Chinese view their bodies as a gift given to them by their parents and forebears. A person's body is not his or her personal property. It must be cared for and well maintained. Confucius taught that "only those shall be truly revered who at the end of their lives will return their physical bodies whole and sound."

The body is composed of 5 solid organs (*ts'ang*), which collect and store secretions, and 5 hollow organs (*fu*), which excrete. The heart and liver are regarded as the noble organs. The head is the storage chamber for knowledge, the back is the home of the chest, the loins store the kidneys, the knees store the muscles, and the bones store the marrow.

The Chinese view the functions of the various organs as comparable to the functions of persons in positions of power and responsibility in the government. For example, the heart is the ruler over all other civil servants, the lungs are the administrators, the liver is the general who initiates all the strategic actions, and the gallbladder is the decision maker.

The organs have a complex relationship, which maintains the balance and harmony of the body. Each organ is associated with a color. For example, the heart—which works in accordance with the pulse, controls the kidneys, and harmonizes with bitter flavors—is red. In addition, the organs have what is referred to as an "aura," the meaning of which, in the medical context, is HEALTH. The aura is determined by the color of the organ. In the balanced, healthy body, the colors look fresh and shiny.

Disease is caused by an upset in the balance of *yin* and *yang*. The weather, too, has an effect on the body's balance and the body's relationship to *yin* and *yang*. For example, heat can be injurious to the heart, and cold is injurious to the lungs. Overexertion is harmful to the body. Prolonged sitting is harmful to the flesh and spine, and prolonged lying in bed can be harmful to the lungs.

Disease is diagnosed by the Chinese physician through inspection and palpation. During inspection, the Chinese physician looks at the tongue (glossoscopy), listens and smells (osphretics), and asks questions (anamnesis). During palpation, the physician feels the pulse (sphygmopalpation).

The Chinese believe that there are many different pulse types, which are all grouped together and must be felt with the 3 middle fingers. The pulse is considered the storehouse of the blood, and a person with a strong, regular pulse is considered to be in good health. By the nature of the pulse, the physician is able to determine various illnesses. For example, if the pulse is weak and skips beats, the person may have a cardiac problem. If the pulse is too strong, the person's body is distended (Wallnöfer & von Rottauscher, 1972).

There are 6 different pulses, 3 in each hand. Each pulse is specifically related to various organs, and each pulse has its own characteristics. According to ancient Chinese sources, there are 15 ways of characterizing the pulses. Each of these descriptions accurately determines the diagnosis. There are 7 *piao* pulses (superficial) and 8 *li* pulses (sunken). An example of an illness that manifests with a *piao* pulse is headache; anxiety manifests with a *li* pulse. The pulses also take on a specific nature with various conditions. For example, specific pulses are associated with epilepsy, pregnancy, and the time just before death.

The Chinese physician is aided in making a diagnosis by the appearance of the patient's tongue. More than 100 conditions can be determined by glossoscopic examination. The color of the tongue and the part of the tongue that does not appear normal are the essential clues to the diagnosis.

Breast cancer has been known to the Chinese since early times. "The disease begins with a knot in the breast, the size of a bean, and gradually swells to the size of an egg. After seven or eight months it perforates. When it has perforated, it is very difficult to cure" (Wallnöfer & von Rottauscher, 1972).

■ Traditional Methods of HEALTH Maintenance and Protection

There are countless ways by which HEALTH is maintained. One example is the practices involved in daily nutrition. Foods, such as thousand-year eggs, are ingested on a daily basis. There are strict rules governing food combinations and foods that must be eaten preceding and after life events, such as childbirth and surgery. Daily exercise is also important, and many people participate in formal exercise programs, such as tai chi.

The Chinese often prepare amulets to prevent evil spirits and protect HEALTH. These amulets consist of a charm with an idol or a Chinese character painted in red or black ink and written on a strip of yellow paper. These amulets are hung over a door or pasted on a curtain or wall, worn in the hair, or placed in a red bag and pinned on clothing. The paper may be burned and the ashes mixed in hot tea and swallowed to ward off evil. Jade is believed to be the most precious of all stones because it is seen as the giver of children, HEALTH immortality, wisdom, power, victory, growth, and food. Jade charms are worn to bring HEALTH and, should they turn dull or break, the wearer will surely meet misfortune. The charm prevents harm and accidents. Children are kept safe with jade charms, and adults are made pure, just, humane, and intelligent by wearing them (Morgan, 1942 [1972], pp. 133–134).

■ Traditional Methods of HEALTH Restoration

Just as there are countless methods used to maintain and protect HEALTH, there are countless ways to restore HEALTH. The following discussion describes traditional methods of restoring HEALTH.

Acupuncture

Acupuncture is an ancient Chinese practice of puncturing the body to cure disease or relieve pain. The body is punctured with special metal needles at points that are precisely predetermined for the treatment of specific symptoms. According to one source, the earliest use of this method was recorded between 106 B.C. and A.D. 200. According to other sources, however, it was used even earlier. This treatment modality stems from diagnostic procedures described earlier. The most important aspect of the practice of acupuncture is the acquired skill and ability to know precisely where to puncture the skin. Nine needles are used in acupuncture, each with a specific purpose. The following is a list of the needles and their purposes (Wallnöfer & von Rottauscher, 1972):

- superficial pricking: arrowhead needle
- massaging: round needle
- knocking or pressing: blunt needle
- venous pricking: sharp 3-edged needle
- evacuating pus: swordlike needle
- rapid pricking: sharp, round needle
- puncturing thick muscle: sharp, round needle
- puncturing thick muscle: long needle
- treating arthritis: large needle
- most extensively used: filiform needle

The specific points of the body into which the needles are inserted are known as *meridians*. Acupuncture is based on the concept that certain meridians extend internally throughout the body in a fixed network. There are 365 points on the skin where these lines emerge. Since all the networks merge and have their outlets on the skin, the way to treat internal problems is to puncture the meridians, which are also categorically identified in terms of *yin* and *yang*, as are the diseases. The treatment goal is to restore the balance of *yin* and *yang* (Wallnöfer & von Rottauscher, 1972). The practice of this art is far too complex to explain in great detail in these pages.

Readers may find it interesting to visit acupuncture clinics in their area. After the therapist carefully explains the art and science of acupuncture, one may be able to grasp the fundamental concepts of this ancient treatment. The practice of acupuncture is based in antiquity, yet it took a long time for it to be accepted as a legitimate method of healing by practitioners of the Western medical system. Currently, numerous acupuncture clinics attract a fair number of non-Asians, and acupuncture is being used as a method of anesthesia in some hospitals.

Moxibustion, Cupping, Bleeding, and Tui Na

Moxibustion has been practiced for as long as acupuncture. Its purpose, too, is to restore the proper balance of *yin* and *yang*. Moxibustion is based on the therapeutic value of heat, whereas acupuncture is a cold treatment. Acupuncture is used mainly in diseases in which there is an excess of *yang*, and moxibustion is used in diseases in which there is an excess of *yin*. Moxibustion is performed by heating pulverized wormwood and passing this concoction above the skin, but not touching it, over certain specific meridians. Great caution must be used in this application because it cannot be applied to all the meridians that are used for acupuncture. Moxibustion is believed to be most useful during the period of labor and delivery, if applied properly.

Other important traditional HEALTH restoring practices are cupping, bleeding, and a form of traditional massage, *Tui Na*.

■ Cupping, as seen in Figures 10–5A and 10–5B, involves creating a vacuum in a small glass by burning the oxygen out of it, then promptly placing the glass on the person's skin surface. Cupping draws blood and lymph to the body's surface that is under the cup. This increases the local circulation. The purpose for doing this is to remove cold and damp "evils" from the body and/or to assist blood circulation. The procedure is frequently used to treat lung congestion.

■ Bleeding, often done with the use of leeches, is performed to "remove heat from the body." Only small amounts of blood are removed.

■ Massage, *Tui Na*, "pushing and pulling," is a complex system of massage or manual acupuncture point stimulation that is used on orthopedic and neurological conditions (Ergil, 1996, pp. 208–209).

Herbal Remedies

Medicinal herbs were used widely in the practice of ancient Chinese healing. Many of these herbs are available and in use today.

Herbology is an interesting subject. The gathering season of an herb was important for its effect. It was believed that some herbs were more effective if gathered at night and that others were more effective if gathered at dawn. The ancient sages understood quite well the dynamics of growth. It is known today that a plant may not be effective if the dew has been allowed to dry on its leaves. The herbalist believes that the ginseng root must be harvested only at midnight in a full moon if it is to have therapeutic value. Ginseng's therapeutic value is due to its nonspecific action. The herb, which is derived from the root of a plant that resembles a person, is recommended for use in more than 2 dozen ailments, including anemia, colics, depression, indigestion, impotence, and rheumatism (Wallnöfer & von Rottauscher, 1972). It has maintained its reputation for centuries and continues to be a highly valued and widely used substance.

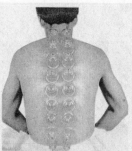
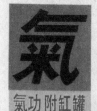
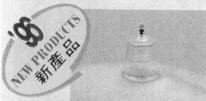
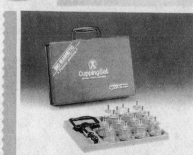
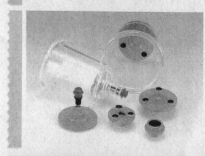

Figure 10-5A   Cupping.

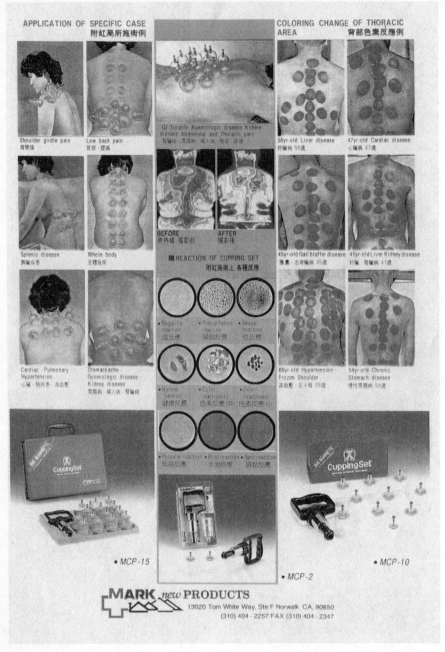

Figure 10-5B Cupping.

To release all the therapeutic properties of ginseng and to prepare it properly are of paramount importance. Ginseng must not be prepared in anything made of metal because it is believed that some of the necessary constituents are leeched out by the action of the metal. It must be stored in crockery. It is boiled in water until only a sediment remains. This sediment is pressed into a crock and stored. Following are some of the specific uses of ginseng (Wallnöfer & von Rottauscher, 1972):

- To stimulate digestion: rub ginseng to a powder, mix with the white of an egg, and take 3 times per day.
- As a sedative: prepare a light broth of ginseng and bamboo leaves.
- For faintness after childbirth: administer a strong brew of ginseng several times a day.
- As a restorative for frail children: give a dash of raw, minced ginseng several times per day.

There are many Chinese medicinal herbs, but none is as famous as ginseng.

I had the opportunity to visit, with one of my Asian American students, an import-export store in Boston's Chinatown where they sell Chinese herbs—if one has the proper prescriptions. The front of the store is a gift shop that attracts tourists. A room in the back is separated from the rest of the store. We were allowed to enter this room when the student explained to the proprietor, in Cantonese, that I was her teacher and that she had brought me to the store to purchase herbs. We stayed there for quite a long time, observing the people who came in with prescriptions. The man carefully weighed different herbs, mixed them together, and dispensed them.

Figures 10–6A and 10–6B illustrate the interior of a Chinese pharmacy, the drawers containing herbs, and the method by which the herbs are weighed in the preparation of a prescription. The herbs necessary to fill the prescription are laid out on the paper in Figure 10–6A, and the directions for preparing them are carefully given to the patient. In general, the herbs are wrapped in cheesecloth and placed in a determined amount of boiling water for a determined amount of time. The resulting liquid is then ingested in specific amounts, at specific times each day. The amount of time that the herbs are boiled determines the concentration of the medicine. Thus, the directions for preparation are carefully followed.

The Chinese doctor who practices in the pharmacy writes the prescription, and the cost of filling a prescription varies from nominal ($5.00) to quite expensive (several hundred dollars), depending on the herbs that are used.

We asked to purchase some of the herbs that he took from the drawers lining the entire wall behind him. He refused to sell us anything except some of the preparations that were on the counter because a prescription was necessary to purchase any of the herbal compounds that he prepared. Undaunted, we purchased a wide variety of herbs that could be used for indigestion, in addition to ointments and liniments used for sore muscles and sprains.

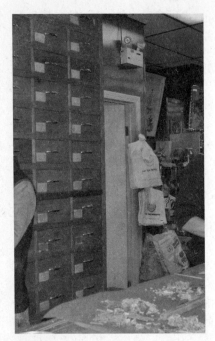

Figure 10-6A Interior of a Chinese pharmacy.

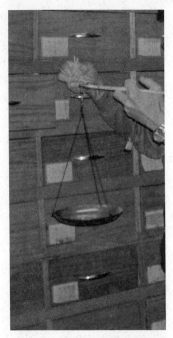

Figure 10-6B Weighing herbs for a prescription.

In addition to herbs and plants, the Chinese use other products with medicinal and healing properties. Some of these products were also used in ancient Europe and are still used today. For example, in China, boys' urine was used to cure lung diseases, soothe inflamed throats, and dissolve blood clots in pregnant women. In Europe, it was used during the 2 world wars as emergency treatment for open wounds. Urea is still used today as a treatment that promotes the healing of wounds. Other popular Chinese remedies include:

- deer antlers—used to strengthen bones, increase a man's potency, and dispel nightmares
- lime calcium—used to clear excessive mucus
- quicksilver—used externally to treat venereal diseases
- rhinoceros horns—highly effective when applied to pus boils; an antitoxin for snakebites
- turtle shells—used to stimulate weak kidneys and to remove gallstones
- snake flesh—eaten as a delicacy to keep eyes healthy and vision clear
- seahorses—pulverized and used to treat gout

Traditional HEALERS

The physician was the primary HEALER in Chinese medicine. Physicians who had to treat women encountered numerous difficulties because men were not allowed to touch women directly who were not family members. Thus, a diagnosis might be made through a ribbon that was attached to the woman's wrist. As an alternative to demonstrating areas of pain or discomfort on a woman's body, an alabaster figure was substituted. The area of pain was pointed out on the figurine (Dolan, 1973, p. 30).

Not much is known about women doctors except that they did exist. Women were known to possess a large store of medical talent. There were also midwives and female shamans. The female shamans possessed gifts of prophecy. They danced themselves into ecstatic trances and had a profound effect on the people around them. As the knowledge that these women possessed was neither known nor understood by the general population, they were feared rather than respected. They were said to know all there was to know about life, death, and birth.

Chinese Pediatrics

Babies are generally breast-fed because neither cow's milk nor goat's milk is acceptable to the Chinese. Sometimes, children are nursed for as long as 4 or 5 years. However, the practice is now varying as more women are working.

Since early time the Chinese have known about and practiced immunization against smallpox. A child was inoculated with the live virus from the crust of a pustule from a smallpox victim. The crust was ground into a powder, and this powder was subsequently blown into the nose of the healthy child through the lumen of a small tube. If the child was healthy, he or she did not generally develop a full-blown case of smallpox but, instead, acquired immunity to this dreaded disease (Wallnöfer & von Rottauscher, 1972).

Box 10–1 presents an overview of Ayurvedic Medicine.

 Box 10–1

Ayurvedic Medicine

Ayurveda is the science of life.
—Deepak Chopra, M.D.

Deepak Chopra introduced Ayurvedic medicine to the United States in 1984. He has emerged as one of the world's leading proponents of the innovative combination of Eastern and Western healing.

(continued)

Box 10–1 *Continued*

Ayurvedic medicine (also called Ayurveda) is one of the world's oldest, and many credit it with being the oldest, medical system. It originated in India and has evolved there over thousands of years. It developed from Hinduism, one of the world's oldest and largest religions and ancient Persian thoughts about HEALTH and HEALING. *Ayurveda* means "the science of life" and is built on theories of HEALTH and ILLNESS and on ways to prevent, manage, or treat HEALTH problems. It is holistic, as it integrates and balances the body, mind, and spirit. The balance is believed to lead to contentment and HEALTH and to help prevent ILLNESS, and it treats specific health problems, whether they are physical or mental. One goal of Ayurvedic practice is to cleanse the body of substances that can cause disease to reestablish harmony and balance (Fugh-Berman, 1996, pp. 36–38).

In the Ayurvedic philosophy, people, HEALTH, and the universe are said to be related, and HEALTH problems can result when the relationships are out of balance. Herbs, metals, massage, and other products and techniques are used with the intent of cleansing the body and restoring balance. Many of the Ayurvedic practices were handed down by word of mouth and were used before there were written records. Two ancient books, written in Sanskrit on palm leaves more than 2,000 years ago, are thought to be the first texts on Ayurveda: *Caraka Samhita* and *Susruta Samhita*. They cover many topics, including

- Pathology (the causes of illness)
- Diagnosis
- Treatment
- How to care for children
- Advice for practitioners, including ethics

Ayurveda is the main system of health care in India, and variations of it have been practiced for centuries in Pakistan, Nepal, Bangladesh, Sri Lanka, and Tibet. About 70% of India's population lives in rural areas and about two thirds of rural people still use Ayurveda and medicinal plants to meet their primary health care needs. In addition, most major Indian cities have an Ayurvedic college and hospital.

The following is a summary of major beliefs in Ayurveda that pertain to HEALTH and disease.

- All things in the universe (both living and nonliving) are joined together.
- Every human being contains elements that can be found in the universe.
- All people are born in a state of balance within themselves and in relation to the universe.
- Disease arises when a person is out of harmony with the universe.

Traditional Definitions of HEALTH and ILLNESS

Basic HEALTH and ILLNESS beliefs include the following.

The constitution, or HEALTH, is called the *prakriti*. The *prakriti* is thought to be a unique combination of physical and psychological characteristics and the way the body functions. It is influenced by such factors as digestion and how the body deals with waste products. The *prakriti* is believed to be unchanged over a person's lifetime.

Three qualities, called *doshas*, form important characteristics of the constitution and control the activities of the body. Practitioners of Ayurveda call the *doshas* by their original Sanskrit names: *vata*, *pitta*, and *kapha*. It is also believed that

1. Each *dosha* is made up of 1 or 2 of the 5 basic elements: space, air, fire, water, and earth.
2. Each *dosha* has a particular relationship to body functions and can be upset for different reasons.
3. A person has his or her own balance of the 3 *doshas*, although one *dosha* usually is prominent. *Doshas* are constantly being formed and reformed by food, activity, and bodily processes.

The *vata dosha* is thought to be a combination of the elements space and air, and it controls very basic body processes, such as cell division, the heart, breathing, and the mind. *Vata* can be thrown out of balance by, for example, staying up late at night, eating dry fruit, or eating before the previous meal is digested. People with *vata* as their main *dosha* are thought to be especially susceptible to skin, neurological, and mental diseases.

The *pitta dosha* represents the elements fire and water. *Pitta* is said to control hormones and the digestive system. When *pitta* is out of balance, a person may experience negative emotions (such as hostility and jealousy) and have physical symptoms (such as heartburn within 2 or 3 hours of eating). *Pitta* is upset by, for example, eating spicy or sour food; being angry, tired, or fearful; or spending too much time in the sun. People with a predominantly *pitta* constitution are thought to be susceptible to heart disease and arthritis.

The *kapha dosha* combines the elements water and earth. *Kapha* is thought to help keep up strength and immunity and to control growth. An imbalance in the *kapha dosha* may cause nausea immediately after eating. *Kapha* is aggravated by, for example, sleeping during the daytime, eating too many sweet foods, eating after one is full, and eating and drinking foods and beverages with too much salt and water (especially in the springtime). Those with a predominant *kapha dosha* are thought to be vulnerable to diabetes, gallbladder problems, stomach ulcers, and respiratory illnesses, such as asthma (Roy, 1999, pp. 96–97).

Traditional Methods of HEALTH Restoration
In diagnosing a patient, the practitioner will

- Ask about diet, behavior, lifestyle practices, and the reasons for the most recent illness and symptoms the patient had
- Carefully observe such physical characteristics as teeth, skin, eyes, and weight
- Take a person's pulse, because each *dosha* is thought to make a particular kind of pulse

In addition to questioning, Ayurvedic practitioners use observation, touch, therapies, and advising. During an examination, the practitioner checks the patient's urine, stool, tongue, bodily sounds, eyes, skin, and overall appearance. The practitioner will also consider the person's digestion, diet, personal habits, and

(continued)

Box 10–1 *Continued*

resilience (ability to recover quickly from illness or setbacks). As part of the effort to find out what is wrong, the practitioner may prescribe some type of treatment. The treatment is generally intended to restore the balance of a particular *dosha*.

The practitioner will develop a treatment plan and may work with people who know the patient well and can help. This helps the patient feel emotionally supported and comforted, which is considered important.

Patients are expected to be active participants in their treatment, because many Ayurvedic treatments require changes in diet, lifestyle, and habits. In general, treatments use several approaches, often more than one at a time. The following are the goals of treatment:

- *Eliminate impurities.* A process called *panchakarma* is intended to be cleansing; it focuses on the digestive tract and the respiratory system. For the digestive tract, cleansing may be done through enemas, fasting, or special diets. Some patients receive medicated oils through a nasal spray or an inhaler. This part of treatment is believed to eliminate worms or other agents thought to cause disease.
- *Reduce symptoms.* The practitioner may suggest various options, including yoga exercises, stretching, breathing exercises, meditation, and exposure to the sun. The patient may take herbs (usually several), often with honey, with the intent to improve digestion, reduce fever, and treat diarrhea. Sometimes, foods such as lentil beans or special diets are also prescribed. Very small amounts of metal and mineral preparations also may be given, such as gold or iron. Careful control of these materials is intended to protect the patient from harm.
- *Reduce worry and increase harmony in the patient's life.* The patient may be advised to seek nurturing and peacefulness through yoga, meditation, exercise, or other techniques.
- *Help eliminate both physical and psychological problems.* Vital points therapy and/or massage may be used to reduce pain, lessen fatigue, or improve circulation. Ayurveda proposes that there are 107 "vital points" in the body where life energy is stored, and these points may be massaged to improve health. Other types of Ayurvedic massage use medicinal oils.

In Ayurveda, the distinction between food and medicine is not as clear as in Western medicine. Food and diet are important components of Ayurvedic practice, so there is a heavy reliance on treatments based on herbs and plants, oils (such as sesame oil), common spices (such as turmeric), and other naturally occurring substances.

Currently, some 5,000 products are included in the "pharmacy" of Ayurvedic treatments. The following are a few examples of how some botanicals (plants and their products) have been or are currently used in treatment. In some cases, these may be mixed with metals.

- The spice turmeric has been used for various diseases and conditions, including rheumatoid arthritis, Alzheimer's disease, and wound healing.
- A mixture (*Arogyawardhini*) of sulfur, iron, powdered dried fruits, tree root, and other substances has been used to treat problems of the liver.

- An extract from the resin of a tropical shrub (*Commiphora mukul*, or guggul) has been used for a variety of illnesses. In recent years, there has been research interest in its possible use to lower cholesterol.

Traditional HEALERS

One example of a traditional Indian HEALER was *Sai Baba*, known as the God that descended to earth. *Sri Sai Baba*, who left his mortal body in 1918, is the living spiritual force that is drawing people from all walks of life, from all parts of the world, into his fold. It is believed that he came to serve humankind and to free them from the clutches of fear. He lived his message through the "Essence of His Being." His life and relationship with the common people was his teaching. He lived with the common people as a penniless *fakir*, wearing a torn *kafni*, sleeping over a mat while resting his head on a brick, and begging for his food. He radiated a mysterious smile and a deep, inward look, of a peace that was all-understanding. One story about him was that he saved a child from drowning. One report has it that word had spread that the 3-year-old daughter of a poor man called Babu Kirwandikar had fallen into a well and had drowned. When the villagers rushed to the well, they saw the child suspended in midair, as if some invisible hand was holding her up! She was quickly pulled out. *Sai Baba* was fond of that child, who was often heard to say, "I am *Baba's* sister!" After this incident, the villagers took her at her word. "It is all *Baba's Leela*," the people would say philosophically. It is from stories such as this that the people who believe in *Sri Sai Baba* gather strength.

Source: Sai Movement. (2002). *Shri SaiBaba of Shirdi* the Perfect Master of the Age. Shirdi, India: Shri SaiBaba Trust. Retrieved from http://www.shrisaibabasansthan.org/, June 29, 2011.

Hay, V. (1994). An Interview with Deepak Chopra. A Magazine of People and Possibilities online. Retrieved from http://www.intouchmag.com/chopra.html, June 28, 2011.

■ Current Health Problems

In many instances, people who were born in the United States into families established here for generations are largely indistinguishable from the general population in their health care beliefs. Other groups, however, especially new immigrants, differ from the general population on many social and health-related issues. Table 10–3 compares selected health indicators in the Asian/Pacific Islander population with people of all races. In most of the selected categories, the rates for the Asian/Pacific Islander population are lower than those for the general population. For example, Asians/Pacific Islanders have a lower rate of births to women receiving third trimester or no prenatal care; a lower rate of live births to teenagers, lower infant mortality, a lower incidence of cancer, and lower rates of homicide and suicide. Table 10–4 compares the causes of death in the Asian population with that of all persons in 2007.

Poor health, however, continues to be found among some Asians partly because of poor working and crowded living conditions. Many people work

Table 10-3 Comparison of Selected Health Status Indicators, All Races and Asian/Pacific Islander: 2007

Health Indicator	All Races	Asian/Pacific Islander[1]
Crude birth rate per 1,000 population by race of mother, 2007	14.3	17.2
Percentage of live births of women receiving prenatal care first trimester, 2007	67.5	69.8
Percentage of live births of women receiving third trimester or no prenatal care, 2007	8.4	7.7
Percentage of live births to teenage childbearing women—under 18, 2007	3.4	0.9
Percentage of low birth weight per live births >2,500 grams, 2007	8.22	8.10
Infant mortality per 1,000 live births, 2006	6.7	4.5
Cancer—all sites per 100,000 population, 2007	446.7	322.0
Lung cancer incidence per 100,000 population, 2007	Men: 65.4 Women: 47.4	Men: 52.4 Women: 27.0
Breast cancer incidence per 100,000, 2007	122.5	98.0
Prostate cancer incidence per 100,000, 2007	158.3	93.3
Male death rates from suicide, all ages, age adjusted per 100,000 resident population, 2007	11.3	9.0
Male death rates from homicide, all ages, age adjusted per 100,000 resident population, 1999/2003	6.1	3.3

[1]Pacific Islanders are clustered with Asian health statistics when indicated.
Source: National Center for Health Statistics. (2010). Health, United States, 2010: With Special Feature on Death and Dying. Hyattsville, MD. 2011: Author. pp. 102,106, 107, 110,124, 137, 180–181, 184–185, and 204. Retrieved from www.cdc.gov/nchs/data/hus/hus10.pdf, November 15, 2011.

long hours in restaurants and laundries and receive the lowest possible wages for their hard work. Many cannot afford even minimal, let alone preventive, health care. Americans of Asian heritage frequently experience unique barriers, including linguistic and cultural differences, when they try to access the unfamiliar health care system.

Language difficulties and adherence to native Chinese culture compound problems already associated with poverty, crowding, and poor health. Many people still prefer the traditional forms of Chinese medicine and seek help from Chinatown "physicians" who treat them with traditional herbs and other methods. Often, Asian people do not seek help from the Western system at all. Others use Chinese methods in conjunction with Western methods of health care, although the Chinese find many aspects of Western medicine distasteful. For example, they cannot understand why so many diagnostic tests, some of which are painful, are necessary. They do, however, accept the practice of immunization and the use of x-rays. An example of a modern health care practice that may cause a problem is the drawing of blood.

Table 10-4 **Comparison of the 10 Leading Causes of Death for Asian Americans/Pacific Islanders and for All Persons: 2007**

Asian Americans	All Persons
1. Malignant neoplasms	Diseases of heart
2. Diseases of heart	Malignant neoplasms
3. Cerebrovascular diseases	Cerebrovascular diseases
4. Unintentional injuries	Chronic lower respiratory diseases
5. Diabetes mellitus	Unintentional injuries
6. Influenza and pneumonia	Alzheimer's disease
7. Chronic lower respiratory diseases	Diabetes mellitus
8. Suicide	Influenza and pneumonia
9. Nephritis, nephrotic syndrome, and nephrosis	Nephritis, nephrotic syndrome, and nephrosis
10. Alzheimer's disease	Septicemia

Source: National Center for Health Statistics. (2010). Health, United States, 2010: With Special Feature on Death and Dying. Hyattsville, MD. 2011: Author, pp. 145–146. Retrieved from www.cdc.gov/nchs/data/hus/hus10.pdf, November 15, 2011.

Chinese people may not understand why the often frequent taking of blood samples, considered routine in Western medicine, is necessary. Blood is seen as the source of life for the entire body, and it is believed that blood is not regenerated. The Asian reluctance to have blood drawn for diagnostic tests may have its roots in the revered teachings of Confucius. The Chinese people also believe that a good physician should be able to make a diagnosis simply by examining a person. Consequently, they do not react well to the often painful procedures used in Western diagnostic workups. Some people—because of their distaste for the drawing of blood—leave the Western system rather than tolerate the pain. The Chinese have deep respect for their bodies and believe that it is best to die with their bodies intact. For this reason, many people refuse surgery or consent to it only under the most dire circumstances. This reluctance to undergo intrusive surgical procedures has deep implications for those concerned with providing health care to Asian Americans.

The hospital is an alien place to many of the Asian people. Not only are the customs and practices strange but also the patients often are isolated from the rest of their people, which enhances the language barrier and feelings of helplessness. Something as basic as food creates another problem. Hospital food is strange to Asian patients and is served in an unfamiliar manner. The typical Asian patient rarely complains about what bothers him or her. Often the only indication that there may be a problem is an untouched food tray and the silent withdrawal of the patient. Unfortunately, the silence may be regarded by the nurses as reflecting good, complacent behavior, and the health care team exerts little energy to go beyond the assumption. The Asian patient who says little and complies with all treatment is seen as stoic, and there is little awareness that deep problems may underlie this "exemplary" behavior. Ignorance on the part of health care workers may cause the patient a great deal of suffering.

Much action has been taken in recent years to make Western health care more available and appealing to the Asian populations. In Boston, for example, there is a health clinic staffed primarily by Chinese dialects–speaking, and other Asian languages nurses and physicians who work as paid employees and as volunteers. Most of the common health-related pamphlets have been translated into Chinese languages and into Vietnamese, Cambodian, and Laotian, and they are distributed to the patients. Booklets on such topics as breast self-examination and smoking cessation are available. Since the languages spoken in the clinic are Mandarin Chinese, other dialects and languages the problem of interpreters has been largely eliminated. The care is personal, and the patients are made to feel comfortable. Unnecessary and painful tests are avoided as much as possible. In addition, the clinic, which is open for long hours, provides social services and employment placements and is quite popular with the community. Although it began as a part-time, storefront operation, the clinic is now housed in its own building.

The following is a synopsis of cultural beliefs regarding mental health and illness, possible causes of mental illness, and methods of preventing mental illness among people of Asian origin. Lack of knowledge or skills in mental health therapy is seen in the Asian communities, as mental illness is much ignored in medical classics. Two points must be noted: the importance placed on the family in caring for the mentally ill and the tendency to identify mental illness in somatic terms. There is a tremendous amount of stigma attached to mental illness. Asian patients tend to come to the attention of mental health workers late in the course of their illness, and they come with a feeling of hopelessness (Lin, 1982, pp. 69–73).

One example of cross-cultural therapy is the Japanese practice of Morita therapy. This 70-year-old treatment originated from a treatment for shinkeishitsu, a form of compulsive neurosis with aspects of neurasthenia. The patient is separated from the family for 1 to 2 weeks and taught that one's feelings are the same as the Japanese sky and instantly changeable. One cannot be responsible for how one feels, only for what one does. At the end of therapy, the patient focuses on what is being done and less on his or her inner feelings, symptoms, concerns, or obsessive thoughts (Yamamoto, 1982, p. 50). In addition, there are countless culture-bound mental HEALTH syndromes that may be identified in the Asian communities:

- Korea—*Hwa-byung*—a syndrome attributed to the suppression of anger is known as "anger syndrome"; symptoms include insomnia, indigestion, and dyspnea.
- China—*Koro*—the occurrence of sudden, intense anxiety when a man believes his penis is folding into his body (Fontaine, 2003, p. 119).
- Japan—*Taijin kyofusho*—intense anxiety about possibly offending others (Office of the Surgeon General (U.S.); Center for Mental Health

Services (U.S.); National Institute of Mental Health (U.S.). Mental Health: Culture, Race, and Ethnicity: A Supplement to Mental Health: A Report of the Surgeon General. Rockville (MD): Substance Abuse and Mental Health Services Administration (U.S.); 2001 Aug. Chapter 1. Introduction).

Asian American Health Care Manpower

Asian Americans, a group that constituted 4.8% of the resident U.S. population in the 2010 census, are for the most part well represented in the enrollment in health professions, as illustrated in Table 10–5. Today, persons who desire to be physicians in China have the option of studying either Chinese or Western medicine. If they select Western medicine, a limited amount of Chinese medicine is also taught. As Chinese traditional medicine is becoming better recognized and better understood in the United States, more doors are being opened to those who prefer or understand this mode of treatment.

The National Sample Survey of Registered Nurses 2008, prepared by the Bureau of Health Professions of the Health Resources Administration, estimates that the registered nurse population in the United States in 2008 numbered 3,063,162; and 2,596,599 were actively employed in nursing positions. Of this number, 83.2% were White (non-Hispanic) and 5.8% were Asian (non-Hispanic). Given that in 2010 people of Asian (non-Hispanic) populations comprised 4.80% of the resident population (see Table 3–2 from Chapter 3), this is a clear indication that there is demographic parity in the percentage of Asian (non-Hispanic) people in nursing.

This chapter has presented an introductory overview of selected cultural phenomena, HEALTH traditions, and health issues of people from Asian heritages. Needless to say, a bigger picture of the phenomenon could fill many books. However, given the significant number of new Asians immigrants, especially from China and India, this beginning discussion is very necessary.

Table 10–5   Percentage of Asians Enrolled in Selected Health Professions Schools Compared with Non-Hispanic Whites: 2007–2008

	Number Enrolled	Non-Hispanic Whites (%)	Asians (%)
Dentistry	19,342	60.6	22.7
Allopathic medicine	74,518	62.4	21.5
Osteopathic medicine	15,634	70.5	17.4
Optometry	5,556	60.3	25.1
Pharmacy	50,691	59.5	21.6
Podiatry	2,095	62.2	11.8
Public health	22,604	59.3	12.5

Source: National Center for Health Statistics. Health, United States, 2010: With Special Feature on Death and Dying. Hyattsville, MD. 2011: Author, pp. 352–353. Retrieved from www.cdc.gov/nchs/data/hus/hus10.pdf, November 15, 2011.

RESEARCH ON CULTURE

A large amount of research has been conducted among members of the Asian American populations. The study described in the following article is one example:

Lee, J and Bell, K. (2011) The Impact of Cancer on Family Relationships Among Chinese Patients. Journal of Transcultural Nursing, 22(3), 225–234.

This qualitative research study examined the impact of cancer on family relationships among members of a Chinese cancer support group. There were 96 participants at group meetings over an 8-month span of time—40% of whom were family members. The methods used included participant observation and in-depth interviews with 7 group members were held. The interview schedule is published in the article.

The findings were that family members were an integral part of the support group. Patients expressed concern about family members and family members identified "equal suffering" when they cared for patients. There was a strong emphasis on the need to conceal emotion. Patients were also anxious about burdening their family members.

The authors concluded that the findings highlight the need for practitioners to focus on the entire family when they develop interventions to help cancer patients cope. They recommend that research should focus on gender differences in Chinese families' experiences of cancer as well as possible differences that may be found based on length of immigration.

Explore 🌐 MediaLink

Go to the Student Resource Site at nursing.pearsonhighered.com for chapter-related review questions, case studies, and activities. Contents of the CULTURALCARE Guide and CULTURALCARE Museum can also be found on the Student Resource Site. Click on Chapter 10 to select the activities for this chapter.

Keeping Up

It goes without saying that much of the data presented in this chapter may be out of date when you read this text. However, at this final stage of writing, it is the most recent information available. The following resources will be most helpful in keeping you abreast of the frequent changes in health care events, costs, and policies:

1. The National Center for Health Statistics publishes Health, United States an annual report on trends in health statistics. It can be retrieved from http://www.cdc.gov/nchs/hus.htm. Health United States 11 is not available, and Health United States 12 will be published in May, 2012.

2. Health related data and other statistics are available from http://www.cdc.gov/DataStatistics/.

3. To follow immigration information—U.S. Department of Commerce Economics and Statistics Administration Office of Homeland Security Office of Immigration Statistics, (2011). Monger, R., & Yankay, J. (2010). Annual Flow Report. U.S. Legal Permanent Residents: 2010. Retrieved from http://www.dhs.gov/files/statistics/publications/gc_1301497627185.shtm.

■ Internet Sources

Hay, V. (1994). An Interview with Deepak Chopra. A Magazine of People and Possibilities online. Retrieved from http://www.intouchmag.com/chopra. html, June 28, 2011.

Humes, K. R., Nicholas, A. J., & Ramirez, R. (2011). Overview of Race and Hispanic Origin: 2010. Census Briefs. P. 4. Retrieved from http://2010. census.gov/2010census/data/, June 26, 2011.

National Center for Alternative and Complimentary Medicine. (2007). Backgrounder: What is Ayurvedic Medicine? Bethesda, Maryland: Author. Retrieved from http://nccam.nih.gov/health/ayurveda/, June 28, 2011.

Office of the Surgeon General (U.S.); Center for Mental Health Services (U.S.); National Institute of Mental Health (U.S.). November 15, 2011. Mental Health: Culture, Race, and Ethnicity: A Supplement to Mental Health: A Report of the Surgeon General. Rockville (MD): Substance Abuse and Mental Health Services Administration (U.S.); Chapter 1. Introduction. Retrieved from http:// www.ncbi.nlm.nih.gov/books/NBK44246/#A1022, March 13, 2011.

Sai Movement. (2002). Shri SaiBaba of Shirdi the Perfect Master of the Age. Shirdi, India: Shri SaiBaba Trust. Retrieved from http://www.shrisaibabasansthan. org/, June 28, 2011.

United States Department of Commerce, U.S. Census Bureau. Census 2010. (2011). Retrieved from http://www.census.gov/, June 27, 2011.

U.S. Department of Commerce Economics and Statistics Administration Office of Homeland Security Office of Immigration Statistics (2011) Monger, R. and Yankay, J. Annual Flow Report. U.S. Legal Permanent Residents: 2010. Retrieved from http://www.dhs.gov/files/statistics/publications/ gc_1301497627185.shtm, June 1, 2011.

U.S. Department of Commerce Economics and Statistics Administration Office of Homeland Security Office of Immigration Statistics (2011) Lee, J. Annual Flow Report U.S. Naturalizations: 2010. Retrieved from http://www.dhs. gov/files/statistics/publications/gc_1302103955524.shtm, June 1, 2011.

U.S. Department of Health and Human Services. (2010). National Center for Health Statistics. Health, United States, 2010: With Special Feature on Death and Dying. Hyattsville, MD. 2011. Author. Retrieved from www.cdc.gov/ nchs/data/hus/hus10.pdf, 2011.

U.S. Department of Health and Human Services, Health Resources and Services. (2010). The National Survey of Registered Nurses 2008 Documentation for the General Public Use File, 2006, Bureau of Health Professions Health Resources and Services Administration. HRSA/BHPr and the National Sample Survey of Registered Nurses. Retreived from http://www.hrsa.gov/ data-statistics/index.html, June 28, 2011.

■ References

Barnes, J. S., & Bennett, C. E. (2002). *The Asian population: 2000.* Washington, DC: U.S. Department of Commerce.

Chan, P. K. (1988, August 3). Herb specialist, interview by author. New York City. Dr. Chan prepared a supplemental written statement in Chinese and English for inclusion in this text.

Dolan, J. (1973). *Nursing in society: A historical perspective.* Philadelphia: W. B. Saunders. National Center for Health Statistics.

Ergil, K. V. (1996). China's traditional medicine. In M. S. Micozzi (Ed.), *Fundamentals of complementary and alternative medicine*, New York: Churchill Livingstone.

Fontaine, K. L. (2003). *Mental health nursing* (5th ed.). Upper Saddle River, NJ: Prentice Hall.

Fugh-Berman, A. (1996). *Alternative medicine: What works.* Tucson, AZ: Odonian Press.

Lee, J., & Bell, K. (2011). The impact of cancer on family relationships among chinese patients. *Journal of Transcultural Nursing, 22*(3), 225–234.

Lin, K. M. (1982). Cultural aspects in mental health for Asian Americans. In A. Gaw (Ed.), *Cross-cultural psychiatry.* Boston: John Wright.

Mann, F. (1972). *Acupuncture.* New York: Vintage Books.

Martin, J. A. (1995). Birth characteristics for Asian or Pacific Islander subgroups, 1992. Monthly vital statistics report, *National Center for Health Statistics, 43*(10), 1.

Morgan, H. T. (1942 [1972]). *Chinese symbols and superstitions.* Detroit, MI: Gale Research. Reprint, S. Pasadena, CA: Ione Perkins.

National Center for Health Statistics. Health, United States, 2010: With Special Feature on Death and Dying. Hyattsville, MD. 2011. Author.

Romo, R. G. (1995, May 3). *Hispanic health traditions and issues.* Paper presented at the Minnesota Health Educators Conference.

Roy, C. (1999). Nurse's handbook of alternative and complementary therapies. Springhouse, PAS: Springhouse.

Smith, H. (1958). *The religions of man.* New York: Harper & Row.

Spector, R. (1992). Culture, ethnicity, and nursing. In P. Potter & A. Perry (Eds.), *Fundamentals of nursing.* St. Louis: Mosby-Year Book.

Wallnöfer, H., & von Rottauscher, A. (1972). *Chinese folk medicine.* M. Palmedo (Trans.), New York: American Library.

Yamamoto, J. (1982). Japanese Americans. In A. Gaw (Ed.), *Cross-cultural psychiatry.* Boston: John Wright.

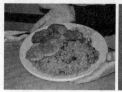

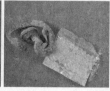
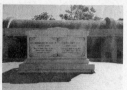

Figure 11–1   **Figure 11–2**   **Figure 11–3**   **Figure 11–4**

Chapter 11

HEALTH and ILLNESS
in the Black Population

God speed the day when human blood shall cease to flow!
In every clime be understood, the claims of human brotherhood,
And each return for evil, good, not blow for blow;
That day will come all feuds to end, and change into a faithful friend each foe.

—Frederick Douglas' 4th of July Speech (1852)

■ Objectives

1. Discuss the background of members of the Black population.
2. Discuss the demographic and new immigrant profiles of members of the Black population.
3. Describe the traditional definitions of HEALTH and ILLNESS of members of the Black population.
4. Describe the traditional methods of HEALTH maintenance and protection of selected communities of the Black population.
5. Describe the traditional methods of HEALING of selected communities of the Black population.
6. Describe current health care problems of members of the Black population.
7. Describe demographic disparity as it is seen in health manpower distribution of the Black population as represented in the health care delivery system.

The opening images for this chapter depict objects symbolic of items used to maintain, protect, and/or restore HEALTH for people in the Black American communities. Figure 11–1 is a typical Haitian meal—it consists of rice, beans, plantains, and chicken—a well-balanced, nutritious meal for health maintenance. Figure 11–2 is a beaded neckpiece that may be worn for protection. Beads carry with them centuries of history and are symbols of wealth and social rank. Their many uses include protection from evil spirits, symbols of stages of growth through life, and symbols of health, fertility, and beauty. Figure 11–3 is that of a dried garden snake and the powder derived from grinding it. The powder is dissolved in water and the solution is used to treat skin maladies, such as rashes and insect bites. Figure 11–4 is the grave monument for Dr. Martin Luther King, Jr., and his wife Coretta Scott King. They are located on the grounds of the King Center in Atlanta, Georgia. The King Center is the official, living memorial dedicated to the advancement of the legacy of Dr. Martin Luther King, Jr., leader of America's greatest nonviolent movement for justice, equality, and peace. More than 1 million visitors from all over the world are drawn annually to the King Center to pay homage to Dr. King. The Memorial attempts to meet with uncompromising insistence, the problems, and needs that face Black people today.

■ Background

"Black or African American" in the 2010 census refers to a person having origins in any of the Black racial groups of Africa. The Black racial category includes people who marked the "Black, African American, or Negro" check-box on the census form. It also includes respondents who marked Sub-Saharan African entries, for example Kenyan and Nigerian; and Afro-Caribbean entries, for example Haitian and Jamaican. The 2010 census showed that the United States population on April 1, 2010, was 308.7 million people. Out of the total population, 38.9 million, or 13%, identified as Black alone. In addition, 3.1 million people, or 1%, reported Black in combination with one or more other races. The Black alone-or-in-combination population grew by 15%, which was more growth than the total population and the Black alone population. Both groups (Black alone-or-in-combination) grew at a slower rate than most other major races and ethnic groups in the country. The majority of Blacks or African Americans alone in the United States in 2010 lived in the South, 56.5%; 16.8% lived in the Northeast; 17.9% in the Midwest; and 8.8% in the West. The states with the highest population of Blacks or African Americans in 2010 were New York, 7.9%; Florida, 7.7%; Texas, 7.6%; Georgia, 3.1%; and California, 7.7% (Rastogi, Johnson, Hoeffel, & Drewery, 2011, pp. 4–9). In 2010, 84.2% of Blacks were high school graduates and for persons over 25, 19.8% were college graduates (U.S. Census Bureau, 2012, p. 151).

"Black" is used in this chapter's text to refer to the Black or African American population, but "Black or African American" is used in tables and figures. This follows the pattern used in Census 2010. Most members of the present Black American community have their roots in Africa, and the majority descend from people who were brought here as slaves from the west coast of Africa (Bullough & Bullough, 1972, pp. 39–41). The largest importation of slaves occurred during the 17th century, which means that Black people have been living in the United States for many generations. Today, a number of Blacks have immigrated to the United States voluntarily—from African countries, the West Indian islands, the Dominican Republic, Haiti, and Jamaica.

Blacks are represented in every socioeconomic group; however, the 1 year estimate released by the United States Census Bureau American Community Survey for 2010 revealed there were over 10 million Blacks or African Americans below the poverty level 27.1% of the Black or African American population (2011). Furthermore, over half of Black Americans live in urban areas surrounded by the symptoms of poverty—crowded and inadequate housing, poor schools, and high crime rates.

For example, Kotlowitz (1991) described the Henry Horner Homes in Chicago as "16 high-rise buildings which stretch over eight blocks and at last census count housed 6,000 people, 4,000 of whom are children." The degree of social and economic change between 1990 and 2000 has been minimal. He presented 2 facts about public housing: "Public housing served as a bulwark to segregation and as a kind of anchor for impoverished neighborhoods" and "It was built on the cheap—the walls are a naked cinder block with heating pipes snaking through the apartment; instead of closets, there are 8-inch indentations in the walls without doors; and the heating system so storms out of control in the winter that it is 85 degrees." Situations similar to this prevail presently.

In 2010, there were a total of 1,042,635 Legal Permanent Residents (LPRs) in the United States, 46% of whom were new arrivals. People from Africa comprised 9.7% of this population of LPRs and people from the Caribbean, 13.4%. The nations that the LPRs were from included Ethiopia, 1.4%; Nigeria, 1.3%; Haiti, 2.2%; and Jamaica, 1.9%. California, New York, Florida, and Texas had the largest populations of LPRs (Monger, & Yankay, 2011, p. 4).

In 2010, there were 619,913 people who naturalized—became citizens of the United States. Of this number, 10.3% were born in Africa and 10.1% were from the Caribbean. Of the African population, 1.5% were from Nigeria and 1.4% from Ethiopia; from the Caribbean, 2.0% were from Haiti and 1.9% from Jamaica. Close to half of the nation's naturalized citizens lived in the metropolitan areas of New York, Los Angeles, or Miami. The median number of years that the people were LPRs was 5 (Lee, 2011, p. 2).

According to some sources, the first Black people to enter this country arrived a year earlier than the Pilgrims, in 1619. Other sources claim that Blacks arrived with Columbus in the 15th century (Bullough & Bullough, 1972, pp. 39–41). In any event, the first Blacks who came to the North American continent did not come as slaves, but, between 1619 and 1860, more than 4 million people were transported here as slaves. One need read only a sampling of the many accounts of slavery to appreciate the tremendous hardships that the captured and enslaved people experienced during that time. Not only was the daily life of the slave very difficult, but the experience of being captured, shackled, and transported in steerage was devastating. Many of those captured in Africa died before they arrived here. The strongest and healthiest people were snatched from their homes by slave dealers and transported en masse in the holds of ships to the North American continent. In general, Black captives were not taken care of or recognized as human beings and treated accordingly. Once here, they were sold and placed on plantations and in homes all over the country—it was only later that the practice was confined to the South. Families were separated; children were wrenched from their parents and sold to other buyers. Some slave owners bred their slaves much as farmers breed cattle today, purchasing men to serve as studs, and judging women based on whether they would produce the desired stock with a particular man (Haley, 1976). However, in the midst of all this inhuman and inhumane treatment, the Black family grew and survived. Gutman (1976), in his careful documentation of plantation and family records, traces the history of the Black family from 1750 to 1925 and points out the existence of families and family or kinship ties before and after the Civil War, dispelling many of the myths about the Black family and its structure. Despite overwhelming hardships and enforced separations, the people managed in most circumstances to maintain both family and community awareness.

The people who came to America from West Africa brought a rich variety of traditional beliefs and practices and came from religious traditions that respected the spiritual power of ancestors. They worshiped a diverse pantheon of gods, who oversaw all aspects of daily life, such as the changes of the seasons, the fertility of nature, physical and spiritual personal health, and communal success. Initiation rites and naming rituals, folktales, and healing practices, dance, song, and drumming were a part of the religious heritage. Many aspects of today's Christian religious practices are believed to have originated in these practices. In addition, it has been estimated that between 10% and 30% of the slaves brought to America between 1711 and 1808 were Muslim. The people brought their prayer practices, fasting and dietary practices, and their knowledge of the Qur'an (Eck, 1994).

Ostensibly, the Civil War ended slavery but in many ways it did not emancipate Blacks. Daily life after the war was fraught with tremendous difficulty, and Black people—according to custom—were stripped of their civil rights. In the South, Black people were overtly segregated, most living in conditions of extreme hardship and poverty (Blackmon, 2008). Those who migrated to the North over the years were subject to all the problems of fragmented urban life: poverty, racism, and covert segregation (Bullough & Bullough, 1972, p. 43; Kain, 1969, pp. 1–30).

The historic problems of the Black community need to be appreciated by the health care provider who attempts to juxtapose modern practices and traditional health and illness beliefs. In addition, health care providers must be aware of the ongoing and historical events in the struggle for civil rights that affect people's lives. Box 11–1 highlights several events in the early history of this struggle. In 2007, the Supreme Court ruled in *Parents v. Seattle Schools* and *Meredith v. Jefferson Schools* that public schools can't consider race when making student school assignments. This may be viewed as an effort to strike down *Brown v. Board of Education*, the landmark ruling of 1956. Also, in 2007, James Ford Seale, a Mississippi Klansman was sentenced to 3 life terms in prison for the Moore/Dee murder of 1964.

Box 11–1

Highlights of the Civil Rights Movement

1954	*Brown v. Board of Education*—segregation in public schools found to be illegal by this landmark Supreme Court ruling
1955	Rosa Parks refuses to give up her seat on a bus in Montgomery, Alabama, and the bus boycott in Alabama begins
	Emmett Till murdered in Mississippi
1957	Central High School, Little Rock, Arkansas, integrated by the "Little Rock Nine"
1959	Sit-ins at lunch counters
1961	Segregation of interstate bus terminals ruled unconstitutional
	Freedom Riders attacked
	James Meredith is the first Black student to enroll in the University of Mississippi
1962	Civil Rights Movement formally organized
1963	Dr. Martin Luther King, Jr., writes the seminal "Letter from Birmingham Jail," in which he argues that people have the moral duty to disobey unjust laws
	March on Washington led by Dr. Martin Luther King, Jr.
1964	Killing of Charles Moore and Henry Dee
	Civil Rights Act passed
1965	Malcolm X assassinated
1965–1968	Over 100 race riots in American cities
1968	Dr. Martin Luther King, Jr., assassinated
1991	Beating of Rodney King
1992	Major race riots in Los Angeles
1995	Million Man March
2007	*Parents v. Seattle Schools and Meredith v. Jefferson Schools*
	Jena, Louisiana—Black high school students held for beating a White student and tried as adults
2008	James Ford Seale convicted and sentenced to three life prison terms for his role in the Moore/Dee murders in 1964
	Senator Edward Kennedy (D-MA) introduces the Civil Rights Act of 2008 that includes provisions that ensure federal funds are not used to subsidize discrimination, holding employers accountable for age discrimination and improving accountability for other violations of civil rights and workers' rights
2009	In the Supreme Court case *Ricci v. DeStefano*, a lawsuit brought against the city of New Haven where firefighter tests to determine promotions were discarded, the Supreme Court ruled (5–4) in favor of the firefighters, saying New Haven's "action in discarding the tests was a violation of Title VII of the Civil Rights Act of 1964"

Source: Brunner, B. and Haney, E., Civil Rights Timeline: Milestones in the modern civil rights movement. © 2000–2012. Reprinted by permission of Pearson Education, Inc., Upper Saddle River, New Jersey.

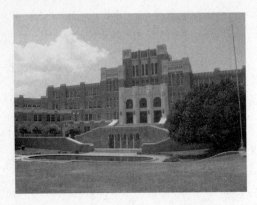

Figure 11-5   Central High School, Little Rock, Arkansas.

It is hard to believe that more than a half-century has passed since the teenage students known today as the "Little Rock Nine" integrated Central High School in Little Rock, Arkansas (Figure 11-5). I vividly remember the scenes on television in 1957 of 9 brave teenagers, my age at the time, trying to enter the school, the cadre of hostile, angry White people spitting at them and hollering epitaphs, and the heavily armed soldiers protecting the teens. These images seared my consciousness and left an indelible imprint on my life. The activities that I accomplished each day—getting up in the morning, walking to school, attending classes, being with my friends, and so forth—were completely disrupted for the students. I remember thinking that this was not Europe; this was not Armenia or Spain, or Russia, or Germany; this was happening in "my backyard," in the United States. People who could be my neighbors violated everything that I had been taught about human dignity and respect. Two years later, my "little sister" in nursing school was one of the Little Rock Nine—I learned firsthand the damage this event wrought on her life and, I believe, on the lives of all of us. Central High School had acquired a most personal meaning. As I write this chapter in 2011, celebrations are being held nationally to recognize and honor the integration of Central High School and the Little Rock Nine. Ostensibly, Central High School and many other schools were integrated, the practices of separate water fountains and "back of the bus" were over and life moved on.

■ Traditional Definitions of *Health* and *Illness*

According to Jacques (1976), the traditional definition of *HEALTH* stems from the African belief about life and the nature of being. To the African, life was a process rather than a state. The nature of a person was viewed in terms of energy force rather than matter. All things, whether living or dead, were believed to influence one another. Therefore, one had the power to influence one's destiny and that of others through the use of behavior, whether proper or otherwise, as well as through knowledge of the person and the world. When one possessed HEALTH, one was in harmony with nature; ILLNESS was a state of disharmony. Traditional Black belief regarding HEALTH did not separate the mind, body, and spirit.

Disharmony—that is, ILLNESS—was attributed to a number of sources, primarily demons and evil spirits. These spirits were generally believed to act of their own accord, and the goal of treatment was to remove them from the body of the ILL person. Several methods were employed to attain this result, in addition to voodoo, which is discussed in the next section. The traditional healers, usually women, possessed extensive knowledge of the use of herbs and roots in the treatment of ILLNESS. Apparently, an early form of smallpox immunization was used by slaves. Women practiced inoculation by scraping a piece of cowpox crust into a place on a child's arm. These children appeared to have a far lower incidence of smallpox than those who did not receive the immunization.

The old and the young were cared for by all members of the community. The elderly were held in high esteem because African people believed that the living of a long life indicated that a person had the opportunity to acquire much wisdom and knowledge. Death was described as the passing from one realm of life to another (Jacques, 1976, p. 117) or as a passage from the evils of this world to another state. The funeral was often celebrated as a joyous occasion, with a party after the burial. Children were passed over the body of the deceased, so that the dead person could carry any potential illness of the child away with him or her.

Many of the preventive and treatment practices of Black people have their roots in Africa but have been merged with the approaches of Native Americans, to whom the Blacks were exposed, and with the attitudes of Whites, among whom they lived and served. Then, as today, ILLNESS was treated in a combination of ways. Methods found to be most useful were handed down through the generations.

■ Traditional Methods of HEALTH Maintenance and Protection

The following sections present examples of practices employed presently or in earlier generations to maintain and protect HEALTH and to treat various types of maladies to restore HEALTH. This discussion cannot encompass all the types of care given to and by the members of the Black community but instead presents a sample of the richness of the traditional HEALTH practices that have survived over the years.

Essentially, HEALTH is maintained with proper diet—that is, eating 3 nutritious meals a day, including a hot breakfast. Rest and a clean environment also are important. Laxatives were and are used to keep the system "running" or "open."

Asafetida—rotten flesh that looks like a dried-out sponge—is worn around the neck to prevent the contraction of contagious diseases. Cod liver oil is taken to prevent colds. A sulfur and molasses preparation is used in the spring because it is believed that at the start of a new season, people are more susceptible to illness. This preparation is rubbed up and down the back, not taken internally. A physician is not consulted routinely and is not generally regarded as the person to whom one goes for the prevention of disease.

Copper or silver bracelets may be worn around the wrist from the time a woman is a baby or young child. These bracelets are believed to protect the wearer as she grows. If for any reason these bracelets are removed, harm befalls the owner. In addition to granting protection, these bracelets indicate when the wearer is about to become ill: the skin around the bracelet turns black, alerting the woman to take precautions against the impending illness. These precautions consist of getting extra rest, praying more frequently, and eating a more nutritious diet.

■ Traditional Methods of HEALTH Restoration

The most common method of treating ILLNESS is prayer. The laying on of hands is described quite frequently. Rooting, a practice derived from voodoo, also is mentioned by many people. In rooting, a person (usually a woman who is known as a "root-worker") is consulted as to the source of a given ILLNESS, and she then prescribes the appropriate treatment. Magic rituals often are employed (Davis, 1998).

The following home remedies have been reported by some Black people as being successful in the treatment of disease:

1. Sugar and turpentine are mixed together and taken by mouth to get rid of worms. This combination can also be used to cure a backache when rubbed on the skin from the navel to the back.

2. Numerous types of poultices are employed to fight infection and inflammation. The poultices are placed on the part of the body that is painful or infected to draw out the cause of the affliction. One type of poultice is made of potatoes. The potatoes are sliced or grated and placed in a bag, which is placed on the affected area of the body. The potatoes turn black; as this occurs, the disease goes away. It is believed that, as these potatoes spoil, they produce a penicillin mold that is able to destroy the infectious organism. Another type of poultice is prepared from cornmeal and peach leaves, which are cooked together and placed either in a bag or in a piece of flannel cloth. The cornmeal ferments and combines with an enzyme in the peach leaves to produce an antiseptic that destroys the bacteria and hastens the healing process. A third poultice, made with onions, is used to heal infections, and a flaxseed poultice is used to treat earaches.

3. Herbs from the woods are used in many ways. Herb teas are prepared—for example, from goldenrod root—to treat pain and reduce fevers. Sassafras tea frequently is used to treat colds. Another herb boiled to make a tea is the root or leaf of rabbit tobacco.

4. Bluestone, a mineral found in the ground, is used as medicine for open wounds. The stone is crushed into a powder and sprinkled on the affected area. It prevents inflammation and is used to treat poison ivy.

5. To treat a "crick" in the neck, 2 pieces of silverware are crossed over the painful area in the form of an X.

6. Nine drops of turpentine 9 days after intercourse act as a contraceptive.

7. Cuts and wounds can be treated with sour or spoiled milk that is placed on stale bread, wrapped in a cloth, and placed on the wound.

8. Salt and pork (salt pork) placed on a rag can be used to treat cuts and wounds.

9. A sprained ankle can be treated by placing clay in a dark leaf and wrapping it around the ankle.

10. A remedy for treating colds is hot lemon water with honey.

11. When congestion is present in the chest and the person is coughing, the chest is rubbed with hot camphorated oil and wrapped with warm flannel.

12. An expectorant for colds consists of chopped raw garlic, chopped onion, fresh parsley, and a little water, all mixed in a blender.

13. Hot toddies are used to treat colds and congestion. These drinks consist of hot tea with honey, lemon, peppermint, and a dash of brandy or whatever alcoholic beverage the person likes and is available. Vicks Vaporub also is swallowed.

14. A fever can be broken by placing raw onions on the feet and wrapping the feet in warm blankets.

15. Boils are treated by cracking a raw egg, peeling the white skin off the inside of the shell, and placing it on the boil. This brings the boil to a head.

16. Garlic can be placed on the ill person or in the room to remove the "evil spirits" that have caused the illness.

Folk Medicine

In many traditional Black communities, folk medicine previously practiced in Africa may still be employed. The methods have been tried and tested and are still relied on. Healers or voodoo practitioners make no class or status distinctions among their patients, treating everyone fairly and honestly. This tradition of equality of care and perceived effectiveness accounts for the faith placed in the practices of the HEALER and in other methods. In fact, the home remedies used by some members of the Black community have been employed for many generations. Another reason for their ongoing use is that hospitals are distant from people who live in rural areas. By the time they might get to the hospital, they would be dead, yet many of the people who continue to use these remedies live in urban areas close to hospitals—sometimes even world-renowned hospitals. Nonetheless, the use of folk medicine persists, and many people avoid the local hospital except in extreme emergencies.

Traditional Methods of HEALING

Voodoo, or Voudou.   Voodoo, or American voudou, is a belief system often alluded to but rarely described in any detail (Davis, 1998). At various times, patients may mention terms such as *fix*, *hex*, or *spell*. It is not clear whether voodoo is fully practiced today, but there is some evidence in the literature that there are people who still believe and practice it to some extent (Wintrob, 1972). It also has been reported that many Black people continue to fear voodoo and believe that when they become ILL they have been "fixed." Voodoo involves 2 forms of magic: white magic, described as harmless, and black magic, which is quite dangerous. Belief in magic is, of course, ancient (Hughes & Bontemps, 1958, pp. 184–185).

Voodoo came to this country about 1724, with the arrival of slaves from the West African coast, who had been sold initially in the West Indies. The people who brought voodoo with them were "snake worshippers." Vodu, the name of their god, with the passage of time became *voodoo* (also *hoodoo*), an all-embracing term that included the god, the sect, the members of the sect, the priests and priestesses, the rites and practices, and the teaching (Tallant, 1946, p. 19).

Tallant goes on to explain that the sect spread rapidly from the West Indies. In 1782, the governor of Louisiana prohibited the importation of slaves from Martinique because of their practice of voodoo. (Despite the fact that gatherings of slaves were forbidden in Louisiana, small groups persisted in practicing voodoo.) In 1803, the importation of slaves to Louisiana from the West Indies was finally allowed, and with them came the strong influence of voodoo. The practice entailed a large number of rituals and procedures. The ceremonies were held with large numbers of people, usually at night and in the open country. Sacrifice and the drinking of blood were integral parts of all the voodoo ceremonies. There were those who believed that this blood was from children. However, it was most commonly thought to be the blood of a cat or young goat. Such behavior evolved from primitive African rites, to which Christian rituals were added to form the ceremonies that exist today. Leaders of the voodoo sect tended to be women, and stories abound in New Orleans about the workings of the sect and the women who ruled it—such as Marie Laveau.

In 1850, the practice of voodoo reached its height in New Orleans. At that time, the beliefs and practices of voodoo were closely related to beliefs about HEALTH and ILLNESS. For example, many ILLNESSES were attributed to a "fix" that was placed on one person out of anger. Gris-gris, the symbols of voodoo, were used to prevent ILLNESS or to give ILLNESS to others. Some examples of commonly used gris-gris follow (Tallant, 1946, p. 226):

1. **Good gris-gris:** powders and oils that are highly and pleasantly scented. The following are examples of good gris-gris: love powder, colored and scented with perfume; love oil, olive oil to which gardenia

perfume has been added; luck water, ordinary water that is purchased in many shades (red is for success in love, yellow for success in money matters, blue for protection and friends).

2. **Bad gris-gris:** oils and powders that have a vile odor. The following are examples of bad gris-gris: anger powder, war powder, and moving powder, which are composed of soil, gunpowder, and black pepper, respectively.

3. **Flying devil oil:** olive oil that has red coloring and cayenne pepper added to it.

4. **Black cat oil:** machine oil.

In addition to these oils and powders, a variety of colored candles, as in Figure 11–6, are used; the color of the candle symbolizes the intention. For example, white symbolizes peace; red, victory; pink, love; yellow, driving off enemies; brown, attracting money; and black, doing evil work and bringing bad luck (Tallant, 1946, p. 226).

The following story exhibits the profound influence that belief in voodoo can have on a person. It was reported in Baltimore, Maryland, in 1967.

> The patient was a young, married black woman who was admitted to the hospital for evaluation of chest pain, syncope, and dyspnea. Her past history was one of good health. However, she had gained over 50 pounds in the past year and was given to eating Argo starch. She began to have symptoms 1 month before she was admitted. Her condition grew worse once in the hospital, and she was treated for heart failure and also for pulmonary embolism. She revealed that she had a serious problem. She had been born on Friday, the thirteenth, in the Okefenokee Swamp and was delivered by a midwife who delivered three children that day. The midwife told the mothers that the children were hexed and that the first would die before her 16th

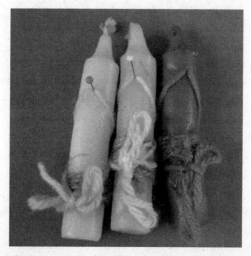

Figure 11–6   Voodoo candles.

birthday, the second before her 21st birthday, and the third (the patient) before her 23rd birthday. The first girl was a passenger in a car involved in a fatal crash the day before her 16th birthday, the second girl was celebrating her 21st birthday in a saloon when a stray bullet hit and killed her. This patient also believed she was doomed. She, too, died—on August 12—a day before her 23rd birthday. (Webb, 1971, pp. 1–3)

There are a number of Catholic saints or relics to whom or to which the practitioners of voodoo attribute special powers. Portraits of Saint Michael, who makes possible the conquest of enemies; Saint Anthony de Padua, who brings luck; Saint Mary Magdalene, who is popular with women who are in love; the Virgin Mary, whose presence in the home prevents illness; and the Sacred Heart of Jesus, which cures organic illness, may be prominently displayed in the homes of people who believe in voodoo (Tallant, 1946, p. 228). These gris-gris are available today and can be purchased in stores in many American cities.

Other Practices.　Many Blacks believe in the power of some people to HEAL and help others, and there are many reports of numerous HEALERS among the communities. This reliance on HEALERS reflects the deep religious faith of the people. (Maya Angelou vividly describes this phenomenon in her book *I Know Why the Caged Bird Sings.*) For example, many Blacks followed the Pentecostal movement long before its present more general popularity. Similarly, people often went to tent meetings and had an all-consuming belief in the HEALING powers of religion.

Another practice takes on significance when one appreciates its historical background: the eating of Argo starch. "Geophagy," or eating clay and dirt, occurred among the slaves, who brought the practice to this country from Africa. In *Roots*, Haley mentions that pregnant women were given clay because it was believed to be beneficial to both the mother and the unborn child (Haley, 1976, p. 32). In fact, red clays are rich in iron. When clay was not available, dirt was substituted. In more modern times, when people were no longer living on farms and no longer had access to clay and dirt, Argo starch became the substitute (Dunstin, 1969). The following was reported by a former student:

> It was my fortune, or misfortune to be born into a family that practiced geophagy (earth eating) and pica (eating Argo laundry starch). Even before I became pregnant I showed an interest in eating starch. It was sweet and dry, and I could take it or leave it. After I became pregnant, I found I wanted not only starch, but bread, grits, and potatoes. I found I craved starchy substances. I stuck to starchy substances and dropped the Argo because it made me feel sluggish and heavy.

It is believed that anemia arose from this practice of substituting non–iron-rich clays or starch for red clays that contain iron. Table 11–1 illustrates examples of cultural phenomena that affect health care among Blacks. Many Black Americans and new immigrants from African countries are Muslims. Box 11–2 presents an overview of Islam and information that must be known in health care settings.

Table 11–1 Examples of Cultural Phenomena Affecting Health Care Among Black or African Americans

Nations of Origin	Many West African countries (as slaves) Ethiopia Nigeria West Indian Islands Dominican Republic Haiti Jamaica
Environmental Control	Traditional HEALTH and ILLNESS beliefs may continue to be observed by "traditional" people and new immigrants
Biological Variations	Sickle-cell anemia Hypertension Cancer of the esophagus Stomach cancer Coccidioidomycosis Lactose intolerance
Social Organization	Family: many single-parent households headed by females Large, extended family networks Strong church affiliations within community Community social organizations
Communication	National languages Dialect: Pidgin French, Spanish, Creole
Space	Close personal space
Time Orientation	Present over future

Source: Spector, R. (1992). Culture, ethnicity, and nursing. In P. Potter & A. Perry (Eds.), *Fundamentals of Nursing* (3rd ed.). St. Louis, MO: Mosby-Year Book. Reprinted with permission. This material was published in Potter & Perry's Fundamentals of Nursing, Jackie Crisp and Catherine Taylor (Eds), Copyright Elsevier (2009).

 Box 11–2

Black Muslims

Today, there about five and one-half million Muslims in the United States and many members of the Black community are practicing Muslims. The religion of Islam is the acceptance of and obedience to the teachings of God, which He revealed to His last prophet, Muhammad. The Five Pillars of Islam are the framework of Muslim life. They are the testimony of faith, prayer, giving *zakat* (support of the needy), fasting during the month of Ramadan, and the pilgrimage to Mecca once in a lifetime for those who are able (see Figure 11–7).

The people may be descendants of the earlier people who were Muslims and came to America as slaves, or they have chosen to convert to Islam. However, it is difficult to generalize in any way about American Muslims because the people come from all walks of life—converts, immigrants, factory workers,

(continued)

Box 11–2 *Continued*

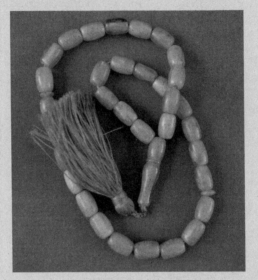

Figure 11–7   Islamic prayer beads.

doctors, professionals, and so forth. In addition, there are many African immigrants from countries, such as the Sudan, who are practicing Muslims, and countless people from Islamic countries are seeking health care services in the United States. The community is unified by a common faith.

Religious beliefs are an important part of the Muslim lifestyle, and health care providers should be familiar with them:

- Muslims are taught that a "person is what he or she eats." Islamic dietary restrictions consist of eating a strictly Halal diet, and a newly admitted patient who refuses to eat should be asked if the hospital's ordinary diet interferes with his or her religious beliefs. The rules of a Halal diet include not eating pork or any pork products (such as nonbeef hamburger and ham). Islamic law teaches that certain foods affect the way a person thinks and acts. Therefore, one's diet should consist of food that has a clean, positive effect. Muslims do not drink alcohol because they feel that it dulls the senses and causes illness. Halal foods are produced using equipment that is cleansed according to Islamic law.
- Muslims pray 5 times a day. Each prayer does not take more than a few minutes and is offered at dawn, noon, mid-afternoon, sunset, and night in almost any setting, such as in fields, offices, factories, universities, or hospitals. Prayer in Islam is a direct link between the worshipper and God. Before a person prays, he or she must be clean and the hands and feet are washed. Prayers are generally said in a prostrate position on a carpet on the floor.
- Muslims fast for a 30-day period during the year (fast of Ramadan). Ramadan is a special time—a month of prayer and repentance. Nothing is taken

by mouth from just before sunrise until after sundown. Ill Muslims, small children, and pregnant women are exempt from this rule. When a person is following the fast, institutions must provide the environment for the safe observance of the practice.

There is also a practice of modesty, with women covering their heads with scarves, *hijabs*, and wearing long dresses, *jibabs*. The need for gender-specific care—that is, males caring for male patients and females caring for female patients, must be adhered to.

The Muslim lifestyle is strictly regulated. According to those who have practiced the religion for many generations, this stems in part from the need for self-discipline, which many Black people have not had because of living conditions associated with urban decay and family disintegration. Muslims believe in self-help and assist in uplifting each other. The Muslim lifestyle is not so rigid that the people do not have good times. Good times, however, are tempered with the realization that too much indulgence in sport and play can present problems. To Muslims, life is precious: if a person needs a transfusion to live, it will be accepted. Because of the avoidance of pork or pork products, however, it is important to understand that a diabetic Muslim will refuse to take insulin that has a pork base. If the insulin is manufactured from the pancreas of a pig, it is considered unclean and will not be accepted. There are preparations of insulin and/or other products that can be prescribed.

Many Muslim communities differ in their practice and philosophy of Islam. Members of some communities dress in distinctive clothing—for example, the women wear long skirts and a covering on the head at all times. Other communities are less strict about dress. Some adherents do not follow the Halal diet and are allowed to drink alcoholic beverages in moderation.

Sources: Ibrahim, I. A. (1996) A Brief Illustrated Guide to Understanding Islam. Houston, Texas: Darussalam. Retrieved from http://www.islam-guide.com/, July 6, 2011; Office of Dawah. (2006–2008). The Religion of Islam. Rawdah: Author. Retrieved from http://www.islamreligion.com/, July 6, 2011.

■ Current Health Problems

Health Differences between Black and White Populations

Morbidity.   Many Black people experience wide, deep health disparities—factors such as the lack of access to health services, low income, and a tendency to self-treat illness and to wait until symptoms are so severe that a doctor must be seen (Weissman, Betancourt, Green, et al. 2011). When statistical adjustments are made for age, Blacks exceed Whites in the average number of days spent in acute care settings, on bed rest, and in restricted activity. Adolescent pregnancy is a major concern with the population. The risk of infant mortality and low birth weight are also greater in the community, as is the rate of low-birth-weight babies. Table 11–2 compares selected health status indicators for Blacks and all races. It illustrates that the birth rate is higher, that the percentages of women not getting early prenatal care and third-trimester or

Table 11-2 Comparison of Selected Health Status Indicators—All Races and Black or African American: 2007

Health Indicator	All Races	Black or African Americans
Crude birth rate per 1,000 population by race of mother	14.3	16.6
Percentage of live births to women receiving prenatal care first trimester	67.5	57.0
Percentage of live births to women receiving third-trimester prenatal care or no prenatal care	8.4	12.6
Percentage of live births to teenage childbearing women under 18	3.4	6.1
Percentage of low birth weight per live births <2,500 grams	8.22	13.55
Infant mortality per 1,000 live births (2006)	6.7	12.9
Cancer—all sites per 100,000 population	446.7	470.0
Lung cancer incidence per 100,000 population	Men: 65.4 Women: 47.4	Men: 87.2 Women: 51.2
Breast cancer incidence per 100,000	122.5	120.5
Prostate cancer incidence per 100,000	158.3	152.0
Male death rates from suicide, all ages, age adjusted per 100,000 resident population	11.3	8.8
Male death rates from homicide, all ages, age adjusted per 100,000 resident population	6.1	37.1

Source: National Center for Health Statistics. Health, United States, 2010: With Special Feature on Death and Dying. Hyattsville, MD. 2011: Author, pp. 102, 106, 107, 110, 124, 137, 180–181, 184–185, and 204. Retrieved from http://www.cdc.gov/nchs/, June 9, 2011.

no prenatal care are higher, and that the percentage of teenage births to women under 18 is nearly double, as is the infant mortality rate.

Sickle-Cell Anemia.   The sickling of red blood cells is a genetically inherited trait that is hypothesized to have originally been an African adaptation to fight malaria. This condition occurs in Africans/Blacks and causes the normal, disk-like red blood cell to assume a sickle shape. Sickling results in hemolysis and thrombosis of red blood cells because these deformed cells do not flow properly through the blood vessels. Sickle-cell disease comprises the following blood characteristics:

1. The presence of 2 hemoglobin-S genes (Hb SS)
2. The presence of the hemoglobin-S gene with another abnormal hemoglobin gene (Hb SC, Hb SD, etc.)
3. The presence of the hemoglobin-S gene with a different abnormality in hemoglobin synthesis

Some people (carriers) have the sickle-cell trait (Hb SS, Hb SC, or others) but do not experience symptoms of the disease.

The clinical manifestations of sickle-cell disease include hemolysis, anemia, and states of sickle-cell crises, in which severe pain occurs in the areas of the body where the thrombosed red cells are located. The cells also tend to clump in abdominal organs, such as the liver and the spleen. At present, statistics indicate that only 50% of children with sickle-cell disease live to adulthood. Some children die before the age of 20, and some suffer chronic, irreversible complications during their lifetime (A.D.A.M. Medical Encyclopedia, 2012).

Sickle-cell anemia can only occur when 2 people who carry sickle-cell trait have a child together. It is possible to detect the sickle-cell trait in healthy adults and to provide genetic counseling about their risk of bearing children with the disease. However, for many people, this is not an option. The cost of genetic counseling, for example, may be prohibitive (A.D.A.M. Medical Encyclopedia, 2012).

Mortality. Blacks born in 2000 in the United States will live, on average, 5.7 fewer years than Whites. The life expectancy for a Black person born in 2007 was 73.6 years, whereas for a White person born in 2007 it was 78.4 years.

The leading 3 chronic diseases that are causes of death for African Americans are the same as those for Whites, but the rates are greater in other diseases. For example:

■ The number of people living with end-stage renal disease per million on December 31, 2007, was 1,698.2—of this total, the prevalence was 4,122.8, Black, and 1,294.6, White.

■ Coronary heart disease death rates are higher for Blacks—305.9/100,000 age adjusted, than for Whites—234.8/100,000 age adjusted.

■ Among women, non-Hispanic Black women had the highest obesity rates.

■ Black men experience a higher risk of cancer of the prostate than White men do.

■ Homicide is the most frequent cause of death for Black American men between the ages of 25 and 34. The rate in 2007 was 82.5 per 100,000 resident population, whereas for White males of the same age it was 9.9 per 100,000.

■ The rate of HIV/AIDS among Black American men is generally higher than that for White men and the mortality rate for Black men, all ages, age adjusted, is 24.5/100,000; for ages 45–64, the rate is 58.3/100,000 and this is the highest rate (NCHS, 2011).

Table 11–3 lists the 10 leading causes of death for Black Americans and compares them with the causes of death for the general population in 2007.

Mental Health Traditions

The family often has a matriarchal structure, and there are many single-parent households headed by females, but there are strong and large extended family networks. There is a continuation of tradition and a strong church affiliation

Table 11-3 **Comparison of the 10 Leading Causes of Death for Black or African American and for All Persons: 2004**

Black or African American	All Persons
1. Diseases of heart	Diseases of heart
2. Malignant neoplasms	Malignant neoplasms
3. Cerebrovascular diseases	Cerebrovascular diseases
4. Unintentional injuries	Chronic lower respiratory diseases
5. Diabetes mellitus	Unintentional injuries
6. Homicide	Alzheimer's disease
7. Nephritis, nephrotic syndrome, and nephrosis influenza and pneumonia	Diabetes mellitus
8. Chronic lower respiratory diseases	Influenza and pneumonia
9. Human immunodeficiency virus (HIV) disease	Nephritis, nephrotic syndrome, and nephrosis
10. Septicemia	Septicemia

Source: National Center for Health Statistics. Health, United States, 2010: With Special Feature on Death and Dying. Hyattsville, MD. 2011: Author, pp. 146–147. Retrieved from http://www.cdc.gov/nchs/, June 9, 2011.

within the families and community. Members of the community may be treated by a traditional Voodoo priest, the "Old Lady" ("granny" or "Mrs. Markus"), or other traditional healers, and herbs are frequently used to treat mental symptoms. Several diagnostic techniques include the use of biblical phrases and/or material from old folk medical books, observation, and/or entering the spirit of the patient. The therapeutic measures include various rituals, such as the reading of bones, the wearing of special garments, or some rituals from voodoo (Spurlock, 1988, p. 173). In addition, there are countless culture-bound mental HEALTH syndromes that may be identified in the Black community:

- West Africa and Haiti—*Boufée delirante*—the sudden outburst of agitated and aggressive behavior, confusion, or occasional hallucinations
- Southern United States and Caribbean groups—Falling-Out—sudden collapse without warning
- North African countries—Zar—person is possessed by a spirit and may shout, weep, laugh, hit his or her head against the wall, or sing
- West Africa—Brain Fog—physical and mental exhaustion, difficulty concentrating, memory loss, irritability, and sleeping and appetite problems (Fontaine, 2003, p. 119).

Blacks and the Health Care System

To some, receiving health care is all too often a degrading and humiliating experience. In many settings, Black patients continue to be viewed as beneath the White health caregiver. Quite often, the insult is a subtle part of experiencing the health care system. The insult may be intentional or unintentional.

An intentional insult is, of course, a blatant remark or mistreatment. An unintentional insult is more difficult to define. A health care provider may not intend to demean a person, yet an action or a tone of voice may be interpreted as insulting. The provider may have some covert, underlying fears or difficulties in relating to Blacks, but the patient quite often senses the difficulty. An unintentional insult may occur because the provider is not fully aware of the patient's background and is unable to comprehend many of the patient's beliefs and practices. The patient, for example, may be afraid of the impending medical procedures and the possibility of misdiagnosis or mistreatment. It is not a secret among the people of the Black community that those who receive care in public clinics and hospitals—and even in clinics of private institutions—are the "material" on whom students practice and on whom medical research is done.

Some Blacks fear or resent health clinics. When they have a clinic appointment, they usually lose a day's work because they have to be at the clinic at an early hour and often spend many hours waiting to be seen by a physician. They often receive inadequate care, are told what their problem is in incomprehensible medical jargon, and are not given an identity, being seen rather as a body segment ("the appendix in treatment room A"). Such an experience creates a tremendous feeling of powerlessness and alienation from the system. In some parts of the country, segregation and racism are overt. There continue to be reports of hospitals that refuse admission to Black patients. In one case, a Black woman in labor was not admitted to a hospital because she had not "paid the bill from the last baby." There was not enough time to get her to another hospital, and she was forced to deliver in an ambulance. In light of this type of treatment, it is no wonder that some Black people prefer to use time-tested home remedies rather than be exposed to the humiliating experiences of hospitalization.

Another reason for the ongoing use of home remedies is poverty. Indigent people cannot afford the high costs of American health care. Quite often—even with the help of Medicaid and Medicare—the hidden costs of acquiring health services, such as absence from work, transportation, and/or child care, are a heavy burden. As a result, Blacks may stay away from clinics or outpatient departments or receive their care with passivity while appearing to the provider to be evasive. Some Black patients believe that they are being talked down to by health care providers and that the providers fail to listen to them. They choose, consequently, to "suffer in silence." Many of the problems that Blacks relate in dealing with the health care system can apply to anyone, but the inherent racism within the health system cannot be denied. Currently, efforts are being made to overcome these barriers.

Since the 1960s, health care services available to Blacks and other people of color have improved. A growing number of community health centers have emphasized health maintenance and promotion. Community residents serve on the boards.

Among the services provided by community health centers is an effort to discover children with high blood levels of lead in order to provide early diagnosis of and treatment for lead poisoning. Once a child is found to have lead poisoning, the law requires that the source of the lead be found and eradicated.

Today, only apartments free of lead paint can be rented to families with young children. Apartments that are found to have lead paint must be stripped and repainted with nonlead paint. Another ongoing effort by the community health centers is to inform Blacks who are at risk of producing children with sickle-cell anemia that they are carriers of this genetic disease. This program is fraught with conflict because many people prefer not to be screened for the sickle-cell trait, fearing they may become labeled once the tendency is discovered.

Birth control is another problem that is recognized with mixed emotions. To some, especially women who want to space children or who do not want to have numerous children, birth control is a welcome development. People who believe in birth control prefer selecting the time when they will have children, how many children they will have, and when they will stop having children. To many other people, birth control is considered a form of "Black genocide" and a way of limiting the growth of the community. Health workers in the Black community must be aware of both sides of this issue and, if asked to make a decision, remain neutral. Such decisions must be made by the patients themselves.

Special Considerations for Health Care Providers

White health care providers know far too little about how to care for a Black person's skin or hair, or how to understand both Black nonverbal and verbal behavior.

Physiological Assessment. Examples of possible physiological problems include the following (in observing skin problems, it is important to note that skin assessment is best done in indirect sunlight) (Bloch & Hunter, 1981):

1. **Pallor.** There is an absence of underlying red tones; the skin of a brown-skinned person appears yellow-brown, and that of a black-skinned person appears ashen gray. Mucous membranes appear ashen, and the lips and nailbeds are similar.

2. **Erythema.** Inflammation must be detected by palpation; the skin is warmer in the area, tight, and edematous, and the deeper tissues are hard. Fingertips must be used for this assessment, as with rashes, since they are sensitive to the feeling of different textures of skin.

3. **Cyanosis.** Cyanosis is difficult to observe in dark-colored skin, but it can be seen by close inspection of the lips, tongue, conjunctiva, palms of the hands, and soles of the feet. One method of testing is pressing the palms. Slow blood return is an indication of cyanosis. Another sign is ashen gray lips and tongue.

4. **Ecchymosis.** History of trauma to a given area can be detected from a swelling of the skin surface.

5. **Jaundice.** The sclera are usually observed for yellow discoloration to reveal jaundice. This is not always a valid indication, however, since

carotene deposits can also cause the sclera to appear yellow. The buccal mucosa and the palms of the hands and soles of the feet may appear yellow.

Several skin conditions are of importance in Black patients (Sykes & Kelly, 1979):

1. **Keloids.** Keloids are scars that form at the site of a wound and grow beyond the normal boundaries of the wound. They are sharply elevated and irregular and continue to enlarge.
2. **Pigmentary disorders.** Pigmentary disorders, areas of either postinflammatory hypopigmentation or hyperpigmentation, appear as dark or light spots.
3. **Pseudofolliculitis.** "Razor bumps" and "ingrown hairs" are caused by shaving too closely with an electric razor or straight razor. The sharp point of the hair, if shaved too close, enters the skin and induces an immune response as to a foreign body. The symptoms include papules, pustules, and sometimes even keloids.
4. **Melasma.** The "mask of pregnancy," melasma, is a patchy tan to dark brown discoloration of the face more prevalent in dark pregnant women.

Hair Care Needs. The care of the hair of Blacks is not complicated, but special consideration must be given to help maintain its healthy condition (Bloch & Hunter, 1981):

1. The hair's dryness or oiliness must be assessed, as well as its texture (straight or extra curly) and the patient's hairstyle preference.
2. The hair must be shampooed as needed and groomed according to the person's preference.
3. Hair must be combed well, with the appropriate tools, such as a "pic" or comb with big teeth, before drying to prevent tangles.
4. If the hair is dry and needs oiling, the preparations that the person generally uses for this purpose ought to be on hand.
5. Once dry, the hair is ready to be styled (curled, braided, or rolled) as the person desires.

Additional Considerations. The majority of the members of the health care profession are steeped in a middle-class White value system. In clinical settings, providers are being helped to become familiar with and understand the value systems of other ethnic and socioeconomic groups. They are being taught to recognize the symptoms of illness in Blacks and to provide proper skin and hair care. The following are guidelines that a health care provider can follow in caring for members of the Black community:

1. The education of an ever-increasing number of Blacks in the health professions must continue to be encouraged.

2. The needs of the patient must be assessed realistically.

3. When a treatment or special diet is prescribed, every attempt must be made to ascertain whether it is consistent with the patient's physical needs, cultural background, income, and religious practices.

4. The patient's belief in and practice of folk medicine must be respected; the patient must not be criticized for these beliefs. Every effort should be made to assist the patient to combine folk treatment with standard Western treatment, as long as the two are not antagonistic. Many people who have a strong belief in folk remedies continue to use them with or without medical sanction.

5. Providers should be familiar with formal and informal sources of help in the Black community. The formal sources consist of churches, social clubs, and community groups. The informal ones include the women who provide care for members of their community in an informal way.

6. The beliefs and values of the health care provider should not be forced on the patient.

7. The treatment plan and the reasons for a given treatment must be shared with the patient.

Black American Health Care Manpower

As seen in Table 11–4, it is evident that the numbers of Blacks enrolled in the health professions' schools is well below the percentage (14%) of Black alone-or-in-combination population in the American society at large.

Recent nursing data are not included in the overall health professions' enrollment data in Table 11–4. However, the National Sample Survey of Registered Nurses for 2008 prepared by the United States Department of Health and Human Services (2010) provides relevant information regarding the demographic profile of American Registered Nurses. It estimates that the registered nurse population in the United States in 2008 was 3,063,162, with 2,596,599

Table 11–4 Percentage of Black or African Americans Enrolled in Selected Health Professions Schools Compared with Non-Hispanic Whites: 2007–2008

	Number Enrolled	Non-Hispanic Whites (%)	Black or African American (%)
Dentistry	19,342	60.6	5.9
Allopathic Medicine	74,518	62.4	7.2
Osteopathic Medicine	15,634	70.5	3.8
Optometry	5,556	60.3	3.1
Pharmacy	50,691	59.5	6.4
Podiatry	2,095	62.2	10.7
Public Health	22,604	59.3	11.7

Source: National Center for Health Statistics. Health, United States, 2010: With Special Feature on Death and Dying. Hyattsville, MD. 2011: Author, pp. 352–353. Retrieved from http://www.cdc.gov/nchs/, June 9, 2011.

registered nurses employed in nursing. Of this number, 83.2% were White (non-Hispanic) and 5.4% were Black/African American (non-Hispanic). Given that in 2010 the White alone population was 63% of the total population and Black/African American (non-Hispanic) people comprised 12.6% of the resident population, this is a clear indication that there is no demographic parity in the percentage of Black/African American (non-Hispanic) people in nursing. This demographic picture and the percentages in the tables demonstrate a situation that is an ongoing concern. Somnath and Shipman (2006), who reviewed a total of 55 studies, found that minority patients tend to receive better interpersonal care from practitioners of their own race or ethnicity, particularly in primary care and mental health settings, and that non–English speaking patients experience better interpersonal care, greater medical comprehension, and greater likelihood of keeping follow-up appointments when they see a language-concordant practitioner. They concluded their study by stating that "the findings indicated greater health professions diversity will likely lead to improved public health by increasing access to care for underserved populations, and by increasing opportunities for minority patients to see practitioners with whom they share a common race, ethnicity or language." They also stated that "race, ethnicity, and language concordance, which is associated with better patient-practitioner relationships and communication, may increase patients' likelihood of receiving and accepting appropriate medical care" (p. 17).

RESEARCH ON CULTURE

A large amount of research has been conducted among members of the Black population. The study described in the following article is one example:

> Wilson, D. W. (2007). From their own voices: The lived experience of African American registered nurses. Journal of Transcultural Nursing, 18(2), 142–149.

This phenomenological study describes the lived experiences of African American nurses who provide care to individuals, families, and communities in southeast Louisiana. The sample consisted of 13 nurses whose ages ranged from 40 to 62, with an average age of 49.53. Their nursing experience ranged from 8 to 39 years and they were educated in ad, diploma, and baccalaureate programs. Four of the informants had earned master's degrees in nursing. The essential themes found in the study were that the participants' experiences included connecting with the patients through the delivery of holistic nursing care and "proving yourself." Holistic care included respect for the patients' cultural backgrounds and the realization that in many ways they were vitally important in meeting the needs of the patients and families. They believed that they were also important in meeting the spiritual and religious needs of patients. The nurses also participated in patient teaching and advocacy. The incidental themes included fulfilling a dream, being invisible and voiceless, surviving and persevering, and mentoring and role modeling. The author recommends that, if the nursing profession is to promote nursing care that is congruent with the needs of culturally diverse patients, it must increase the representation of African American registered nurses.

Explore 🌐 MediaLink

Go to the Student Resource Site at nursing.pearsonhighered.com for chapter-related review questions, case studies, and activities. Contents of the CULTURALCARE Guide and CULTURALCARE Museum can also be found on the Student Resource Site. Click on Chapter 11 to select the activities for this chapter.

Box 11–3: Keeping Up

It goes without saying that much of the data presented in this chapter may be out of date when you read this text. However, at this final stage of writing, it is the most recent information available. The following resources will be most helpful in keeping you abreast of the frequent changes in health care events, costs, and policies:

1. The National Center for Health Statistics publishes Health, United States an annual report on trends in health statistics. It can be retrieved from http://www.cdc.gov/nchs/hus.htm. Health, United States, 11 is not available, and Health, United States, 12 will be published in May, 2012.
2. Health-related data and other statistics are available from http://www.cdc.gov/DataStatistics/.
3. The Centers for Disease Control and Prevention aims to eliminate health disparities for vulnerable populations as defined by race/ethnicity, socio-economic status, geography, gender, age, disability status, risk status related to sex and gender, and among other populations identified to be at-risk for health disparities. Current, pertinent information is available at http://www.cdc.gov/omhd/topic/healthdisparities.html.

■ Internet Sources

A.D.A.M. Medical Encyclopedia. (2012). Sickle cell anemia. Retrieved from http://www.ncbi.nlm.nih.gov/pubmedhealth/PMH0001554/, March 12, 2012.

Brunner, B., & Haney, E. (2009). Civil Rights Timeline: Milestones in the Modern Civil Rights Movement. Upper Saddle River, NJ: Pearson Education. Retrieved from http://www.infoplease.com/spot/civilrightstimeline1.html, July 2, 2011.

Ibrahim, I. A. (2002). A Brief Illustrated Guide to Understanding Islam. Houston, Texas: Darussalam. Retrieved from http://www.islam-guide.com/frm-editors.htm, July 6, 2011.

Lee, J. (2011). Annual Flow Report U.S. Naturalizations: 2010. Washington, DC: U.S. Department of Commerce, Economics and Statistics Administration, Office of Homeland Security, Office of Immigration Statistics. Retrieved from http://www.dhs.gov/files/statistics/publications/gc_1302103955524.shtm, June 1, 2011.

Manderschied, R. W., Thomas, D., Wright, D., & Zinder, K. (2010). *Mental health, United States, 2008*. Washington, DC: Center for Mental Health Services and National Institute of Mental Health, DHHS Pub. No. (SMA) 10-4590, U.S. Government Printing Office. Retrieved from http://store.samhsa.gov/product/Mental-Health-United-States-2008/SMA10-4590, July 6, 2011.

Monger, R., & Yankay, J. (2011). U.S. Legal Permanent Residents: 2010 Annual Flow Report. Washington, DC: U.S. Department of Commerce, Economics and Statistics Administration, Office of Homeland Security, Office of Immigration Statistics. Retrieved from http://www.dhs.gov/files/statistics/publications/gc_1301497627185.shtm, June 1, 2011.

National Center for Health Statistics. (2011). Health, United States, 2010: With Special Feature on Death and Dying. Hyattsville, MD: Author. Retrieved from http://www.cdc.gov/nchs/, June 9, 2011.

Office of Dawah. (2006–2008). The Religion of Islam. Rawdah: Author. Retrieved, from http://www.islamreligion.com/, July 6, 2011.

Rastogi, S., Johnson, T., Hoeffel, E., & Drewery, M., Jr. (2011). The Black Population: 2010. Washington, DC: U.S. Department of Commerce. Retrieved from http://2010.census.gov/2010census/data/, December 2, 2011.

Somnath, S., & Shipman, S. (2006). The Rationale for Diversity in the Health Professions: A Review of the Evidence. Washington, DC: U.S. Department of Health and Human Services, Health Resources and Services Administration, Bureau of Health Professions. Retrieved from http://www.hrsa.gov/, July 6, 2011.

United States Census Bureau (2011) American Community Survey 1-year estimates. Retrieved from http://factfinder2.census.gov/faces/tableservices/jsf/pages/productview.xhtml?pid=ACS_10_1YR_S1701&prodType=table, March 13, 2011.

United States Census Bureau. (2012). Statistical Abstract of the United States: 2012. Retrieved from http://2010.census.gov/2010census/data/, December 2, 2011.

United States Department of Health and Human Services. (2010). The Registered Nurse Population Findings from the March 2008 National Sample Survey of Registered Nurses. Washington, DC: Author. Retrieved from ftp://ftp.hrsa.gov/bhpr/workforce/0306rnss.pdf, July 6, 2008.

Weissman, J.S., Betancourt, J. R., Green, A. R., Meyer, G. S., Tan-McGrory, A., Nudel, J.D., Zeidman, J. A., & Carrillo, J. E. (2011) *Commissioned paper: Healthcare Disparities Measurement*. National Quality Forum. Retrieved from http://www2.massgeneral.org/disparitiessolutions/z_files/Disparities%20Commissioned%20Paper.pdf, March 14, 2012.

References

Bass, P. H., & Pugh, K. (2001). *In our own image—Treasured African-American traditions, journeys, and icons*. Philadelphia: Running Press.

Blackmon, D. A. (2008). *Slavery by another name*. New York: Doubleday.

Bloch, B., & Hunter, M. L. (1981, January–February). Teaching physiological assessment of Black persons. *Nurse Educator*, 26.

Bullough, B., & Bullough, V. L. (1972). *Poverty, ethnic identity, and health care.* New York: Appleton-Century-Crofts.

Davis, R. (1998). *American voudou—Journey into a hidden world.* Denton: University of North Texas Press.

Dunstin, B. (1969). Pica during pregnancy. Chap. 26 in *Current concepts in clinical nursing.* St. Louis, MO: Mosby.

Eck, D. (1994). *African religion in America: On common ground.* New York: Columbia University Press.

Fontaine, K. L. (2003). *Mental health nursing* (5th ed.). Upper Saddle River, NJ: Prentice Hall.

Gutman, H. G. (1976). The Black family in slavery and freedom, 1750–1925. New York: Pantheon.

Haley, A. (1976). *Roots.* New York: Doubleday.

Hughes, L., & Bontemps, A. (Eds.), (1958). *The book of negro folklore.* New York: Dodd, Mead.

Jacques, G. (1976). Cultural health traditions: A Black perspective. In M. Branch & P. P. Paxton (Eds.), *Providing safe nursing care for ethnic people of color.* New York: Appleton-Century-Crofts.

Kain, J. F. (Ed.). (1969). *Race and poverty.* Englewood Cliffs, NJ: Prentice Hall.

Kotlowitz, A. (1991). *There are no children here: The story of two boys growing up in the other America.* New York: Doubleday.

Spector, R. (1992). Culture, ethnicity, and nursing. In P. Potter & A. Perry (Eds.), *Fundamentals of Nursing* (3rd ed.). St. Louis, MO: Mosby-Year Book.

Spurlock, J. (1988). Black Americans. In L. Comas-Diaz & E. E. H. Griffith (Eds.), *Cross-cultural mental health.* New York: John Wiley & Sons.

Sykes, J., & Kelly, A. P. (1979, June). Black skin problems. *American Journal of Nursing,* 1092–1094.

Tallant, R. (1946). *Voodoo in New Orleans* (7th printing). New York: Collier.

Webb, J. Y. (1971). Letter. Dr. J. R. Krevans to Y. Webb, 15 February 1967. Reported in Superstitious influence—Voodoo in particular—Affecting health practices in a selected population in southern Louisiana. Paper. New Orleans, LA.

Wintrob, R. (1972). Hexes, roots, snake eggs? M.D. vs. occults. *Medical Opinion, 1*(7), 54–61.

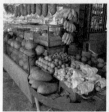
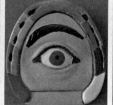
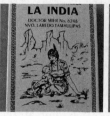
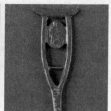

Figure 12-1 **Figure 12-2** **Figure 12-3** **Figure 12-4**

Chapter 12

HEALTH and ILLNESS
in the Hispanic Populations

My heart is in the earth . . .

—*Greenhaw (2000)*

■ Objectives

1. Discuss the background of members of selected communities of the Hispanic populations.
2. Discuss the demographic profile of selected communities of the Hispanic populations.
3. Describe the traditional definitions of *HEALTH* and *ILLNESS* of selected communities of the Hispanic populations.
4. Describe the traditional methods of HEALTH maintenance and protection of selected communities of the Hispanic populations.
5. Describe the traditional methods of HEALING of selected communities of the Hispanic populations.
6. Describe current health care problems of the Hispanic populations.
7. Describe demographic disparity as it is seen in the health manpower distribution of the Hispanic populations as represented in the health care delivery system.

The opening images for this chapter depict a place and objects symbolic of items used to maintain, protect, and/or restore HEALTH for people in the Hispanic communities. Figure 12–1 is a fruit stand where tropical fruits such as papayas are sold—part of a balanced diet for health maintenance. Figure 12–2 is an "eye" from Cuba. This ceramic eye can be hung in the home for protection and would be seen as an object that would protect the family members from the harm that could be caused by jealous neighbors. Figure 12–3 is a box that contains an herbal preparation to treat a kidney malady. It can be purchased in a grocery store or *botanica*. Figure 12–4 is a crutch, or *milagro*, that could be brought to a church and placed on a statue of a saint, usually Saint Lazarus.

■ Background

The largest emerging majority group in the United States is composed of the Hispanic or Latino populations. According to the 2010 Census, of the 308.7 million people who resided in the United States on April 1, 2010, 50.5 million—16%—were of Hispanic or Latino origin. The Hispanic population was 13% of the total population in 2000. In fact, more than half of the growth in the total population of the United States between 2000 and 2010 was due to the increase in the Hispanic population. About three-quarters of Hispanics reported as Mexican, Puerto Rican, or Cuban origin. More than three-quarters of the Hispanic population lived in the West or South; 41% of Hispanics lived in the West and 36% lived in the South. The Northeast and Midwest accounted for 14% and 9%, respectively, of the Hispanic population.

The terms *Hispanic* and *Latino* are used interchangeably in Census 2010 and refer to a person of Cuban, Mexican, Puerto Rican, South or Central American, or other Spanish culture or origin regardless of race (Ennis, Rios-Vargas, & Albert, 2011, p. 2). The term will be used accordingly in this chapter. Figure 12–5 and Table 12–1 display the population distribution in 2010. They are the youngest population group with a mean age of 27.2 years.

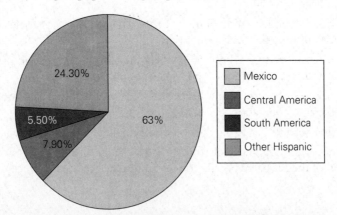

Figure 12–5   Origins of the Hispanic populations: 2010.
Source: Ennis, S. R., Rios-Vargas, M., & Albert, N. G. (2011). *The Hispanic population: 2010.* Retrieved from http://2010.census.gov/2010census/data/, December 4, 2011, p. 3.

Table 12–1 Percent Distribution of the Hispanic Population by Type of Origin: 2010

Central American	70.9%
Mexican	63.0%
South American	5.5%
Caribbean	15.5%
Cuban	3.5%
Dominican	2.8%
Puerto Rican	9.2%
All other Hispanic	8.1%

Source: Ennis, S. R., Rios-Vargas, M., & Albert, N. G. (2011). *The Hispanic population: 2010.* Retrieved from http://2010.census.gov/2010census/data/, December 4, 2011, p. 4.

Other relevant demographic data include:

■ Hispanics are more geographically concentrated than non-Hispanic Whites, with 27.8% of the population living in California, 18.7% living in Texas, 8.4% in Florida, and 6.8% in Florida (Ennis, Rios-Vargas, & Albert, 2011, p. 7).

■ Hispanics are more likely than non-Hispanic Whites to be less than 18 years old, as 34.4% of Hispanics are younger than 5 and 22.8% of the non-Hispanic White population are younger than 5.

■ Of the 1,042,625 persons who became Legal Permanent Residents in 2010, 13.3% were from Mexico, 3.2% from Cuba, 2.1% from Columbia, and 1.8% from El Salvador (Monger & Yankay, 2011, p. 4).

■ Of the 619,913 persons naturalizing in 2010, 10.8% were from Mexico, 3.0% from Colombia, 2.5% from the Dominican Republic, 2.3% from Cuba, and 1.7% from El Salvador (Lee, 2011, p. 2).

■ Hispanics were more likely than non-Hispanic Whites to live in poverty—25.3% of the Hispanic population and 9.4% of the White alone population (DeNavas-Walt, Procter, & Smith, 2010, p. 15).

■ Between 2008 and 2009, the poverty rate increased for non-Hispanic Whites (from 8.6% to 9.4%), and for Hispanics (from 23.2% to 25.3%) (DeNavas-Walt, Proctor, & Smith, 2010, p. 5).

■ The total percentage of Hispanic people over 25 who graduated from high school in 2010 was 62.9 and 13.9% graduated from college (U. S. Census Bureau, 2011, p. 151).

This section has presented a descriptive overview of the Hispanic populations as a whole; the next 2 sections describe the Mexican, or Mesoamerican, population and the Puerto Rican groups. The term *Mesoamerican* is inclusive in that it describes peoples with Mexican and Central and South American origins

(Carmack, Gasco, & Gossen, 1996, p. xvii). There is much confusion as to what their proper name is and, for the purposes of this chapter, overall government designations of *Hispanic* or *Latino* will be used for the aggregate populations and Spanish or Iberian origins and *Mexican* or *Mesoamerican* to refer to people who have a history and origins south of the United States/Mexico border.

■ Mexicans

The United States shares a 2,000-mile-long border with Mexico, which, in spite of walls and tightened security, remains easily crossed in both directions. The flow of people, goods, and ideas across it has a powerful impact on both countries.

Figure 12–6 is the fence, or wall, as it appears in Nogales, Arizona. It is an enormous structure that will eventually hug all 2,000 miles of the U.S./Mexico border. Here, you can see that it abuts the yards of families residing on the Mexican side of the border. The United States federal government is planning to complete building a wall such as this across the entire 2,000 miles of the United States/Mexico border.

Americans of Hispanic origin, according to the 2010 census, numbered at least 308.7 million people; of this number, 63.0% were of Mexican origin (Ennis, Rios-Vargas, & Albert, 2011, p. 3). The Mexicans have been in the United States for a long time, moving from Mexico and later intermarrying with Indians and Spanish people in the southwestern parts of what is now the United States. Santa Fe, New Mexico, was settled in 1609. Most of the

Figure 12-6 The fence along the United States/Mexico border; Mexico is on the right side.

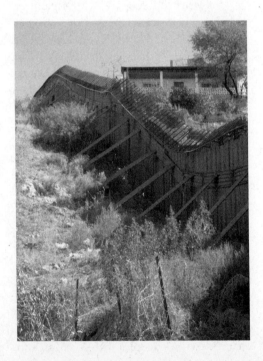

descendants of these early settlers now live in Arizona, California, Colorado, New Mexico, and Texas. A large number of Mexicans also live in Illinois, Indiana, Kansas, Michigan, Missouri, Nebraska, New York, Ohio, Utah, Washington, and Wisconsin, where most arrived as migrant farm workers. While located there as temporary farm workers, they found permanent jobs and stayed. Contrary to the popular views that Mexicans live in rural areas, most live in urban areas. Mexicans are employed in all types of jobs. Few, however, have high-paying or high-status jobs in labor or management. The majority work in factories, mines, and construction; others are employed in farm work and service areas. At present, only a small—though growing—number are employed in clerical and professional areas. The number of unemployed in this group is high, and the earnings of those employed are well below the national average. The education of Mexicans, like that of most minorities in the United States, lags behind that of most of the population. Many Mexicans fail to complete high school. In the past few years, this situation has begun to change, and Mexican children are being encouraged to stay in school, go on to college, and enter the professions.

Traditional Definitions of HEALTH and ILLNESS

There are conflicting reports about the traditional meaning of HEALTH among Mexicans. Some sources maintain that HEALTH is considered to be purely the result of "good luck" and that a person loses his or her health if that luck changes (Welch, Comer, & Steinman, 1973, p. 205). Some people describe HEALTH as a reward for good behavior. Seen in this context, HEALTH is a gift from God and should not be taken for granted. People are expected to maintain their own equilibrium in the universe by performing in the proper way, eating the proper foods, and working the proper amount of time. The protection of HEALTH is an accepted practice that is accomplished with prayer, the wearing of religious medals or amulets, and the keeping of relics in the home. Herbs and spices can be used to enhance this form of prevention, as can exemplary behavior (Lucero, 1975).ILLNESS is seen as an imbalance in an individual's body or as punishment meted out for wrongdoing. The causes of ILLNESS can be grouped into 5 major categories:

1. **The body's imbalance.** Imbalance may exist between "hot" and "cold" or "wet" and "dry." The theory of hot and cold was taken to Mexico by Spanish priests and was fused with Aztec beliefs. The concept actually dates to the early Hippocratic theory of disease and 4 body humors. The disrupted relationship among these humors is often mentioned by Mexicans as the cause of disease (Lucero, 1975).

   There are 4 body humors, or fluids: (1) blood, hot and wet; (2) yellow bile, hot and dry; (3) phlegm, cold and wet; and (4) black bile, cold and dry. When all four humors are balanced, the body is HEALTHY. When any imbalance occurs, an ILLNESS is manifested (Currier, 1966). These concepts, of course, provide one way of determining the remedy for a particular ILLNESS. For example, if an

ILLNESS is classified as hot, it is treated with a cold substance. A cold disease, in turn, must be treated with a hot substance. Food, beverages, animals, and people possess the characteristics of hot and cold to various degrees. Hot foods cannot be combined; they are to be eaten with cold foods. There is no general agreement as to what is a hot disease or food and what is a cold disease or food. The classification varies from person to person, and what is hot to one person may be cold to another (Saunders, 1958, p. 13). Therefore, if a Mexican patient refuses to eat the meals in the hospital, it is wise to ask precisely what the person can eat and what combinations of foods he or she thinks would be helpful for the existing condition. It is important to note that *hot* and *cold* do not refer to temperature but are descriptive of a particular substance itself.

For example, after a woman delivers a baby, a hot experience, she cannot eat pork, which is considered a hot food. She must eat something cold to restore her balance. Penicillin is a hot medication; therefore, it may be believed that it cannot be used to treat a hot disease. The major problem for the health care provider is to know that the rules, so to speak, of hot and cold vary from person to person. If health care providers understand the general nature of the hot and cold imbalance, they will be able to help the patient reveal the nature of the problem from the patient's perspective and manage it accordingly.

2. **Dislocation of parts of the body.** Two examples of "dislocation" are *empacho* and *caida de la mollera* (Nall & Spielberg, 1967). *Empacho* is believed to be caused by a ball of food clinging to the wall of the stomach. Common symptoms of this illness are stomach pains and cramps. This ailment is treated by rubbing and gently pinching the spine. Prayers are recited throughout the treatment. Another, more common, cause of such illness is thought to be lying about the amount of food consumed. A 20-year-old Hispanic woman experienced the acute onset of sharp abdominal pain. She complained to her friend, and together they diagnosed the problem as *empacho* and treated it by massaging her stomach and waiting for the pain to dissipate. It did not, and they continued folk treatment for 48 hours. When the pain did not diminish, they sought help in a nearby hospital. The diagnosis was acute appendicitis. The young woman nearly died and was quite embarrassed when she was scolded by the physician for not seeking help sooner.

Caida de la mollera is a more serious illness. It occurs in infants and young children aged under 1 year who are dehydrated (usually because of diarrhea or severe vomiting) and whose anterior fontanelle is depressed below the contour of the skull (Dorsey & Jackson, 1976, p. 56). Much superstition and mystery surround this problem. Some of the poorly educated and rural people, in particular, may believe that it is caused by a nurse's or physician's having touched the baby's head. This can be understood if we take into account that (1) an infant's fontanelle becomes depressed if the infant is dehydrated and (2) when physicians or nurses measure an infant's head they touch this area. If a mother takes her baby to a physician for an examination and sees the physician touch the child's head, and if the baby gets sick thereafter with *caida de la mollera*, it might be very easy for the woman to believe it is the fault of the physician's or nurse's touch. Unfortunately, epidemics of diarrhea are common in the rural and urban areas of the Southwest, and a number of children tend to be affected. One case of severe dehydration that leads to *caida de la mollera* may create quite a stir among the people. The folk treatment of this illness has not been found to be effective. Unfortunately, babies are rarely taken to the hospital in time, and the mortality rate for this illness is high (Lucero, 1975).

3. **Magic or supernatural causes outside the body.** Witchcraft or possession is considered to be culturally patterned role-playing, a safe vehicle for restoring oneself. Witchcraft or possession legitimizes acting out bizarre behavior or engaging in incoherent speech. Hispanic tradition, especially in the borderlands (the geographic area along the United States/Mexico border), blends the medieval heritage of medieval Castilian and English traditions with Mexican Indian folk beliefs (Kearney & Medrano, 2001, p. 119). *Brujas* (witches) use black, or malevolent, magic, while *curanderos* use white, or benevolent, magic. Spells may be cast to influence a lover or to get back at a rival, and cards are read to tell the future. *Herbrias* sell herbs, amulets, and talismans (Kearney & Medrano, p. 117).

   A lesser disease that is caused from outside the body is *mal ojo*. *Mal ojo* means "bad eye," and it is believed to result from excessive admiration on the part of another. General malaise, sleepiness, fatigue, and severe headache are the symptoms of this condition. The folk treatment is to find the person who has caused the illness by casting the "bad eye" and having him or her care for the afflicted person (Nall & Spielberg, 1967). The belief in the evil eye, *mal de ojo*, can be traced back to the mid-1400s and Spain (Kearney & Medrano, 2001, p. 118). It has origins that go back even further in many parts of the world. This belief is common today.

4. **Strong emotional states.** *Susto* is described as an illness arising from fright. It afflicts many people—males and females, rich and poor, rural dwellers and urbanites. It involves soul loss: The soul is able to leave the body and wander freely. This can occur while a person is dreaming or when a person experiences a particularly traumatic event. The symptoms of the disease are (1) restlessness while sleeping; (2) listlessness, anorexia, and disinterest in personal appearance when awake, including disinterest in both clothing and personal

hygiene; and (3) loss of strength, depression, and introversion. The person is treated by *curandero* (a folk healer, discussed earlier and in the section on *curanderismo*), who coaxes the soul back into the person's body. During the healing rites, the person is massaged and made to relax (Rubel, 1964).

5. *Envidia.* *Envidia*, or envy, is also considered to be a cause of illness and bad luck. Many people believe that to succeed is to fail. That is, when one's success provokes the envy of friends and neighbors, misfortune can befall the person and his or her family. For example, a successful farmer, just when he is able to purchase extra clothing and equipment, is stricken with a fatal illness. He may well attribute the cause of this illness to the envy of his peers. A number of social scientists have, after much research, concluded that the "low" economic and success rates of Mexicans can ostensibly be attributed to belief in *envidia* (Lucero, 1975).

Religious Rituals

Magico-religious practices are quite common among the Mexican population. The more severe an illness, the more likely these practices will be used. There are 4 types of practices:

1. **Making promises.** A *promesa* may be made to God or to a saint; for example, a person may promise to donate money to a cause if he or she recovers from an ILLNESS.
2. **Visiting shrines.** Many people make pilgrimages to shrines to offer prayers and gifts. This practice has origins in Jerusalem, and later Spain, with the visits to Santiago de Compostela starting in the 11th century (Kearney & Medrano, 2001, p. 110).
3. **Offering medals and candles**.
4. **Offering prayers** (Nall & Spielberg, 1967).

It is not unusual for the Mexico people residing near the southern border of the continental United States to return home to Mexico on religious pilgrimages. The film *We Believe in Niño Fedencio*, demonstrates how these pilgrimages are conducted. The lighting of candles also is a frequently observed practice. Beautiful candles made of beeswax and tallow can be purchased in many stores, particularly grocery stores and pharmacies such as Sr. Garcia's *Yerberia*, located in Mexican neighborhoods (Figures 12–7, 12–8, and 12–9). Many homes have shrines with statues and pictures of saints. The candles are lit here and prayers are recited. Some homes have altars with statues and pictures on them and are the focal point of the home. Some Mexicans are devoted to the Virgin de San Juan del Valle and make pilgrimages to the shrine in San Juan, Texas. Figure 12–10 is a *retalbo*—a painting on wood or a piece of metal that illustrates a HEALING miracle. You can see the ill person lying in bed, the person praying, and the Virgin.

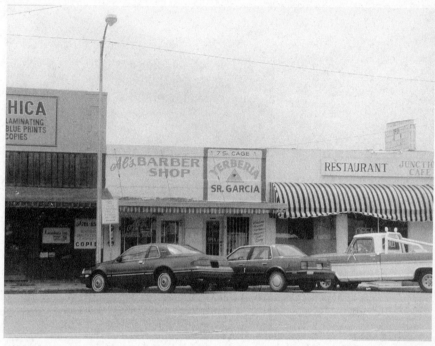

Figure 12-7   A traditional community resource *Yerberia* in Mission, Texas.

In Catholic churches in communities with Hispanic populations, such as San Antonio, Texas, or Chimayo, New Mexico (Figure 12–11), it is not unusual to see statues covered with flowers and votive figures, such as those in Figures 12–12 and 12–13. These miniature articles are known in Spanish as *milagros*, meaning "miracles," *ex-votos*, or *promesas*. They are offered to a saint in thanks for answering a person's prayers for HEALING, success, a good marriage, and so forth. The *milagros* are made from wax, wood, bone, or a variety of metals and are an integral part of an ancient folk tradition found in many cultures (Egan, 1991, pp. 1–2). This practice, too, originated in Spain and even today one can see and purchase these objects in countless churches (Kearney & Medrano, 2001, p. 115).

Curanderismo

There are no specific rules for knowing who in the community uses the services of folk healers. Not all Mexicans do, and not all Mexicans believe in their precepts. Initially, it was thought that only the poor used a folk healer, or *curandero*, because they were unable to get treatment from the larger, institutionalized health care establishments. It now appears, however, that the use of HEALERS occurs widely throughout the Mexican population. Some people try to use HEALERS exclusively, whereas others use them along with modern medical care. The HEALERS do not usually advertise, but they are well known throughout the population because of informal community and kinship networks.

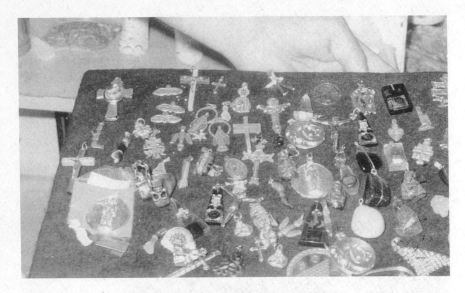

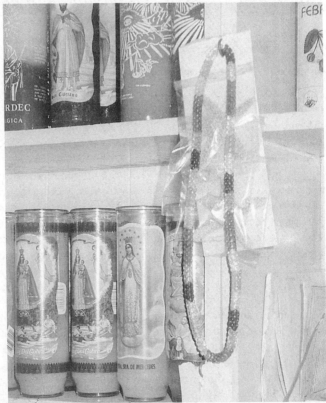

Figures 12-8 and 12-9   **Samples of amulets and candles sold in Sr. Garcia's *Yerberia.***

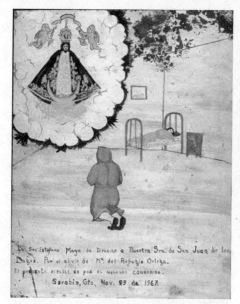

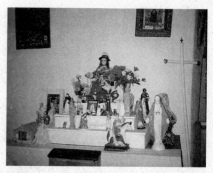

Figure 12-11 An altar in *El Santuario de Chinmayo*, Chinmayo, New Mexico.

Figure 12-10 A *retalbo* that depicts a person praying to the Virgin of San Juan de la Valle for the HEALING of a loved one.

Curanderismo is defined as a medical system (Maduro, 1976). It is a coherent view with historical roots that combine Aztec, Spanish, spiritualistic, homeopathic, and scientific elements. There are *curanderos* practicing in Spain, and there is an established community of *curanderos* in close proximity to Granada.

The *curandero(a)* is a holistic healer. The people who seek help from him or her do so for social, physical, and psychological purposes. The *curandero(a)* can be either a "specialist" or a "generalist," a full-time or part-time practitioner. Mexicans who believe in *curanderos* consider them to be religious figures.

A *curandero(a)* may receive the "gift of healing" through 3 means:

1. He or she may be "born" to heal. In this case, it is known from the moment of a *curandero(a)*'s birth that something unique about this person means that he or she is destined to be a healer.

2. He or she may learn by apprenticeship—that is, the person is taught the ways of healing, especially the use of herbs.

3. He or she may receive a "calling" through a dream, trance, or vision by which contact is made with the supernatural by means of a "patron" (or "caller"), who may be a saint. The "call" comes either during adolescence or during the midlife crisis. This "call" is resisted at first. Later, the person becomes resigned to his or her fate and gives in to the demands of the "calling."

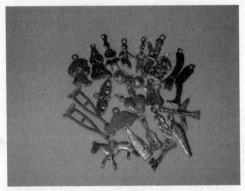

Figure 12-12 *Milagros.* This photograph is an example of the assortment of various miniature articles that may be purchased for the nominal cost of $1.00 in *botanicas* or in a marketplace from traditional people. In this image are crutches, a head, a woman, children and a baby, an arm, a leg, eyes, breasts, a torso, a heart, a car, a horse, a key, a whisky bottle, and others. When a person is experiencing a problem with one of these anatomical areas or objects, he or she may pray for recovery; make a *promesa* to a saint; and when the person's prayer is answered, take the *milagro* to a church and place it near the saint the person prayed to.

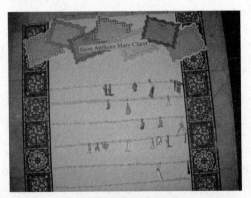

Figure 12-13 *Milagros* placed at the Shrine of Saint Anthony in the Church of the Sacred Heart of Mary in San Antonio, Texas.

Other folk healers include the *materia*, or spirit channeler, and the *partera*, or lay midwife. The *parteras* continue to practice today, but their numbers are dwindling. Box 12–1 describes the scope of the *partera*'s practice.

Box 12–1

Parteras

In Mexico and South Texas, there is a long history of the use of midwives, or *parteras*. The practice of midwifery predates Cortes. The goddess Tlozoteotl was the goddess of childbirth, and the midwives were known as *Tlamatqui-Tuti*. A *partera* is viewed as a HEALER by many members of the Mexican American and Mexican communities. She (most are women, although currently obstetricians from Mexico are providing this service in South Texas) is described as an individual who has the ability to HEAL and is outgoing, warm, gentle, caring, and cooperative. The *partera*'s duties include (1) giving advice to the pregnant woman, (2) giving physical aid, such as treating any illness the woman experiences during pregnancy, (3) guiding the woman through her pregnancy in terms of nutrition or activities she can and cannot do, and (4) being in attendance during labor and delivery.

Patients are most often referred to *parteras* by their friends or relatives, and a *partera* with a good reputation is always busy. Some *parteras* receive referrals from the health department with which they register, some advertise in the local newspaper or telephone book, and some have signs on their homes or clinics (Figure 12–14).

The *parteras* avoid delivering women with high blood pressure, anemia, a history of diabetes, multiple babies, and transverse presentations. Some *parteras* also prefer to send women with breech presentations to the hospital. If an unfamiliar woman in labor appears at their door in the middle of the night who is very poor with no place to go to deliver, most claim they will take her in.

Most *parteras* keep records of their deliveries. Included in these records are such data as the name of the mother, date, time of admission, stage of labor, time in labor, contractions, time of delivery, presenting part, time of delivery and condition of the placenta, and physical condition of the mother and baby.

The amount of prenatal care the *parteras* deliver ranges from a lot to a little. In general, the mothers seek assistance during their third or fourth month of pregnancy. When the *partera*'s assistance is sought, the mother is sent either to the health department or to a doctor for routine blood work. The *partera* is able to follow the mother's case and gives her advice and massages. One important service that the *partera* performs is the repositioning of the fetus in the womb through massage.

A *partera* may give several forms of advice to the pregnant woman. For example, she may advise the woman who is experiencing pica (the craving for and ingestion of nonfood substances, such as clay and laundry starch) to purchase solid milk of magnesia in Mexico. The milk of magnesia tastes like clay,

(continued)

Box 12–1   *Continued*

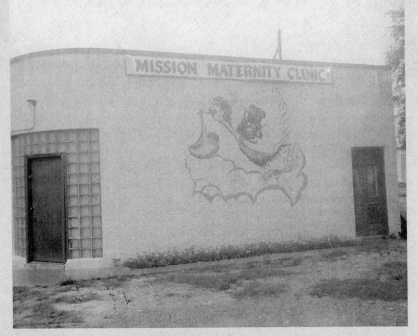

Figure 12-14   Sign for a *partera*.

thereby satisfying the pica, and is not considered harmful. The mother with food cravings is advised to satisfy them. The mothers are also instructed:

1. not to lift heavy objects,
2. to take laxatives to prevent constipation,
3. to exercise often by walking frequently,
4. not to cross their legs, and
5. not to bathe in hot water. The reason for the last two admonitions is the belief that crossing the legs and taking hot baths can cause the baby to assume the breech position.

If the *partera* knows the exact date of the mother's last period, she is able to estimate accurately when the woman is going to deliver by calculating 8 lunar months and 27 days from the onset of the last period.

With the onset of labor, the mother contacts the *partera*. She goes to the birthing place—the home or clinic of the *partera*—or the *partera* goes to her home. The mother is examined vaginally to determine how far along in labor she is and the position of the baby. She is instructed to shower and to empty her bowels—with an enema, if necessary—and she is encouraged to walk and move around until the delivery is imminent. Once the mother is ready to deliver, she is put to bed. Most of the mothers are delivered lying down in bed. If the mother chooses to do so, however, she is delivered in a squatting or sitting position. Several home remedies may be used during labor, including *comino* (cumin seed) tea or *canela* (cinnamon) tea to stimulate labor.

The baby is stimulated if needed, and the mucus is removed from the mouth and nose as needed with the use of a bulb syringe. The cord is clamped, tied with cord ties, and cut with scissors that have been boiled and soaked in alcohol. The stump is then treated with merbromin (Mercurochrome), alcohol, or a combination of the two. The baby is weighed, and some time after the delivery it is bathed. Most *parteras* bind both the mother and the baby. The baby may be fed oregano or cumin tea right after birth or later to help it spit up the mucus. Eyedrops are instilled in the baby's eyes, in compliance with state laws (silver nitrate is used most frequently).

The *partera* stays at the mother's home for several hours after the delivery and then returns to check the mother and the baby the next day. If the mother delivers at the home of the *partera*, she generally stays 12 to 14 hours.

There are several ways of disposing of the placenta. It may just be placed in a plastic bag and thrown in the trash, or it may be buried in the yard. Some placentas are buried with a religious or folk ceremony. There are several folk reasons for the burial of the placenta. The placenta must be buried so that the animals will not eat it. If it is eaten by a dog, the mother will not be able to bear any more children. If it is thrown in the trash, the mother's womb may become "cold." If the baby is a girl, the placenta is buried near the home, so the daughter will not go far away. If it is a boy, it is buried far away from the home to ensure the child's independence.

The practice of the *partera* continues today. *Parteras* in the state of Texas are licensed and registered as direct entry midwives. They are not certified as nurse midwives. In Hidalgo County in the Rio Grande Valley, there are now 10 registered *parteras* remaining and who continue to practice in the traditional manner. Table 12–2 presents several aspects of the demographic and health situation in the 5 counties that border Mexico in the southern part of the state along the Rio Grande River where the *parteras* are practicing (Texas Department of State Health Services, 2011).

The practice of the *partera* in the Rio Grande Valley is the life of the past, the present, and the future: "a way of life *de ayer, hoy y mañana*" (Castillo, 1982).

Sources: Adapted from Spector, R. (1996). *Cultural diversity in health and illness* (4th ed.) Stamford, CT: Appleton & Lange, pp. 305–325;

Castillo, J. Former director, Division of Health Related Professions. (1982, April 6). *Personal Letter.* Brownsville: Texas Southmost College.

Health Restoration

The most popular form of HEALTH restoration used by folk healers involves herbs, especially when used as teas. The *curandero* knows what specific herbs to use for a problem. This information is revealed in dreams, in which the "patron" gives suggestions.

Because the *curandero* has a religious orientation, much of the treatment includes elements of both the Catholic and Pentecostal rituals and artifacts: offerings

Table 12-2 Selected Health Facts in Selected Counties along the U.S./Mexico Border, Rio Grande Valley, Texas: 2008

County	Population	Hispanic (%)	Per capita Income ($)	Below Poverty Level (%)	Live Births	Licensed Lay Midwives (2010)	Fetal Deaths
Cameron	393,355	87.1	21,387	33.5	8,153	4	47
Hidalgo	724,971	91.2	19,721	34.8	17,137	10	114
Starr	62,648	97.9	15,452	36.8	1,343	0	6
Zapata	14,314	89	18,849	26.2	318	0	2
Webb	238,269	95.2	22,831	26.6	5,933	3	29

Source: Texas Department of State Health Services. (2011). 2008 Health Facts Profiles for Texas. Retrieved from http://www.dshs.state.tx.us/chs/cfs/2008/2008-Health-Facts-Profiles-for-Texas/, July 11, 2011; Texas Department of State Health Services. (2011). Midwife, Direct Entry (DEM) by County of Residence 2010. Retrieved from http://www.dshs.state.tx.us/chs/hprc/tables/Midwife,-Direct-Entry-%28DEM%29-by-County-of-Residence—September,-2010/, December 4, 2011.

of money, penance, confession, the lighting of candles, *milagros*, and the laying on of hands. Massage is used in illnesses such as *empacho*.

Cleanings, the removal of negative forces or spirits, or *limpias*, are done in two ways. The first is by passing an unbroken egg over the body of the ILL person. The second method entails passing herbs tied in a bunch over the body. The back of the neck, which is considered a vulnerable spot, is given particular attention.

In contrast to the depersonalized care Mexicans expect to receive in medical institutions, their relationship with and care by the *curandero(a)* are uniquely personal, as described in Table 12–3. This special relationship between Mexicans and the *curanderos* may well account for folk healers' popularity. In addition to the close, personal relationship between patient and healer, other factors may explain the continuing belief in *curanderismo*:

1. The mind and body are inseparable.
2. The central problem of life is to maintain harmony, including social, physical, and psychological aspects of the person.
3. There must be harmony between the hot and cold, wet and dry. The treatment of ILLNESS should restore the body's harmony, which has been lost.
4. The patient is the passive recipient of disease when the disease is caused by an external force. This external force disrupts the natural order of the internal person, and the treatment must be designed to restore this order. The causes of disharmony are evil and witches.
5. A person is related to the spirit world. When the body and soul are separated, soul loss can occur. This loss is sometimes caused by *susto*, a disease or illness resulting from fright, which may afflict individuals from all socioeconomic levels and lifestyles.

Table 12-3 Comparison between *Curanderos, Parteras,* and Other Traditional Healers and Allopathic Health Care Providers

Curanderos, Parteras, and Other Traditional Healers	Allopathic Health Care Providers
1. Maintain informal, friendly, affective relationship with entire family	1. Businesslike, formal relationship; deal only with the patient
2. Make house calls day or night	2. Patient must go to physician's office or clinic, and only during the day; may have to wait for hours to be seen; home visits are rarely made
3. For diagnosis, consult with head of house, create a mood of awe, talk to all family members; are not authoritarian, have social rapport, build expectation of cure	3. Rest of family is usually ignored; deal solely with the ill person, and may deal only with the sick part of the patient; authoritarian manner creates fear
4. Are generally less expensive than physicians	4. More expensive than *curanderos*
5. Have ties to the "world of the sacred"; have rapport with the symbolic, spiritual, creative, or holy force	5. Secular; pay little attention to the religious beliefs or meaning of an illness
6. Share the world view of the patient—that is, speak the same language, live in the same neighborhood or in some similar socioeconomic conditions, may know the same people, understand the patient's lifestyle	6. Generally do not share the world view of the patient—that is, may not speak the same language, do not live in the same neighborhood, do not understand the patient's socioeconomic conditions or lifestyle

6. The responsibility for recovery is shared by the ILL person, the family, and the *curandero(a)*.

7. The natural world is not clearly distinguished from the supernatural world. Thus, the *curandero(a)* can coerce, curse, and appease the spirits. The *curandero(a)* places more emphasis on his or her connections with the sacred and the gift of healing than on personal properties. (Such personal properties might include social status, a large home, and expensive material goods.)

Several types of emotional illnesses are found among the traditional people from Hispanic communities. These are further divided into **mental illness** (in which the illness is not judged) and **moral illness** (in which others can judge the victim). The causes of mental illness and examples of the illness they cause are as follows:

- heredity—epilepsy (*epilepsia*)
- hex—evil eye (*mal ojo*)
- worry—anxiety (*tirisia*)

- fright—hysteria (*histeria*)
- blow to the head—craziness (*locura*)

The causes of moral illness and examples of the illness they cause are as follows:

- vice—use of drugs (*drogadicto*)
- character weakness—alcoholism (*alcoholismo*)
- emotions—jealousy (*celos*) and/or rage (*coraje*) (Spencer, Nichols, Lipkin, et al., 1993, p. 133)

Ethnopharmacologic teas may be used to treat these maladies and amulets may be worn or religious rituals followed to prevent or treat them. The following are examples of herbs that may be purchased in grocery stores, markets, and *botanicas*, and are used as teas to treat the listed maladies:

- camomile tea, *Manzanilla*, used to cure fright
- spearmint tea, *Yerb Buena*, used to treat nervousness
- orange leaves, *Te de narranjo*, used as a sedative to treat nervousness
- sweet basil, *Albacar*, used to treat fright and to ward off evil spirits (Spencer, Nichols, Lipkin, et al., 1993, p. 133)

The HEALTH beliefs and practices discussed here are prevalent today (2012). I recently spoke with an immigrant from a small village in Mexico and inquired about *curanderismo*. He was excited to know that I was familiar with the practice and was proud to share his knowledge and experiences.

■ Puerto Ricans

Puerto Rican migrants to the United States mainland are American citizens, albeit with a different language and culture. They are neither immigrants nor aliens. According to the 2010 census, 9.2% of the Hispanic population are Puerto Ricans (Ennis, Rios-Vargas, & Albert, 2011, p. 3). Most live on the East Coast, with the greatest number living in New York City and metropolitan New Jersey. Most Puerto Ricans migrate to search for a better life or because relatives, particularly spouses and parents, have migrated previously. Life on the island of Puerto Rico is difficult because there is a high level of unemployment. Puerto Ricans are not well known or understood by the majority of people in the continental United States. Little is known about their cultural identity. Mainlanders tend to forget that Puerto Rico is, for the most part, a poor island whose people have many problems. When many Puerto Ricans migrate to the mainland, they bring many of their problems—especially those with poor health and social circumstance (Cohen, 1972).

Puerto Ricans, along with Cubans, constitute the most recent major immigration group to these shores. They cover the spectrum of racial differences and have practiced racial intermarriage. Many are Catholic, but some belong to Protestant sects.

Many people from Puerto Rico perceive HEALTH and ILLNESS and use folk healers and remedies in ways similar to those used by other Hispanics, whereas others practice *santeria*. Most studies on HEALTH and ILLNESS beliefs and HEALING have been conducted on Mexicans. It is not easy to find information about the beliefs of Puerto Ricans. Much of the information presented here was gleaned from students and patients. Both groups feel that their beliefs should be known by health care deliverers. One student, whose mother is a healer and is teaching her daughter the art, corroborated much of the following material.

Common Folk Diseases and Their Treatment

Table 12–4 lists a number of folk diseases and the usual source and type of treatment as reported to me by several Puerto Ricans. Many of these diseases or disharmonies were mentioned in the section on Mexican approaches. Nonetheless, there are subtle differences in the ways folk diseases are perceived by Mexicans and Puerto Ricans. For example, although diseases are classified as hot and cold, treatments—that is, food and medications—are categorized as hot (*caliente*), cold (*frio*), and cool (*fresco*). Cold illnesses are treated with hot remedies; hot diseases are treated with cold or cool remedies. Table 12–5 lists the major illnesses, foods, and medicines and herbs associated with the hot-cold system as it is applied among Puerto Ricans in the United States.

A number of activities are carried out to maintain the proper hot-cold balance in the body. Examples are as follows:

1. *Pasmo*, a form of paralysis, usually is caused by an upset in the hot-cold balance. For example, if a woman is ironing (hot) and then steps out into the rain (cold), she may get facial or other paralysis.

Table 12–4 Folk Diseases Among Puerto Rican and Other Hispanic People

Name	Description	Treatment	Source of Treatment
Susto	Sudden fright, causing shock	Relaxation	Relative or friend
Fatigue	Asthma-like symptoms	Oxygen; medications	Western health care system
Pasmo	Paralysis-like symptoms, face or limbs	Prevention; massage	Folk
Empacho	Food forms into a ball and clings to the stomach, causing pain and cramps	Strong massage of the stomach; medication; gentle pinching and rubbing of the spine	Folk
Mal ojo	Sudden, unexplained illness in a usually well child or person	Prevention; babies wear a special charm	Depends on the severity of the symptoms: usually home or folk
Ataque	Screaming; falling to the ground; wildly moving arms and legs; hysterical crying	None—ends spontaneously	

Table 12-5 The Hot-Cold Classification Among Puerto Ricans and Other Hispanic People

	Frio (Cold)	*Fresco* (Cool)	*Caliente* (Hot)
Illness or bodily condition	Arthritis Menstrual period Joint pain	Colds	Constipation Diarrhea Pregnancy Rashes Ulcers
Medicines and herbs		Bicarbonate of soda Linden flowers Milk of magnesia Nightshade Orange flower water Sage Tobacco	Anise Aspirin Castor oil Cinnamon Cod-liver oil Iron tablets Penicillin Vitamins
Foods	Avocado Banana Coconut Lima beans Sugar cane White beans	Barley water Whole milk Chicken Fruits Honey Raisins Salt cod Watercress Onions Peas	Alcoholic beverages Chili peppers Chocolate Coffee Corn meal Evaporated milk Garlic Kidney beans

Source: Schilling, B., & Brannon, E. (1986, September). Health-related dietary practices. In *Cross-cultural counseling— a guide for nutrition and health counselors,* p. 5. Alexandra, VA: U.S. Department of Health and Human Services. Nutrition and Technical Services Division. Reprinted with permission.

2. A person who is hot cannot sit under a mango tree (cold) because he or she can get a kidney infection or "back problems."

3. A baby should not be fed a formula (hot), as it may cause rashes; whole milk (cold) is acceptable.

4. A man who has been working (hot) must not go into the coffee fields (cold), or he could contract a respiratory illness.

5. A hot person must not drink cold water, as it could cause colic.

There is often a considerable time lag between disregarding these precautions and the occurrence of illness. A patient who had injured himself while lifting heavy cartons in a factory revealed that the "true" reason he was now experiencing prolonged back problems was because as a child he often sat under a mango tree when he was "hot" after running. This childhood habit had significantly damaged his back, so that, as an adult, he was unable to lift heavy objects without causing injury. Table 12–5 provides additional examples of this phenomenon.

The following are examples of selected behaviors a patient may manifest with an illness thought to be caused by an imbalance of hot and cold:

- During pregnancy a woman may avoid hot-classified foods and medicines and take cool-classified medicines.
- During the postpartum period or during menstruation a woman may avoid cool-classified foods and medicines.
- Infant formulas containing evaporated milk, which are hot-classified, may be avoided as the baby is fed cold-classified whole milk.
- Penicillin, a hot-classified prescription, may not be taken for diarrhea, constipation, or a rash, as these are hot-classified symptoms.
- When a diuretic is prescribed that needs to be supplemented with cold-classified bananas or raisins, the bananas or raisins may not be eaten when the disease is a cold-classified condition.

These examples illustrate the use of foods or medicines to restore a sense of balance (Harwood, 1971).

Puerto Ricans also share with others of Hispanic origin a number of beliefs in spirits and spiritualism. They believe that mental illness is caused primarily by evil spirits and forces. People with such disorders are preferably treated by a "spiritualist medium" (Cohen, 1972). The psychiatric clinic is known as the place where *locos*, mentally ill people, go. This attitude is exemplified in the Puerto Rican approach to visions and the like. The social and cultural environment encourages the acceptance of having visions and hearing voices. In the dominant culture of the continental United States, when one has visions or hears voices, one is encouraged to see a psychiatrist. When a Puerto Rican regards this experience as a problem, he or she may seek help through *Santeria* (Mumford, 1973).

Santeria is the form of Latin American magic that had its birth in Nigeria, the country of origin of the Yoruba people, who were brought to the New World as slaves over 400 years ago. The *Santeria*, or *santero*, may use storytelling as a way of helping people cope with day-to-day difficulties (Flores-Peña, 1991). They brought with them their traditional religion, which was in time synthesized with Catholic images. The believers continue to worship in the traditional way, especially in Puerto Rico, Cuba, and Brazil. The Yorubas identified their gods—*Orishas*—with the Christian saints and invested in these saints the same supernatural powers of gods. The *orishas*/saints related to health situations are listed in Table 12–6.

Santeria is a structured system consisting of *espiritismo* (spiritualism), which is practiced by gypsies and mediums who claim to have *facultades* (sacred abilities). These special *facultades* provide them with the "license" to practice. The status or positions of the practitioners form a hierarchy: The head is the *babalow*, a male; second is the *presidente*, the head medium; and third are the *santeros*. Novices are the "believers." The *facultades* are given to the healer from protective Catholic saints, who have African names and are known as *protecciones*. *Santeria* can be practiced in storefronts, basements, homes, and even college dormitories. *Santeros* dress in white robes for ceremonies and wear special beaded bracelets as a sign of their identity.

Table 12-6 **Selected *Orishas*, the Corresponding Saints, and Related Health Problems**

Orisha	Saint	Health Problem
Obatala	Crucified Christ	Bronchitis
Chango	Saint Barbara	Violent death
Babalu-Aye	Saint Lazarus	Sickness
Bacoso	Saint Christopher	Infections
Ibeyi	Saints Cosmos and Damian	Infant illnesses
Ifa	Saint Anthony	Fertility
Yemaya	Our Lady of Regla	Maternity

Sources: Gonzalez-Wippler, M. (1987). *Santeria—African magic in Latin America*. Bronx, New York: Original Publications, pp. 1–30; Riva, A. (1990). *Devotions to the Saints*. Los Angeles: International Imports, pp. 91–93.

Puerto Ricans are able to accept much of what Anglos may judge to be idiosyncratic behavior. In fact, behavioral disturbances are seen as symptoms of illness that are to be treated, not judged. Puerto Ricans make a sharp distinction between "nervous" behavior and being *loco*. To be *loco* is to be bad, dangerous, evil. It also means losing all one's social status. Puerto Ricans who seek standard American treatment for mental illness are castigated by the community. They understandably prefer to get help for the symptoms of mental illness from the *santero*, who accepts the symptoms and attributes the cause of the illness to spirits outside the body. Puerto Ricans have great faith in this system of care and maintain a high level of hope for recovery.

The *santero* is an important person, respecting the patient and not gossiping about either the patient or his or her problems. Anyone can pour his or her heart out with no worry of being labeled or judged. The *santero* is able to tell a person what the problem is, prescribe the proper treatment, and tell the person what to do, how to do it, and when to do it. A study in New York found that 73% of the Puerto Rican patients in an outpatient mental health clinic reported having visited a *santero*. Often, a sick person is taken to a psychiatrist by his or her family to be "calmed down" and prepared for treatment by a *santero*. Families may become angry if the psychiatrist does not encourage belief in God and prayer during work with the patient. Because of cultural differences and beliefs, a psychiatrist may diagnose as illness what Puerto Ricans may define as health. Frequently, a spiritualist treats the "mental illness" of a patient as *facultades*, which makes the patient a "special person." Thus, esteem is granted to the patient as a form of treatment. I visited a *santero* in Los Angeles with the hope of his granting me an interview. Instead, he argued that if I wanted to know about his practice I should "sit," so I did. He proceeded to examine my head and palms, throw and read cowrie shells, tell me a story, and asked me to interpret it. Once this was accomplished, he recommended certain interventions. His manner was extremely calming and, when he interpreted the story with me, I discovered his uncanny ability to read habits and behavior

Table 12-7 Examples of Cultural Phenomena Affecting Health and Health Care among Hispanic Americans

Nations of Origin	Hispanic countries: Spain, Cuba, Mexico, Central and South America, Puerto Rico
Environmental Control	Traditional health and illness beliefs may continue to be observed by "traditional" people Folk medicine tradition Use of herbs, teas, lotions, and candles Traditional healers: *curandera, espiritista, partera, senoria*
Biological Variations	Diabetes mellitus Parasites Coccidiodomycosis Lactose intolerance
Social Organization	Nuclear families Large, extended family networks *Compadrazzo* (godparents) Strong church affiliations within community Community social organizations
Communication	Primary language: Spanish or Portuguese
Space	Tactile relationships: touch, handshakes, embrace Value physical presence
Time Orientation	Present

Source: Spector, R. (1992). Culture, ethnicity, and nursing. In P. Potter & A. Perry (Eds.), *Fundamentals of nursing* (3rd ed.). St. Louis, MO: Mosby-Year Book. Reprinted with permission. This material was published in Potter & Perry's Fundamentals of Nursing, Jackie Crisp and Catherine Taylor (Eds), Copyright Elsevier (2009).

(Flores-Peña, 1991). A number of cultural phenomena affect the health and health care of Hispanic Americans (Table 12–7) (Mumford, 1973).

Entry into Mainland Health Systems

Puerto Ricans living in New York City and other parts of the northern United States experience a high rate of illness and hospitalization during their first year on the mainland, as do other people of Hispanic origin. It is worthwhile considering the vast differences between living in New York and living in Puerto Rico. In Puerto Rico, there is no winter weather. The winters in the North can be bitterly cold, and adjustment to climate change in itself is extremely difficult. Migrant people may be forced to live in crowded living quarters with poor sanitation.

Puerto Ricans seeking health care may go to a physician, a folk practitioner, or both. The general progression of seeking care is as follows:

1. The person seeks advice from a daughter, mother, grandmother, or neighbor woman. These sources are consulted because the women of this culture are the primary healers and dispensers of medicine at the family level.

2. If the advice is not sufficient, the person may seek help from a *senoria* (a woman who is especially knowledgeable about the causes and treatment of illness).

3. If the *senoria* is unable to help, the person goes to a more sophisticated folk practitioner, an *espiritista* or a *curandera*. If the problem is "psychiatric," a *santero* may be consulted. These names describe similar people—those who obtain their knowledge from spirits and treat illness according to the instructions of the spirits. Herbs, lotions, creams, and massage often are used.

4. If the person is still not satisfied, he or she may go to a physician.

5. If the results are not satisfactory, the person may return to a folk practitioner. He or she may seek medical help sooner than step 4 or may go back and forth between the two systems.

Not all people from Puerto Rico use the folk system. Health care providers should remember that people who appear to have delayed seeking health care have most likely counted on curing their illness through the culturally known and well-understood folk process. Often when people disappear (or "elope") from the established health system, they may have elected to return to the folk system. Those who elope from the larger, institutionalized medical system may visit a *botanica* (Figures 12–15 and 12–16). In these small *botanicas*, one can

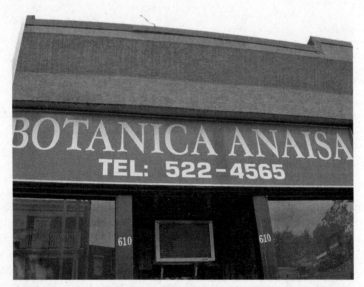

Figure 12-15 A *botanica* in Boston, Massachusetts. There are several *botanicas* in the Boston metropolitan area. The *botanicas* are visited primarily by people from Puerto Rico, the Dominican Republic, Mexico, and other Hispanics residing in the area. They sell numerous herbs and herbal preparations, amulets of all sorts, *milagros*, and statues of saints. A *santera* works in this *botanica*, and she is available to people to give advice and sell herbal remedies.

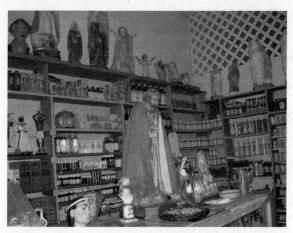

Figure 12–16   Interior of a *botanica* in Boston, Massachusetts.

purchase herbs, potents, Florida water, ointments, and incense prescribed by spiritualists. Some of these *botanicas* are so busy that each customer is given a number and is assisted only after the number is called (Mumford, 1973). There are countless *botanicas* located in one small area of New York City. A Spanish-speaking colleague and I visited a *botanica* in Boston that was similar to a pharmacy. The owner explained the various remedies that were for sale. We were allowed to purchase only a few items because we did not have a spiritualist's prescription for herbs. The store also sold amulets, candles, religious statues, cards, medals, and relics.

A limited number of *santeros* place advertisements in local Spanish daily newspapers. Some of the more industrious ones distribute flyers in the New York City subways. Others maintain a low profile, and patients visit them because of their well-established reputations.

Current Health Problems

The Hispanic health profile is marked by diversity, and people of the Hispanic community experience perhaps the most varied set of health issues encountered by any of the emerging majority populations. The diversity in health problems is intertwined with the effects of socioeconomic status, as well as with geographic and cultural differences. The most important health issues for Hispanics are related to these demographic facts: The population is young and has a high birth rate.

Table 12–8 compares selected health status indicators between all races and Hispanics. The leading causes of death among Hispanic Americans illustrate differences between their health experiences and those of the total population, as can be seen in Table 12–9.

Hispanics experience a number of barriers when seeking health care. The most obvious one is language. In spite of the fact that Spanish-speaking people constitute one of the largest minority groups in this country, very few

Table 12-8   Comparison of Selected Health Status Indicators—All Races and Hispanic or Latino: 2007

Health Indicator	All Races	Hispanic or Latino
Crude birth rate per 1,000 population by race of mother	14.3	23.4
Percentage of live births to women receiving first-trimester prenatal care	67.5	56.1
Percentage of live births to women receiving third-trimester prenatal care or no prenatal care	8.4	12.9
Percentage of live births to teenage childbearing women—under 18	3.4	5.3
Percentage of low birth weight per live births <2,500 grams	8.22	6.93
Infant mortality per 1,000 live births (2006)	6.7	5.4
Cancer—all sites per 100,000 population	446.7	326.5
Lung cancer incidence per 100,000 population	Men: 65.4	38.0
	Women: 47.4	22.5
Breast cancer incidence per 100,000	122.5	83.8
Prostate cancer incidence per 100,000	158.3	116.2
Male death rates from suicide, all ages, age adjusted per 100,000 resident population	11.3	10.1
Male death rates from homicide, all ages, age adjusted per 100,000 resident population	6.1	11.2

Source: U.S. Department of Health and Human Services & National Center for Health Statistics. *Health, United States, 2010*: With Special Feature on Death and Dying. Hyattsville, MD. 2011: Author, pp. 102, 106, 107, 110, 124, 137, 180–181, 184–185, and 204. Retrieved from www.cdc.gov/nchs/data/hus/hus10.pdf, December 11, 2011.

Table 12-9   Comparison of the 10 Leading Causes of Death for Hispanic or Latino Americans and for All Persons: 2007

Hispanic or Latino Americans	All Persons
1. Diseases of heart	Diseases of heart
2. Malignant neoplasms	Malignant neoplasms
3. Unintentional injuries	Cerebrovascular diseases
4. Cerebrovascular diseases	Chronic lower respiratory diseases
5. Diabetes mellitus	Unintentional injuries
6. Chronic liver disease and cirrhosis	Alzheimer's disease
7. Chronic lower respiratory diseases	Diabetes mellitus
8. Homicide	Influenza and pneumonia
9. Certain conditions originating in the perinatal period	Nephritis, nephrotic syndrome, and nephrosis
10. Influenza and pneumonia	Septicemia

Source: U.S. Department of Health and Human Services & National Center for Health Statistics. *Health, United States, 2010*: With Special Feature on Death and Dying. Hyattsville, MD. 2011: Author, pp. 146–147. Retrieved from www.cdc.gov/nchs/data/hus/hus10.pdf, December 11, 2011.

health care deliverers speak Spanish. This is especially true in communities in which the number of Spanish-speaking people is relatively small. Hispanics who live in these areas experience tremendous frustration because of the language barrier. Even in large cities, there are far too many occasions when a sick person has to rely on a young child to act not only as a translator but also as an interpreter. One way of sensitizing young nursing students to the pain of this situation is to ask them to present a health problem to a person who does not speak or understand a word of English. Needless to say, this is extremely difficult; it is also embarrassing. People who try this rapidly comprehend and appreciate the feelings of patients who are unable to speak or understand English. (After this experience, 2 of my students decided to take a foreign-language elective.) Language will continue to be a problem until (1) there are more physicians, nurses, and social workers from the Spanish-speaking communities and (2) more of the present deliverers of health care learn to speak Spanish.

A second crucial barrier that Hispanic people encounter is poverty. The diseases of the poor—for example, tuberculosis, malnutrition, and lead poisoning—all have high incidences among Spanish-speaking populations.

A final barrier to adequate health care is the time orientation of Hispanic Americans. To Hispanics, time is a relative phenomenon. Little attention is given to the exact time of day. The frame of reference is wider, and the issue is whether it is day or night. The American health care system, on the other hand, places great emphasis on promptness. Health care providers demand that clients arrive at the exact time of the appointment—despite the fact that clients are often kept waiting. Health system workers stress the client's promptness rather than their own. In fact, they tend to deny responsibility for the waiting periods by blaming them on the "system." Many facilities commonly schedule all appointments for 9:00 A.M. when it is clearly known and understood by the staff members that the doctor will not even arrive until 11:00 A.M. or later. The Hispanic person frequently responds to this practice by arriving late for appointments or failing to go at all. They prefer to attend walk-in clinics, where the waits are shorter. They also much prefer going to traditional healers.

Hispanic American Health Care Manpower

As seen in Table 12–10, it is evident that the numbers of Hispanics or Latinos enrolled in the health professions' schools is well below the percentage (16.3%) of Hispanic or Latino people in the American resident population.

Recent nursing data are not included in the overall health professions enrollment data in Table 12–10. However, the National Sample Survey of Registered Nurses 2008 prepared by the Bureau of Health Professions of the Health Resources Administration provides relevant information regarding the demographic profile of American Registered Nurses. It estimates that the registered nurse population in the United States in 2008 was 3,063,162, with

Table 12-10 **Percentage of Hispanic or Latino Americans Enrolled in Selected Health Professions Schools Compared with Non-Hispanic Whites: 2007–2008**

	Number Enrolled	Non-Hispanic Whites (%)	Hispanic or Latino American (%)
Dentistry	19,342	60.6	6.3
Allopathic medicine	74,518	62.4	3.1
Osteopathic medicine	15,634	70.5	3.6
Optometry	5,556	60.3	4.6
Pharmacy	50,691	59.5	4.0
Podiatry	2,095	62.2	5.4
Public Health	22,604	59.3	8.8

Source: U.S. Department of Health and Human Services & National Center for Health Statistics. *Health, United States, 2010:* With Special Feature on Death and Dying. Hyattsville, MD. 2011: Author, pp. 352–353. Retrieved from www.cdc.gov/nchs/data/hus/hus10.pdf, December 11, 2011.

2,596,599 registered nurses employed in nursing. Of this number, 83.2% were White non-Hispanic and 3.6% were Hispanic or Latino American (United States Department of Health and Human Services, Health Resources and Services, 2010). Given that in 2010 the White alone population was 63% of the total population and Hispanic or Latino American people comprised 16.3% of the resident population, this is a clear indication that there is no demographic parity in the percentage of Hispanic or Latino American people in nursing. This demographic picture and the percentages in the tables demonstrate a situation that is an ongoing concern. Somnath and Shipman (2006), who reviewed a total of 55 studies, found that minority patients tend to receive better interpersonal care from practitioners of their own race or ethnicity, particularly in primary care and mental health settings, and that non–English speaking patients experience better interpersonal care, greater medical comprehension, and greater likelihood of keeping follow-up appointments when they see a language-concordant practitioner. They concluded their study by stating that "the findings indicated greater health professions diversity will likely lead to improved public health by increasing access to care for underserved populations, and by increasing opportunities for minority patients to see practitioners with whom they share a common race, ethnicity or language." They also stated that "race, ethnicity, and language concordance, which is associated with better patient-practitioner relationships and communication, may increase patients' likelihood of receiving and accepting appropriate medical care" (Somnath & Shipman, 2006, p. 17).

RESEARCH ON CULTURE

Much research has been conducted among members of the Hispanic American population. The following article describes one such study:

> Whittemore, R. (2007). *Culturally competent interventions for Hispanic adults with type 2 diabetes: A systemic review.* Journal of Transcultural Nursing, 18 (2), 157–166.

Significant research has been conducted in the past several decades with the goal of reducing health disparities in Hispanic adults with type 2 diabetes. The purpose of this study was to describe and synthesize the research on culturally competent interventions aimed at improving outcomes in the target population. The author used an integrative review method to describe the intervention components of culturally competent interventions; the efficacy of interventions in terms of clinical outcomes, behavioral outcomes, and knowledge; cultural strategies of interventions; and factors associated with attendance and attrition of interventions. She analyzed 11 studies conducted between 1994 and 2005 on this topic and found that most culturally competent interventions were efficacious. The culturally competent interventions included community-based education in the language—Spanish—understood by the patients. Other strategies included family involvement, translation as needed, bilingual professional staff, emphasis on types of food, and support groups.

Other interventions that were examined included the following:

- *Clinical outcomes.* Improvements in glycemic control with education were documented.
- *Behavioral outcomes.* Evaluation of dietary and exercise behaviors and significant improvements were found.
- *Diabetes-related knowledge.* A significant increase in diabetes-related knowledge was reported for participants who received culturally competent interventions.

The author notes that the development of culturally competent interventions requires attention to countless cultural factors, is complex, and requires a multidisciplinary and multifaceted approach.

Explore 🌐 MediaLink

Go to the Student Resource Site at nursing.pearsonhighered.com for chapter-related review questions, case studies, and activities. Contents of the CULTURALCARE Guide and CULTURALCARE Museum can also be found on the Student Resource Site. Click on Chapter 12 to select the activities for this chapter.

Box 12–2 Keeping Up

It goes without saying that much of the data presented in this chapter may be out of date when you read this text. However, at this final stage of writing, it is the most recent information available. The following resources will be most helpful in keeping you abreast of the frequent changes in health care events, costs, and policies:

1. The National Center for Health Statistics publishes *Health, United States*, an annual report on trends in health statistics. It can be retrieved from http://www.cdc.gov/nchs/hus.htm. *Health, United States, 2011* is not available and *Health, United States, 2012* will be published in May, 2012.
2. Health-related data and other statistics are available from http://www.cdc.gov/DataStatistics/.
3. To follow immigration information—U.S. Department of Commerce Economics and Statistics Administration, Office of Homeland Security, http://www.dhs.gov/.

■ Internet Sources

DeNavas-Walt, C., Proctor, B. D., & Smith, J. C. (2010). Income, Poverty, and Health Insurance Coverage in the United States: 2009. United States Census Bureau. Retrieved from http://www.census.gov, July 7, 2011.

Ennis, S. R., Rios_Vargas, M. and Albert, N. G. (2011). The Hispanic population in the United States. Retrieved from http://2010.census.gov/2010census/data/, July 11, 2011, p. 3.

Humes, K. R., Jones, N. A., & Ramirez, R. R. (2011). Overview of Race and Hispanic Origin: 2010. U.S. Department of Commerce, U.S. Census Bureau, Census 2010. Retrieved from http://www.census.gov/, June 27, 2011.

Lee, J. (2011). Annual Flow Report U.S. Naturalizations: 2010. U.S. Department of Commerce, Economics and Statistics Administration, Office of Homeland Security, Office of Immigration Statistics. Retrieved from http://www.dhs.gov/files/statistics/publications/gc_1302103955524.shtm, June 1, 2011.

Monger, R., & Yankay, J. (2011). Annual Flow Report. U.S. Legal Permanent Residents: 2010. U.S. Department of Commerce, Economics and Statistics Administration, Office of Homeland Security, Office of Immigration Statistics. Retrieved from http://www.dhs.gov/files/statistics/publications/gc_1301497627185.shtm, June 1, 2011.

Somnath, S., & Shipman, S. (2006). The Rationale for Diversity in the Health Professions: A Review of the Evidence. Washington, DC: U.S. Department of Health and Human Services, Health Resources and Services Administration, Bureau of Health Professions. Retrieved from http://www.hrsa.gov/, January 5, 2008.

Texas Department of State Health Services. (2011). 2008 Health Facts Profiles for Texas. Retrieved from http://www.dshs.state.tx.us/chs/cfs/2008/2008-Health-Facts-Profiles-for-Texas/, July 11, 2011.

Texas Department of State Health Services. (2011). Midwife, Direct Entry (DEM) by County of Residence 2010. Retrieved from http://www.dshs.state.tx.us/chs/hprc/tables/Midwife,-Direct-Entry-%28DEM%29-by-County-of-Residence—September,-2010/, December 11, 2011.

U.S. Census Bureau. (2011). Statistical Abstract of the United States: 2012. Retrieved from http://2010.census.gov/2010census/data/, December 4, 2011.

U.S. Department of Health and Human Services & National Center for Health Statistics. (2011). Health, United States, 2010: With Special Feature on Death and Dying. Hyattsville, MD: Author, pp. 146–147. Retrieved from www.cdc.gov/nchs/data/hus/hus10.pdf, December 11, 2011.

U.S. Department of Health and Human Services, Health Resources and Services. (2010). The National Survey of Registered Nurses 2008 Documentation for the General Public Use File, 2006. Bureau of Health Professions, Health Resources and Services Administration. BHPr/HRSA and the National Sample Survey of Registered Nurses. Retrieved from http://www.hrsa.gov/data-statistics/index.html, June 28, 2011.

■ References

Carmack, R. M., Gasco, J., & Gossen, G. H. (1996). *The legacy of Mesoamerica*. Upper Saddle River, NJ: Prentice Hall.

Castillo, J. Former director, Division of Health Related Professions. (1982, April 6). *Personal Letter*. Brownsville: Texas Southmost College.

Cohen, R. E. (1972, June). Principles of preventive mental health programs for ethnic minority populations: The acculturation of Puerto Ricans to the United States. *American Journal of Psychiatry, 128*(12), 79.

Currier, R. L. (1966, March). The hot-cold syndrome and symbolic balance in Mexican and Spanish-American folk medicine. *Ethnology, 5*, 251–263.

Dorsey, P. R., & Jackson, H. Q. (1976). Cultural health traditions: The Latino/Mexican perspective. In M. F. Branch & P. P. Paxton (Eds.), *Providing safe nursing care for ethnic people of color*. New York: Appleton-Century-Crofts.

Egan, M. (1991). *Milagros*. Santa Fe: Museum of New Mexico Press.

Flores-Peña, Y., & Evanchuk, R. J. (1994). *Santeria garments and altars*. Jackson: University of Mississippi Press.

Flores-Peña, Y. (1991). Personal interview. Los Angeles, CA.

Gonzalez-Wippler, M. (1987). *Santeria—African magic in Latin America*. New York: Original.

Greenhaw, W. (2000). *My heart is in the earth*. Montgomery, AL: River City.

Harwood, A. (1971). The hot-cold theory of disease: Implications for treatment of Puerto Rican patients. *Journal of the American Medical Association, 216*, 1154–1155.

Kearney, M., & Medrano, M. (2001). *Medieval culture and the Mexican American borderlands*. College Station: Texas A & M University Press.

Lucero, G. (1975, March). *Health and illness in the Mexican community*. Lecture given at Boston College School of Nursing.

Maduro, R. J. (1976, January). *Curanderismo: Latin American folk healing*. Conference, San Francisco.

Mumford, E. (1973, November–December). Puerto Rican perspectives on mental illness. *Mount Sinai Journal of Medicine, 40*(6), 771–773.

Nall, F. C., II, & Spielberg, J. (1967). Social and cultural factors in the responses of Mexican-Americans to medical treatment. *Journal of Health and Social Behavior, 8*, 302.

Riva, A. (1990). *Devotions to the saints*. Los Angeles: International Imports.

Rubel, A. J. (1964, July). The epidemiology of a folk illness: Susto in Hispanic America. *Ethnology, 3*(3), 270–271.

Saunders, L. (1958). Healing ways in the Spanish southwest. In E. G. Jaco (Ed.), *Patients, physicians, and illness*. Glencoe, IL: Free Press.

Schilling, B., & Brannon, E. (1986). Health-related dietary practices. *In Cross-cultural counseling: A guide for nutrition and health counselors*. Alexandria, VA: U.S. Department of Health and Human Services.

Spector, R. (1996). *Cultural diversity in health and illness* (4th ed.). Stamford, CT: Appleton & Lange.

Spencer, R. T., Nichols, L. W., Lipkin, G. B., et al. (1993). *Clinical pharmacology and nursing management* (4th ed.). Philadelphia: Lippincott.

Welch, S., Comer, J., & Steinman, M. (1973, September). Some social and attitudinal correlates of health care among Mexican Americans. *Journal of Health and Social Behavior, 14*, 205.

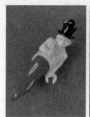
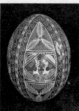
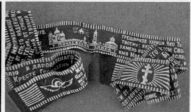
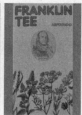

Figure 13-1 Figure 13-2 Figure 13-3   **Figure 13-4**

Chapter 13

HEALTH and ILLNESS
in the White Populations

Labour to keep alive in your Breast that Little Spark of Celestial Fire Called
Conscience.

—*George Washington, in J. Needleman (2003)*

◼ Objectives

1. Discuss the background of the White non-Hispanic populations.
2. Discuss the demographic profile of the White non-Hispanic populations.
3. Describe the traditional definitions of HEALTH and ILLNESS of the White non-Hispanic populations.
4. Describe the traditional methods of HEALTH maintenance and protection of selected communities of the White non-Hispanic populations.
5. Describe the traditional methods of HEALING of the White non-Hispanic populations.
6. Describe health problems of the White non-Hispanic populations.

The opening images for this chapter depict objects symbolic of items used to maintain, protect, and/or restore HEALTH for people in the White European American communities. Figure 13–1 is an Italian horn and worn, carried, or hung in the home for protection and luck. Figure 13–2 is a *pysanka*, or egg. The *pysanka* is a traditional symbol of life, which has evolved over the centuries. It is given as a gift to family and friends to wish them prosperity, strength,

323

health, and happiness. They are mainly painted at Easter and symbolize the renewal of life. Figure 13–3 is a "belt" that was purchased in a Russian Orthodox church in Moscow. The belt is worn under clothing to separate the "clean" upper body from the "dirty" lower body. Figure 13–4 is an example of an over-the-counter herbal remedy. These remedies are sold in homeopathic pharmacies in many European countries. This particular remedy is a laxative and was purchased in Switzerland.

■ Background

The 2010 census showed that the U.S. population on April 1, 2010, was 308.7 million. Out of the total population, 223.6 million people, or 63.7%, identified as White alone and 72.4% reported they were White in combination with one or more other races. The White population increased at a slower rate than the total population. The population of Whites who reported more than 1 race grew in every region between 2000 and 2010, particularly in the South and the Midwest. The following is the regional distribution of the White alone population: Northeast, 18.3%; Midwest, 24.1%; South, 37.7%; and the West, 21.9%. The states with the largest percentage of White alone were California, 7.6%; Texas, 5.8%; Florida, 5.5%; New York, 5.7%; and Pennsylvania, 5.1%. The cities with the largest number of White alone in 2010 were New York, Los Angeles, Chicago, Houston, and San Diego, California. The places with the largest multiple-race White populations were New York and Los Angeles. In 2010, 87.6 million people over 25 graduated high school and 19.8 million were college graduates or more (Hixson, Hepler, & Kim, 2011).

Members of White European American communities have been immigrating to this country since the very first settlers came to the shores of New England. The White non-Hispanic population has diverse and multiple origins. The recent literature in the area of ethnicity and health/HEALTH has focused on people of color, and little has been written about the HEALTH traditions of the White non-Hispanic ethnic communities. In this chapter, an introductory overview of the differences in traditional HEALTH beliefs and practices, by ethnicity, is presented. Given that we are talking about 63.7–70% of the American population, from many diverse countries, and with diverse ethnocultural and religious heritages, the enormity of the task of attempting to describe each difference is readily apparent. Instead, this chapter presents an overview of the relevant demographics of the White non-Hispanic population, highlights some of the basic beliefs of selected groups (those groups with which I have had the greatest exposure), and presents a comparison of the health status of Whites to the whole population as well as the census cohorts. The overview includes not only library research but also firsthand interviews and observations of people in their daily experiences with the health care delivery system, both as inpatients and as community residents receiving home care.

The major groups migrating to this country between 1820 and 1990 included people from Germany, Italy, the United Kingdom, Ireland,

Austria-Hungary, Canada, and Russia; they comprised a majority of the total immigrant population. However, in 1970, the numbers of immigrants from Europe began to decrease.

In 2010, there were a total of 1,042,635 Legal Permanent Residents (LPRs) in the United States, 46% of whom were new arrivals. People from Europe comprised 8.5% of this population. Not one European nation was among the top 20 nations of birth (Monger & Yankay, 2011, p. 4).

In 2010, there were 619,913 people who naturalized—became citizens of the United States. Of this number, 12.6% were born in Europe. Of the European population, 1.4% were from the United Kingdom (Lee, 2011, p. 2).

The 1980 census was the first to include a question about ancestry. The U.S. Census Bureau uses the term ancestry to refer to a person's ethnic origin or descent, roots, heritage, or the place of birth of the person or the person's parents or ancestors before their arrival in the United States. Some ethnic identities, such as "German" can be traced to geographic areas outside the United States, while other ethnicities, such as "Pennsylvania Dutch" or "Cajun," evolved in the United States. Table 13-1 illustrates the numbers of people claiming ancestry from European countries. The responses to the question of ancestry were a reflection of the ethnic group(s) with which persons identified, and respondents were able to indicate their ethnic group regardless of how many generations they were removed from it.

An additional facet to note is that in many states, the non-Hispanic White population is now a minority. States where less than 50% of the population are non-Hispanic Whites are California, Hawaii, New Mexico, and Texas. The District of Columbia has a White non-Hispanic minority of 35% (Humes, Nicholas & Ramirez, 2011, p.18).

The following discussion focuses on selected White ethnic groups and attempts to describe some of the history of their migration to America, the areas where they now live, the common beliefs regarding health/HEALTH and illness/ILLNESS, some kernels of information regarding family and social life, and problems that members from a given group may have in interacting with

Table 13-1 Population by Selected Ancestry Group: 2010

Ancestry	Numbers Identifying Themselves as This Ancestry (millions)
German	47.9
Irish	34.6
English	25.9
Italian	17.2
Polish	9.6
French (except Basque)	8.8
Scottish	5.5

Source: U.S. Census Bureau. (2011). 2005–2009 American Community Survey, B04006 People Reporting Ancestry. 5-Year Estimates (2009). Retrieved from http://search.census.gov/search?q=people+reporting+ancestry+2009&btnG=Search&btnG.x=0&btnG.y=0&entqr=0&ud=1&output=xml_no_dtd&oe=UTF_8&ie=UTF_ December 4, 2011.8&client=default_frontend&proxystylesheet=default_frontend&sort=date%3AD%3AL%3Ad1&site=census.

Table 13-2   **Examples of Cultural Phenomena Affecting Health Care Among European (White) Americans**

Nations of origin	Germany, England, Italy, Ireland, the former Soviet Union, and all other European countries
Environmental control	Primary reliance on "modern, Western" health care delivery system Remaining traditional HEALTH and ILLNESS beliefs and practices may be observed Some remaining traditional folk medicine and practices may be observed Homeopathic medicine resurgent
Biological variations	Breast cancer Heart disease Diabetes mellitus Thalassemia (Southern Europeans)
Social organization	Nuclear families Extended families Judeo-Christian religions Community and social organizations
Communication	National languages Many learned English rapidly as immigrants Verbal, rather than nonverbal
Space	Noncontact people—aloof, distant (Northern European) Southern countries—closer contact and touch
Time orientation	Future over present

Source: Spector, R. (1992). Culture, ethnicity, and nursing. In P. Potter & A. Perry (Eds.), *Fundamentals of nursing* (3rd ed.). St. Louis, MO: Mosby-Year Book. Reprinted with permission. This material was published in Potter & Perry's Fundamentals of Nursing, Jackie Crisp and Catherine Taylor (Eds), Copyright Elsevier (2009).

health care providers. The intention is not to create a vehicle for stereotyping but to whet the reader's appetite to search out more information about the people in their care, given the vast differences among Whites. There are countless cultural phenomena affecting health care; Table 13–2 suggests a few.

■ German Americans

The following material, relating to both the German American and Polish American communities, was obtained from research conducted in southeastern Texas in May 1982 and updated over time. It is by no means indicative of the HEALTH and ILLNESS beliefs of the entire German American and Polish American communities. It is included here to demonstrate the type of data that can be gleaned using an "emic" (a description of behavior dependent on the person's categorization of the action) approach to collecting data. It cannot be generalized, but it allows the reader to grasp the diversity of beliefs that surround us (Lefcowitz, 1990, p. 6).

Since 1830 more than 7 million Germans have immigrated to the United States. There are presently 50.7 million Americans, or 16.4% of the population, who claim German ancestry. California, Texas, and Pennsylvania have the largest numbers of people with German ancestry. The Germans represent a cross section of German society and have come from all social strata and walks of life. Some people have come to escape poverty, others have come for religious or political reasons, and still others have come to take advantage of the opportunity to open up the new lands. Many were recruited to come here, as were the Germans who settled in the German enclaves in Texas. The immigrants represented all religions, including primarily Lutherans, Catholics, and Jews. They represented the rich and the poor, the educated and the ignorant, and were of all ages. Present-day descendants are farmers, educators, and artists. The Germans brought to the United States the cultural diversity and folkways they observed in Germany. The tradition of the Christmas tree and the festivals of Corpus Christi, *Kinderfeste* (children's feast), and *Sangerfeste* (singing festival) all originated in Germany (Conzen, 1980, pp. 405–425). The German Americans introduced the first kindergartens.

The Germans began to migrate to the United States in the 17th century and have contributed 15.2% of the total immigration population. They are the least visible ethnic group in the United States, and people often are surprised to discover that there is such a large Germanic influence in this country. In some places, the German communities maintain strong identification with their German heritage. For example, the city of Fredericksburg, Texas, maintains an ambience of German culture and identity. Some people born there who are fourth-generation and more continue to learn German as their first spoken language (Spector, 1983).

The German ethnic community is the second largest in the state of Texas and is exceeded only by the Mexican community. Germans have been immigrating to Texas since 1840 and continue to arrive. They are predominantly Catholic, Lutheran, and Methodist. Many of these people have maintained their German identity. The major German communities in Texas are Victoria, Cuero, Gonzales, New Braunfels, and Fredericksburg.

During the European freedom revolutions of 1830 and 1848, Texas was quite popular, especially in Germany, and was seen as a "wild and fabulous land." For tradition-bound German families, however, the abandonment of the homeland was difficult. They were enticed, however, by the hopes of economic and social improvement and political idealism. An additional reason for the mass migration was the overpopulation of Germany and the immigrants' desire to escape an imminent European catastrophe. By the 1840s, several thousand northern Germans had come to Texas, and another large migration occurred in 1890. This second cluster of people came because there was severe crop failure in Russian-occupied Germany, and the Russian language had become a required subject in German schools. Other German migrations occurred from 1903 to 1905.

The Germans found pleasure in the small things of everyday life. They were tied together by the German language because it bound them to the past, entertaining them with games, riddles, folk songs and literature, and folk wisdom. The greatest amusement was singing and dancing. Religion for the Lutherans, Catholics, and Methodists was a part of everyday life. The year was measured by the church calendar; observance of church ritual paced the milestones of the life cycle. The Germans believed that each individual was a "part of the fabric of humanity," that "history was a continued process," and "everything had a purpose as mankind strove to something better" (Lich, 1982, pp. 33–72).

The Germans had a penchant for forming societies and clubs, the longest-lasting of which are the singing societies. The first was organized in 1850 and exists still today. The Germans brought with them their customs and traditions; their cures, curses, and recipes; and their tools and ways of building (Lich, 1982).

HEALTH and ILLNESS

Among the Germans, health is described as more than not being ill but as a state of well-being—physically and emotionally—the ability to do your duty, positive energy to do things, and the ability to do, think, and act the way you would like, to go and congregate, to enjoy life. Illness may be described as the absence of well-being: pain, malfunction of body organs, not being able to do what you want, a blessing from God to suffer, and a disorder of body, imbalance.

Causes of ILLNESS

Most German Americans believe in the germ theory of infection and in stress-related theories. Other causes of illness are identified, however, such as drafts, environmental changes, and belief in the evil eye and punishment from God.

The methods of maintaining health include the requirement of dressing properly for the season, proper nutrition, and the wearing of shawls to protect oneself from drafts—also, the taking of cod-liver oil, exercise, and hard work. Methods for preventing illness include wearing an asafetida bag around the neck in the winter to prevent colds, scapulars, religious practices, sleeping with the windows open, and cleanliness.

The use of home remedies to treat illness continues to be practiced. Table 13–3 gives examples of commonly used home remedies. Figure 13–5, is a remedy that may be purchased in Germany and is used to treat colds.

Current Health Problems

There do not appear to be any unusual health problems particular to German Americans.

Table 13-3   ILLNESS Symptoms and Remedies Among German Americans

Gastrointestinal Problems

Symptom	Remedy
Constipation	Castor oil
	Black draught
Diarrhea or vomiting	Do not eat for 24 hours
	Chicken soup
Stomachache	Peppermint tea
	Tea and toast
	Berries, elderberries

Respiratory Problems

Symptom	Remedy
Cold	Wet compress around throat—cover with wool
	Lemon juice and whiskey
	Chopped onions in a sack applied to the soles of the feet
	Olbas (made in Germany)
Cough	Goose fat—rub on chest
	Honey and milk
	Tausend Gülden Krout (thousand golden cabbage)—rum
Earache	Warm oil in ear
	Warm towels
	Bitter geranium leaves
Sore throat	Camphor on a wet rag—wrap around the throat
	Gargle with salt water
	Onion compress
	Chicken soup
	Liniments

Physical Injuries

Symptom	Remedy
Bumps	Hard knife (cold metal), place on bump
Cuts	Iodine—clean well
Puncture wounds (nail)	Soak in kerosene
Wounds	Clean well with water—apply iodine

Miscellaneous Problems

Symptom	Remedy
Aches and pains	Kytle's liniment
	Olbas
	Volcanic oil
	Salves and liniments
Arthritis	Warm-water soaks
	Honey, vinegar, and water soaks
Boils	"Capital water"—sulfur water—drink this (this is available at the Texas capital)

(continued)

Table 13-3 ILLNESS **Symptoms and Remedies Among German Americans (*continued*)**

Clean body after winter	*Kur* (similar to hot springs) drink
Fever	Cold compress on head—fluids
Headache	Iced cloth on head
Menstrual cramps	Cardui
Rheumatism	Aloe vera—rub on sore area
	Cod-liver oil—massage
	Apply fig juice
Ringworm	Chamomile tea compress
Stye	One half of hard-boiled egg—apply warm white on eye
Toothache	Cloves
	Salbec tea
	Olbas
Warts	Apply fig juice and fig leaf milk

Source: Spector, R. E. (1983). *A description of the impact of Medicare on health-illness beliefs and practices of White ethnic senior citizens in Central Texas.* Ph.D. diss. University of Texas at Austin School of Nursing. Ann Arbor, MI: University Microfilms International. Reprinted with permission.

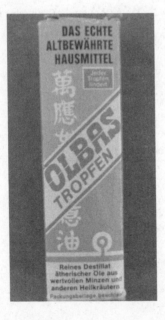

Figure 13-5 *Olbas.*

■ Italian Americans

The Italian American community is made up of immigrants who came here from mainland Italy and from Sicily and Sardinia and other Mediterranean islands that are part of Italy. The number of Americans claiming Italian ancestry is over 18 million. Over 77% of the people, 5 years and older, speak Italian at home and 39.6% speak English less than very well. Fifty-one percent of people of Italian ancestry reside in the Northeast (U.S. Census Bureau, 2001, p. 46).

Italian Americans indeed have a proud heritage in the United States, for America was "founded" by an Italian—Christopher Columbus; named for an Italian—Amerigo Vespucci; and explored by several Italian explorers, including Verrazano, Cabot, and Tonti (Bernardo, 1981, p. 26).

History of Migration

Between 1820 and 1990, over 5 million people from Italy immigrated to the United States (Lefcowitz, 1990, p. 6). The peak years were from 1901 to 1920, and only a small number of people continue to come today. Italians came to this country to escape poverty and to search for a better life in a country where they expected to reap rewards for their hard labor. The early years were not easy, but people chose to remain in this country and not return to Italy. Italians tended to live in neighborhood enclaves, and these neighborhoods, such as the North End in Boston and Little Italy in New York, still exist as Italian neighborhoods. Although the younger generation may have moved out, they still return home to maintain family, community, and ethnic ties (Nelli, 1980, pp. 545–560).

The family has served as the main tie keeping Italian Americans together because it provides its members with the strength to cope with the surrounding world and produces a sense of continuity in all situations. The family is the primary focus of the Italian's concern, and Italians take pride in the family and the home. Italians are resilient, yet fatalistic, and they take advantage of the present. Many upwardly mobile third- and fourth-generation Italian Americans often experience conflict between familial solidarity and society's emphasis on individualization and autonomy (Giordano & McGoldrick, 1996, p. 571). As mentioned, the home is a source of great pride, and it is a symbol of the family, not a status symbol per se. The church also is an important focus for the life of the Italian. Many of the festivals and observances continue to exist today, and in the summer, the North End of Boston, Massachusetts, is alive each weekend with the celebration of a different saint (Figure 13–6). Madonna Della Cava

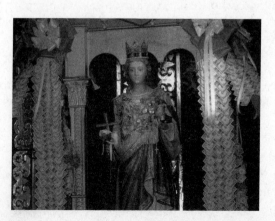

Figure 13–6   Madonna Della Cava.

is an example of one of the saints for whom there is a summer festival. The prayers offered to her include prayers for health. Note the gold and money that has been pinned on the statue's clothes and decorations.

The father traditionally has been the head of the Italian household, and the mother is said to be the heart of the household.

Italian Americans have tended to attain low levels of education in the United States, but their incomes are comparable to or higher than those of other groups.

The Italian population falls into four generational groups: (1) the elderly, living in Italian enclaves; (2) a second generation, living both within the neighborhoods and in the suburbs; (3) a younger, well-educated group, living mainly in the suburbs; and (4) new immigrants (Ragucci, 1981, p. 216). More than 80% of Italian Americans marry people from a different ethnic group (Giordano & McGoldrick, 1996).

HEALTH and ILLNESS

Italians tend to present their symptoms to their fullest point and to expect immediate treatment for ailments. In terms of traditional beliefs, they may view the cause of illness to be one of the following: (1) winds and currents that bear diseases, (2) contagion or contamination, (3) heredity, (4) supernatural or human causes, and (5) psychosomatic interactions.

One such traditional Italian belief contends that moving air, in the form of drafts, causes irritation and then a cold that can lead to pneumonia. A belief an elderly person may express in terms of cancer surgery is that it is not a good idea to have surgery because surgery exposes the inner body to the air, and if the cancer is exposed to the air the person is going to die quicker. Just as drafts are considered to be a cause of illness, fresh air is considered to be vital for the maintenance of health. Homes and the workplace must be well ventilated to prevent illness from occurring.

One sees a belief in contamination manifested in the reluctance of people to share food and objects with people who are considered unclean, and often in not entering the homes of those who are ill. Traditional Italian women have a strong sense of modesty and shame, resulting in an avoidance of discussions relating to sex and menstruation.

Blood is regarded by some, especially the elderly, to be a "plastic entity" that responds to fluids and food and is responsible for many variable conditions. Various adjectives, such as *high* and *low* and *good* and *bad*, are used to describe blood. Some of the "old superstitions" include the following beliefs:

1. Congenital abnormalities can be attributed to the unsatisfied desire for food during pregnancy.
2. If a pregnant woman is not given food that she smells, the fetus will move inside and a miscarriage will result.

3. If a pregnant woman bends, turns, or moves in a certain way, the fetus may not develop normally.

4. A woman must not reach during pregnancy because reaching can harm the fetus.

Italians may also attribute the cause of illness to the evil eye (*malocchio*) or to curses (*castiga*). The difference between these two causes is that less serious illnesses, such as headaches, may be caused by *malocchio* whereas more severe illnesses, which often can be fatal, may be attributed to more powerful *castiga*. Curses are sent either by God or by evil people. An example of a curse is the punishment from God for sins and bad behavior (Ragucci, 1981, p. 216).

Italians recognize that illness can be caused by the suppression of emotions, as well as stress from fear, grief, and anxiety. If one is unable to find an emotional outlet, one well may "burst." It is not considered healthy to bottle up emotions (Ragucci, 1981, p. 232).

Often, the care of the ill is managed in the home, with all members of the family sharing in the responsibilities. The use of home remedies ostensibly is decreasing, although several students have reported the continued use of rituals for the removal of the evil eye and the practice of leeching. One practice described for the removal of the evil eye was to take an egg and olive oil and to drip them into a pan of water, make the sign of the cross, and recite prayers. If the oil spreads over the water, the cause of the problem is the evil eye, and the illness should get better. Mineral waters are also used, and tonics are used to cleanse the blood. There is a strong religious influence among Italians, who believe that faith in God and the saints will see them through the illness. One woman whom I worked with had breast cancer. She had had surgery several years before and did not have a recurrence. She attributed her recovery to the fact that she attended mass every morning and that she had total faith in Saint Peregrine, whose medal she wore pinned to her bra by the site of the mastectomy. Italian people tend to take a fatalistic stance regarding terminal illness and death, believing that it is God's will. Death often is not discussed between the dying person and the family members. I recall when caring for an elderly Italian man at home that it was not possible to have the man and his wife discuss his impending death. Although both knew that he was dying and would talk with the nurse, to each other he "was going to recover," and everything possible was done to that end.

Italian families observe numerous religious traditions surrounding death, and funeral masses and anniversary masses are observed. It is the custom for the widow to wear black for some time after her husband's death (occasionally for the remainder of her life), although this is not as common with the younger generations.

Health-Related Problems

Two genetic diseases commonly seen among Italians are (1) favism, a severe hemolytic anemia caused by deficiency of the X-linked enzyme glucose-6-phosphate dehydrogenase and triggered by the eating of fava beans, and

(2) the thalassemia syndromes, also hemolytic anemias that include Cooley's anemia (or beta-thalassemia) and alpha-thalassemia (Ragucci, 1981, p. 222).

Language problems frequently occur when elderly or new Italian immigrants are seeking care. Often, due to modesty, people are reluctant to answer the questions asked through interpreters, and gathering of pertinent data is very difficult.

Problems related to time also occur. Physicians tend to diagnose emotional problems more often for Italian patients than for other ethnic groups because of the Italian pattern of reporting more symptoms and reporting them more dramatically (Giordano & McGoldrick, 1996, p. 576).

In general, Italian Americans are motivated to seek explanations with respect to their health status and the care they are to receive. If instructions and explanations are well given, Italians tend to cooperate with health care providers. It is often necessary to provide directions in the greatest detail and then to provide written instructions to ensure compliance with necessary regimens.

■ Polish Americans

The first people immigrating to this country from Poland came with Germans in 1608 to Jamestown, Virginia, to help develop the timber industry. Since that time, Poland, too, has given America one of its largest ethnic groups, with over 10.1 million people claiming Polish ancestry. The peak year for Polish immigration was 1921, and well over 578,875 people immigrated here. Many of the people arriving before 1890 came for economic reasons. Those coming here since that time have come for both economic and political reasons and for religious freedom. Polish heroes include Casimir Pulaski and Thaddeus Kosciuszko, who were heroes in the American Revolution. The major influx of Poles to the United States began in 1870 and ended in 1913. The people who arrived were mainly peasants seeking food and release from the political oppression of 3 foreign governments in Poland. The immigrants who came both before and after this mass migration were better educated and not as poor. In the United States, Polish immigrants lived in poor conditions either because they had no choice or because that was the way they were able to meet their own priorities. They were seen by other Americans to live as animals and were often mocked and called stupid. Quite often, the Polish people spoke and understood several European languages but had difficulty learning English and were therefore scorned. Polish people shared the problem as a community and banded together in tight enclaves called "Polonia." They attempted to be as self-sufficient as possible. They worked at preserving their native culture, and voluntary Polish ghettos grew up in close proximity to the parish church (Green, 1980, pp. 787–803). Over 85.5% of those 5 years and older speak Polish at home and 50.3% speak English less than very well. Thirty-seven percent of people of Polish ancestry reside in the Northeast, as well as 37% in the Midwest (U.S. Census Bureau, 2001, p. 46).

An example of the Polish experience in the United States is that of the Polish immigrants in Texas. The first Poles came to Texas in the second half of the 19th century, and most of them settled in Victoria, San Antonio, Houston, and Bandera. The first Polish colonies in America were located in Texas, the oldest being Panna Maria (Virgin Mary) in Karnes County, 50 miles southeast of San Antonio. Unlike other Poles who wanted to return to Poland, the colonists who arrived in Texas after 1850 came to settle permanently and had no intention of returning to their homeland. Although these people came to Texas for economic, political, and religious reasons, severe poverty was their major reason for leaving Poland.

The first collective Polish immigration to America was in 1854, when 100 families came to Texas. They landed in Galveston, where a few in the party remained. The rest traveled in a procession northwestward, taking with them a few belongings, such as featherbeds, crude farm implements, and a cross from their parish church. Their dream was to live on the fertile lands of Texas and raise crops, speak their own language, educate their children, and worship God as they pleased. This dream did not materialize, and members of the band grew discouraged. Some of the immigrants remained in Victoria and others went to San Antonio.

The people who went to San Antonio continued to travel; on Christmas Eve, 1854, they stopped at the junction of the San Antonio and Cibolo Rivers; there, under a live oak tree, they celebrated mass and founded Panna Maria. From 1855 to 1857, others followed this small group in moving to this part of Texas.

These settlers were exposed to many dangers from nature, such as heat, drought, snakes, and insects. The Polish settlers were not accepted by the other settlers in the area because their language, customs, and culture were different, but the immigrants survived and many moved to settle other areas near Panna Maria. Today, the people of Panna Maria continue to live simple lives close to nature and God and speak mainly Polish.

Much of the history of the Polish people in Texas is written around the founding and the location of the various church parishes. For example, in 1873 the Parish of the Nativity of the Blessed Virgin Mary was begun in Cestohowa. Within this church above the main altar is a large picture of the Virgin Mary of Czestochowa. This picture was taken to the church from Panna Maria. It is a copy of the famous Black Madonna of Czestochowa, Poland, a city 65 miles east of where the immigrants to Texas originated. The Black Madonna is a beloved, miraculous image and a source of faith to the Polish people. The Shrine of Our Lady in Czestochowa, Poland, is one of the largest shrines in the world. Since the 14th century, that picture had been the object of veneration and devotion of Polish Catholics. It is claimed to have been painted by Saint Luke the Evangelist. Its origin is traced to the 5th or 6th century and is the oldest picture of the Virgin in the world. The scars on the face date from 1430, when bandits struck it with a sword. The history, traditions, and miracles of Czestochowa are the heritage of the Polish people (Dworaczyk, 1979). One woman I interviewed said she had been ill with a fatal disease. The entire time that she lay close to death she prayed to the Virgin. When she finally did recover, she made a pilgrimage back to her homeland in Poland and visited the shrine to give thanks to the Virgin. The woman was positive that this was the source of her recovery.

HEALTH and ILLNESS

The definitions of HEALTH among the Polish people I interviewed included "feeling okay—as a whole—body, spirit, everything a person cannot separate"; "happy, until war, do not need doctor, do not need medicine"; "active, able to work, feel good, do what I want to do"; and "good spirit, good to everybody, never cross." The definitions of ILLNESS may include "something wrong with body, mind, or spirit"; "one wrong affects them all"; "not capable of working, see the doctor often"; "not right, something ailing you"; "not active"; "feeling bad"; and "opposite of health, not doing what I want to do." The methods for maintaining HEALTH include maintaining a happy home, being kind and loving, eating healthy food, remaining pure, walking, exercising, wearing proper clothing, eating a well-balanced diet, trying not to worry, having faith in God, being active, dressing warmly, going to bed early, and working hard. The methods for preventing ILLNESS include cleanliness, the wearing of scapulars, avoiding drafts, following the proper diet, not gossiping, keeping away from people with colds, and wearing medals because "God is with you all the time to protect you and take care of you." Other ideas about ILLNESS include the beliefs that ILLNESSES are caused by poor diets and that the evil eye may well exist as a causative factor. This belief was attributed to the older generations and is not regarded as prevalent among younger Polish Americans.

The home remedies listed in Table 13–4 were described by informants and are in common use among Polish Americans. One remedy is Swamp Root, a preparation used as a diuretic. Swamp Root is a liquid preparation used to flush the kidneys and bladder, thereby aiding in their work of eliminating waste

Table 13–4 ILLNESS Symptoms and Remedies Among Polish Americans

Gastrointestinal Problems	
Symptom	**Remedy**
Colic	Tea—peppermint or chamomile
	Sugar, water, vinegar, and soda; makes soda water
	Bess-plant tea
	Homemade sauerkraut
Constipation	Epsom salts—teaspoon in water—cleans out stomach
	Cascara
	Castor oil
	Senna-leaf tea
Cramps	Chamomile tea
Diarrhea	Paregoric
	Cinnamon tea
	Dried blueberries
	Coffee beans—to be chewed
Gas	Soda water
Indigestion	*Aloes vulgaris*—juniper and elderberries
	Peppermint and spearmint teas
	Blackberries

Respiratory Problems

Symptom	Remedy
Cold	Castor oil—mentholatum
	Flaxseed or mustard poultice on chest
	Dried raspberries and tea with wine
	Mustard plaster
	Oatmeal poultices—hot bricks to feet
	Cupping
	Camphor salve
	Oxidine
	Goose fat—rub on chest
Cough	Honey and hot water; bedrest
	Hot lemonade with whiskey; honey
	Few drops of turpentine and sugar
	"Gugel Mugel"—warm milk with butter, whiskey, and honey
	Honey and warm milk
	Milk with butter and garlic
	Mustard plaster
	Linden tea
	Onion poultice
Croup	Few drops of kerosene and sugar
Sore throat	Honey
	Warm water, salt—gargle
	Goose grease around throat covered with dry rag
	Paint throat with kerosene
	Goose fat in milk

Physical Injury

Symptom	Remedy
Burns	Aloe vera
Cuts	Vinegar, water, flour paste
	Clean with urine
	Carbolic salve
Puncture wounds (nail)	Turpentine and liniment
	Salt pork—put on wound and soak the wound in hot water
	Hunt's lightning oil
Frostbite	Snow—put on frozen area
Scratches, sores	Liniment
	Moss
	Spider webs
Sprains	Liniments—Sloan's Volcanic

Miscellaneous Problems

Symptom	Remedy
Earache	Hot-water-bottle to ear
	Camphor on cotton—place in ear
Fever	Chamomile tea

(continued)

Table 13-4 ILLNESS **Symptoms and Remedies among Polish Americans (*continued*)**

Miscellaneous Problems	
Symptom	**Remedy**
Flu	Novak Oil—rub on head
	Knorr's Green Drops
Headache	Vinegar—on a cloth, apply to head
	Steam kettle—cover head and inhale
High blood pressure	Cooked garlic
	Garlic oil
Lice	Kerosene—cover hair with kerosene
Toothache	Hot salt compress
Neuralgia	Bedrest
Pyorrhea	Yarrow tea
Rheumatism	Lemon juice—rub on sore places
Trouble urinating	Juice of pumpkin seeds made into a tea
	Swamp Root medicine

Source: Spector, R. E. (1983). *A description of the impact of Medicare on health-illness beliefs and practices of White ethnic senior citizens in Central Texas.* Ph.D. diss. University of Texas at Austin School of Nursing. Ann Arbor, MI: University Microfilms International. Reprinted with permission.

matter. It contains 10.5% alcohol and various herbs such as peppermint, cape aloes, oil of juniper, and buchu leaves incorporated into a syrup. The alcohol is used for the purpose of preserving the ingredients (Figure 13–7).

Health Care Problems

The Polish community has not tended to have any major problems with health care deliverers. Language may be a barrier if members of the older generation

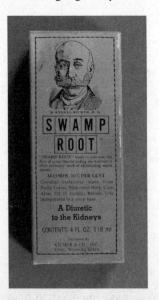

Figure 13-7 Swamp Root.

do not speak English, and the taking of health histories is complicated when the providers cannot communicate directly with the informant. Again, problems may develop when there is difficulty finding someone who is conversant in Polish whom the informant can trust to reveal personal matters and who can translate medical terms accurately.

In Poland, there is a shortage of medical supplies, so the people tend to use faith healers and believe in miracle workers. On the main street of Warsaw, all sorts of folk medicine and miracle-worker paraphernalia are on sale: divining rods, cotton sacks filled with herbs to be worn over an ailing heart or liver, coils of copper wire to be placed under food to rid it of poisons, and pendulums (*Letter from Poland*, 1983).

■ Health Status of the White Population

There are countless health status indicators wherein the White cohort of the population differs from the total population, each of the racial groups, and Hispanics. In each of the preceding 4 chapters, there has been a table comparing the relevant group and all races. In this chapter, it is appropriate to compare the White non-Hispanic population to the total population (Table 13–5) and also to all races (Table 13–6). In spite of the fact that only 13 health indicators

Table 13-5 Comparison of Selected Health Status Indicators—All Races and White non-Hispanic: 2007

Health Indicator	All Races	White Non-Hispanic
Crude birth rate per 1,000 population by race of mother	14.3	11.6
Percentage of live births to women receiving first-trimester prenatal care	67.5	74.9
Percentage of live births to women receiving third-trimester prenatal care or no prenatal care	8.4	5.5
Percentage of live births to teenage childbearing women—under 18	3.4	2.0
Percentage of low birth weight per live births <2,500 grams	8.22	7.28
Infant mortality per 1,000 live births (2006)	6.7	5.6
Cancer—all sites per 100,000 population	446.7	479.4
Lung cancer incidence per 100,000 population	Men: 65.4	69.1
	Women: 47.4	54.5
Breast cancer incidence per 100,000	122.5	133.5
Prostate cancer incidence per 100,000	158.3	158.7
Male death rates from suicide, all ages, age adjusted per 100,000 resident population	11.3	21.9
Male death rates from homicide, all ages, age adjusted per 100,000 resident population	6.1	3.7

Source: National Center for Health Statistics. *Health, United States, 2010*: With Special Feature on Death and Dying. Hyattsville, MD. 2011: Author, pp. 102, 106, 107, 110, 124, 137, 180–181, 184–185, and 204. Retrieved from **www.cdc.gov/nchs/data/hus/hus10.pdf** 2011.

Table 13–6 Comparison of Selected Health Status Indicators—All Races, American Indian and Alaska Native, Asian/Pacific Islander, Black or African American, Hispanic or Latino, and White Non-Hispanic: 2007

Health Indicator	All Races	American Indian and Alaska Native	Asian/Pacific Islander[1]	Black or African American	Hispanic or Latino	White Non-Hispanic
Crude birth rate per 1,000 population by race of mother	14.3	15.3	17.2	16.9	23.4	11.6
Percentage of live births to women receiving first-trimester prenatal care	67.5	53.2	69.8	57.0	56.1	74.9
Percentage of live births to women receiving third-trimester or no prenatal care	8.4	14.0	7.7	12.6	12.9	5.5
Percentage of live births to teenage childbearing women—under 18	3.4	6.1	0.9	6.1	5.3	2.0
Percentage of low-birth- weight per live births <2,500 grams	8.22	7.46	8.10	13.55	6.93	7.28
Infant mortality per 1,000 live births (2006)	6.7	8.3	4.5	12.9	5.4	5.6
Cancer—all sites per 100,000 population	446.7	332.0	322.0	470.0	326.5	479.4

Lung cancer incidence per 100,000 population	Men: 65.4 Women: 47.4	a a	52.4 27.0	87.2 51.2	38.0 22.5	69.1 54.5
Breast cancer incidence per 100,000	122.5	83.4	98.0	120.5	83.8	133.5
Prostate cancer incidence per 100,000	158.3	77.9	93.3	227.4	116.2	158.7
Male death rates from suicide, all ages, age adjusted per 100,000 resident population	11.3	18.1	9.0	8.8	10.1	21.9
Male death rates from homicide, all ages, age adjusted per 100,000 resident population	6.1	9.2	3.3	37.1	11.2	3.7

Source: National Center for Health Statistics. (2006). *Health, United States, 2006 with chartbook on trends in the health of Americans.* Hyattsville, MD: Author, pp. 135, 140, 144, 149, 160, 227, 230, 244.

a: no data available.
[1]Pacific Islanders are clustered with Asian health statistics when indicated.

Table 13-7 **Comparison of the 10 Leading Causes of Death for White Americans and for All Persons: 2007**

White Americans	All Persons
1. Diseases of heart	Diseases of heart
2. Malignant neoplasms	Malignant neoplasms
3. Chronic lower respiratory diseases	Cerebrovascular diseases
4. Cerebrovascular diseases	Chronic lower respiratory diseases
5. Unintentional injuries	Unintentional injuries
6. Alzheimer's disease	Alzheimer's disease
7. Diabetes mellitus	Diabetes mellitus
8. Influenza and pneumonia	Influenza and pneumonia
9. Nephritis, nephrotic/syndrome and nephrosis	Nephritis, nephrotic/syndrome and nephrosis
10. Suicide	Septicemia

Source: National Center for Health Statistics. (2007). Health, United States, 2007 with chartbook on trends in the health of Americans. Hyattsville, MD: Author, p. 187.

are listed as examples in the tables, the health differences and disparities in the overall populations are readily apparent.

Table 13–7 lists the 10 leading causes of death for Whites and compares them with the causes of death for the general population in 2007.

In this chapter, as in this entire book, I have attempted to open the door to the enormous diversity in health and illness beliefs that exists in White (European American) communities specifically and in the entire American population in general. I have only opened the door and invited you to peek inside. There is a richness of knowledge to be gained. It is for you to acquire it as you care for all patients. Ask them what they believe about health/HEALTH and illness/ILLNESS and what their traditional beliefs, practices, and remedies are. The students whom I am working with find this to be a very enlightening experience.

RESEARCH IN CULTURE

A great amount of research has been conducted among members of the White American populations. The following article describes one such study:

Hutson, S. P., Dorgan, K. A., Phillips, A. N., & Behringer, B. (2007, November). *The mountains hold things in: The use of community research review work groups to address cancer disparities in Appalachia.* Oncology Nursing Forum, 34(6), 1133–1139.

The purpose of this research study was to review regional findings about cancer disparities with grass-roots community leaders in Appalachia and to discover what makes the experience of cancer unique in that part of the country. The study was community-based and information was gathered from focus groups. Four major themes emerged from the focus groups:

1. *Cancer storytelling.* One theme was the ubiquitous nature of cancer and that the members of the community expect to get cancer. Many participants believed that "cancer was more a hereditary thing" because of family histories.
2. *Cancer collectiveness.* Rural families tend to rely on themselves.
3. *Health care challenges.* Participants were doubtful about their ability to navigate and trust the health care system. They also told of the state's history of overlooking the people in this community.
4. *Cancer expectations.* Some rural people may not embrace what are seen as basic patients' rights.

The key discoveries were that the cancer experience in Appalachia appears to be affected uniquely by cultural, economic, and geographic influences; that health care professionals and researchers must respect and partner with existing social and familial community networks; and the use of community research review work is a viable method to examine cancer disparities in a marginalized population. Suggestions from this study supported the need for patient navigators and advocate services to reach communities and bridge the gaps between the health care system and laypeople. Cancer information should be tailored to individual patients' attributes, such as education and literacy levels and cultural and familial beliefs.

Explore 🌐 MediaLink

Go to the Student Resource Site at nursing.pearsonhighered.com for chapter-related review questions, case studies, and activities. Contents of the CULTURALCARE Guide and CULTURALCARE Museum can also be found on the Student Resource Site. Click on Chapter 13 to select the activities for this chapter.

■ Internet Sources

Hixson, L., Hepler, B., & Kim, M. (2011). The White Population: 2010. Retrieved from http://www.census.gov/, December 4, 2011.

Humes, K. R., Nicholas, A. J., Ramirez, R. (2011). Overview of Race and Hispanic Origin: 2010. Census Briefs. Retrieved from http://2010.census.gov/2010census/data/, June 26, 2011, p 4.

Lee, J. (2011). Annual Flow Report U.S. Naturalizations: 2010. U.S. Department of Commerce, Economics and Statistics Administration, Office of Homeland Security, Office of Immigration Statistics. Retrieved from http://www.dhs.gov/files/statistics/publications/gc_1302103955524.shtm, June 1, 2011.

Monger, R., & Yankay, J. (2011). Annual Flow Report. U.S. Legal Permanent Residents: 2010. U.S. Department of Commerce, Economics and Statistics Administration, Office of Homeland Security, Office of Immigration Statistics. Retrieved from http://www.dhs.gov/files/statistics/publications/gc_1301497627185.shtm, June 1, 2011.

U.S. Census Bureau. (2011). 2010 American Community Survey, B04003 People Reporting Ancestry. Retrieved from http://factfinder2.census.gov/faces/tableservices/jsf/pages/productview.xhtml?pid=ACS_10_1YR_B04003&prodType=table, March 12, 2012.

U.S. Department of Health and Human Services. (2011). National Center for Health Statistics. Health, United States, 2010: With Special feature on Death and Dying. Hyattsville, MD: Author. Retrieved from www.cdc.gov/nchs/data/hus/hus10.pdf, March 12, 2012.

■ References

Bernardo, S. (1981). *The ethnic almanac.* New York: Doubleday.

Conzen, K. N. (1980). Germans. In S. Thernstrom (Ed.), *Harvard encyclopedia of American ethnic groups.* Cambridge, MA: Harvard University Press.

Dworaczyk, E. J. (1979). *The first Polish colonies of America in Texas.* San Antonio, TX: Naylor.

Giordano, J., & McGoldrick, M. (1996). Italian families. In M. McGoldrick, J. Giordano, & J. K. Pearce (Eds.), *Ethnicity and family therapy* (2nd ed.). New York: Guilford.

Green, V. (1980). Poles. In S. Thernstrom (Ed.), *Harvard encyclopedia of American ethnic groups.* Cambridge, MA: Harvard University Press.

Lefcowitz, E. (1990). *The United States immigration history timeline.* New York: Terra Firma Press.

Letter from Poland—of faith healers and miracle workers. (1983, August 21). *Boston Globe,* p.15.

Lich, G. E. (1982). *The German Texan.* San Antonio: University of Texas Institute of Texan Cultures.

Needleman, J. (2003). *The American soul.* NY: Tarcher/Putman.

Nelli, H. S. (1980). Italians. In S. Thernstrom (Ed.), *Harvard encyclopedia of American ethnic groups.* Cambridge, MA: Harvard University Press.

Ragucci, A. T. (1981). Italian Americans. In A. Harwood (Ed.), *Ethnicity and medical care.* Cambridge, MA: Harvard University Press.

Spector, R. E. (1983). *A description of the impact of Medicare on health-illness beliefs and practices of White ethnic senior citizens in Central Texas.* PhD. diss., University Texas at Austin School of Nursing. Ann Arbor, MI: University Microfilms International.

U.S. Census Bureau. (2001). *Statistical abstract of the United States: 2001.* Washington, DC: Author.

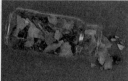 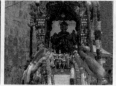 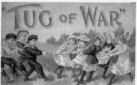

Figure 14-1 Figure 14-2   Figure 14-3   Figure 14-4

Chapter 14

CULTURALCOMPETENCE

The opening images for this chapter bring closure to the process of becoming CULTURALLYCOMPETENT. They both summarize and symbolize many of the concepts presented in the text. Each chapter opened with images representing amulets, remedies, and/or shrines that were related to the content of the chapter. Here, a symbolic image of an amulet, remedy, and shrine are followed by an image of the "tug of war" that one may experience as they embrace the ideas of CULTURALCOMPETENCY. Figure 14–1 is a *Daruma*—a doll—representing the Indian priest Bodhidharma, the founder of Zen Buddhism in China. It was said he lost his arms and legs meditating in a cave. The dolls are made of paper-mache on a bamboo frame. They are used as charms, or amulets, for the fulfillment of special wishes and as a talisman for protection against "small pox." They are popular with Japanese Americans today and can be purchased at Japanese cultural events. Figure 14–2 is an example of an herbal remedy. The use of herbs—often those that can be grown in your own back yard—to treat many maladies is common. Countless people turn to herbs, usually as their first source of medication, and evidence now indicates that the use of herbal remedies is prevalent among many people. Figure 14–3 is a Thai Spirit Shrine located on a street corner in Los Angeles, California. It is a place where passersby are able to stop and meditate for as long as they desire to do so. Figure 14–4, "Tug of War," represents the ongoing tensions between the allopathic and homeopathic philosophies and the conflict you may experience when you encounter people who prefer traditional health and illness beliefs and practices rather than modern health care therapies. Implicit in CULTURALCOMPETENCY is the understanding of a situation from a "person or patient's point of view."

The perplexing questions—

- *Why* must health care deliverers—nurses, physicians, public health and social workers, and other health care professionals—study culture, ethnicity, religion, and become culturally competent?
- *Why* must they know the difference between "hot" and "cold" and *yin* and *yang*?
- *Why* must they be concerned with the patient's failure to practice what professionals believe to be good preventive medicine, with the patient's failure to follow a given treatment regimen, or with the patient's failure to seek medical care during the initial phase of an illness?
- *Why* is there a difference between curing and HEALING?

—have now been explored and selected answers presented.

There is little disagreement that health care services in this country are unevenly distributed and that the poor and the emerging majority get the short end of the stick in terms of the care they receive (or do not receive). The apparent health disparities are a reality, as are the demographic and social disparities in areas of housing, employment, education, and opportunity. Just as there is the need to understand the people who comprise our multicultural society, there is also the need to understand new immigrants as more and more people flock to this country. Yet it is often maintained that when health care is provided, people fail to use it or use it inappropriately. Why is this seeming paradox so?

The major focus of this book has been on the provider's and the patient's differing perceptions of health/HEALTH and illness/ILLNESS. These differences may account for the health care provider's misconception that services are used inappropriately and that people do not care about their health. What to the casual observer appears to be "misuse" may represent our failure to understand and to meet the needs and expectations of the patient. This possibility may well be difficult for health care providers to face, but careful analysis of the available information seems to indicate that this may—at least in part—be the case. How, then, can we, who are health care providers, change our method of operations and provide both safe and effective care for all—the emerging majority and, at the same time, for the population at large? The answer to this question is not an easy one, and some researchers think we are not succeeding. A number of measures can and must be taken to ameliorate the current situation. CULTURALCARE and the educational preparation leading to this is a *process*, one that becomes a way of life and must be recognized as such. This is a philosophical issue. The changing of one's personal and professional philosophies, ideas, and stereotypes does *not* occur overnight, and the process, quite often, is neither direct nor easy. It is a multistep process, in which one must:

- explore his or her own cultural identity and heritage and confront biases and stereotypes;
- develop an awareness and understanding of the complexities of the modern health care delivery system—its philosophy and problems, biases, and stereotypes;

- develop a keen awareness of the socialization process that brings the provider into this complex system; and
- develop the ability to "hear" things that transcend language, foster an understanding of the patient and his or her cultural heritage, and the resilience found within the culture that supports family and community structures.

Given the processes of acculturation, assimilation, and modernism, this is often difficult and painful. Yet, once the journey of exploring one's own cultural heritage and prejudices is undertaken, the awareness of the cultural needs of others becomes more subtle and understandable. This is well accomplished by using the umbrella of HEALTH traditions as the point of entry.

A student I once taught described the journey this way:

> I was born in 1973 to fourth-generation Japanese American parents. I understood Japanese culture and the way of thinking and did not question when my parents told me to eat noodles on New Year's Day to bring long life. Then I changed schools and went to the Caucasian school. I came to hate my heritage and wanted to scream that "I'm as white on the inside as you are." I was bitter and embarrassed by my heritage and blamed my family, who were proud of their ancestry. When my parents tried to teach me about Japanese American history, I was not interested. I came to know, understand, and hate racism. On the inside I felt as "white American" as everyone else but I soon realized what I felt inside was not what other people saw. I now acknowledge who I am and I accept myself.

The voice of this young student speaks for many. In the course of having to explore the family's traditional health beliefs and practices, the student began to see, think through, understand, and accept herself.

Although curricula in professional education are quite full, CULTURALCARE *studies must be taken by all people who wish to deliver health care.* In the wake of September 11, 2001, it is obvious that it is no longer sufficient to teach a student in the health professions to "accept patients for who they are." The question arises: Who is the patient? Introductory sociology and psychology courses fail to provide this information unless tailored to include culture aspects of HEALTH and ILLNESS. It is learned best by meeting with the people themselves and letting them describe who they are from their own perspective. I have suggested 2 approaches to the problem. One is to have people who work as patient advocates or as nurses and physicians come to the class setting and explain how people of their ethnic group view health/HEALTH and illness/ILLNESS and describe the given community's HEALTH traditions. Another approach is to send students out into communities where they will have the opportunity to meet with people in their own settings. It is not necessary to memorize all the available lists of herbs, hot–cold imbalances, folk diseases, and so forth. The objective is to become more sensitive to the crucial fact that multiple factors underlie given patient behaviors. One, of course, is that the patient may well perceive and understand HEALTH from quite a different perspective than that of the health care provider. *Each person comes from a unique culture and a unique socialization process.*

The health care provider must be sensitive to his or her own perceptions of health and illness and the practices he or she employs. Even though the perceptions of most health professionals are based on a middle-class and medical-model viewpoint, providers must realize that there are other ways of regarding health and illness. The early chapters of this book are devoted to consciousness raising about self-treatment. It is always an eye-opening experience to publicly scrutinize ourselves in this respect. Quite often, we are amazed to see how far we stray from the system's prescribed methods of keeping healthy. The journals confirm that we, too, delay in seeking health care and fail to comply with treatment regimens. Often, our ability to comply rests on quite pragmatic issues, such as "What is it doing for me?" and "Can I afford to miss work and stay in bed for two days?" As we gain insight into our own health–illness attitudes and behaviors, we tend to be much more sympathetic to and empathetic with the person who fails to come to the clinic or who hates to wait for the physician or who delays in seeking health care.

The health care provider should be aware of the complex issues that surround the delivery of health care from the patient's viewpoint. Calling the medical society for the name of a physician (because a "family member has a health problem") and visiting and comparing the services rendered in an urban and a suburban emergency room are exercises that can enable us to better appreciate some of the difficulties that the poor, the emerging majority, and the population at large all too often experience when they attempt to obtain health care. Members of the health care team have a number of advantages in gaining access to the health care system. For example, they can choose a physician whom they know because they work with him or her or because someone they work with has recommended this physician. Health care providers must never forget, however, that most people do not have these advantages. It is indeed an unsettling, anxiety-provoking, and frustrating experience to be forced to select a physician from a list. It is an even more frustrating experience to be a patient in an unfamiliar location—for example, an urban emergency room, where, quite literally, anything can happen. The film by Michael Moore, SICKO, paints a most painful picture of the modern health care system. Books, such as J. P. Kassirer's *On the Take* illustrate the complicity of the health care system and big business; and T. R. Reid's, *The Healing of America: A Global Quest for Better and Cheaper, and Fairer Health Care* serve to illustrate other aspects of the complex health care system we live with today. Yet, people entering the system ought to be familiar with all aspects of it and many issues not mentioned, such as the costs of procedures and medications.

Another barrier to adequate health care is the financial burden imposed by treatments and tests. There are other issues as well. For example, a Chinese patient—who traditionally does not believe that the body replaces the blood taken for testing purposes—should have as little blood work as necessary, and the reasons for the tests should be explained carefully. A Hispanic woman who believes that taking a Pap smear is an intrusive procedure that will bring shame to her should have the procedure performed by a female physician or nurse. When this is not possible, she should have a female chaperone with her for the entire time that the male physician or nurse is in the room.

More members of the emerging majority must be represented in the health care professions. Multiple issues are related to the problem of underrepresentation—the demographic disparity—that is ongoing because there are inadequate numbers of people from emerging majorities. Many of the programs designed to increase the number of emerging majority students in the health care team have failed. Difficulties surrounding successful entrance into and completion of professional education programs are complex and numerous, having their roots in impoverished community structures and early educational deprivation. Although society is in some ways dealing with such issues—for example, initiating improvements in early education—we are faced with an *immediate* need to bring more emerging majority people into health care services.

One method would be the more extensive use of patient advocates and outreach workers from the given ethnic community who may be recognized there as healers. The people can provide an overwhelmingly positive service to both the provider and the patient in that they can serve as the bridge in bringing health care services to the target community. The patient advocate can speak to the patient in the language that he or she understands and in a manner that is acceptable. Advocates are also able to coordinate medical, nursing, social, and even educational services to meet the patient's needs as the patient perceives them. In settings where advocates are employed, many problems are resolved to the convenience of both the health care member and, more importantly, the patient!

The nettlesome issue of language bursts forth with regularity. There is always a problem when a non–English-speaking person tries to seek help from the English-speaking majority. The more common languages, French, Italian, and Spanish, ideally should be spoken by at least some of the professional people who staff hospitals, clinics, neighborhood health care centers, and home health agencies. The use of an interpreter or translator is always difficult because the translator generally "interprets" what he or she translates. To bring this thought home, the reader should recall the childhood game of "gossip": A message is passed around the room from person to person, and by the time it gets back to the sender, its content is usually substantially changed. This game is not unlike trying to communicate through a translator, and the situation is even more frustrating when—as can often be the case in urban emergency rooms—the translator is a 6-year-old child. It is, obviously, far more satisfying and productive if the patient, nurse, and physician can all speak the same language. All institutions must follow the mandates of Title VI of the Civil Rights Law. In fact, in many institutions there are professional interpreters available, however, they may not be present 24 hours a day. Telephone devices and some computer-generated programs are available, but costly.

Health services must be made far more accessible and available to members of the emerging majority. I believe that one of the most important events in this modern era of health care delivery is the advent of neighborhood health centers. They are successful essentially because people who work in them know the people of the neighborhood. In addition, the people of the community can contribute to the decision making involved in governing and running the agency so that services are tailored to meet the needs of the patients. Concerned members of the health care team have a moral obligation to support the increased use of health care centers and not their decreased use, as currently tends to occur because of cutbacks in response to allegations (frequently politically motivated) of too-high costs or the misuse of funds. These neighborhood health care centers provide greatly needed personal services in addition to relief from the widespread depersonalization that occurs in larger institutions. When health care providers who are genuinely concerned face this reality, perhaps they will be more willing to fight for the survival of these centers and strongly urge their increased funding rather than acquiesce in their demise. In rural areas, the problem is even greater, and far more comprehensive health planning is needed to meet patient needs.

In the beginning of this text and throughout it, I used the metaphor of climbing stairs to reach CULTURALCOMPETENCY. However, this can be seen, too, as a journey. Thus, the *road*, or ascent, to CULTURALCOMPETENCY is similar to traveling on a road to anywhere. It takes time and thought and active participation. It is a learning experience wherein you discover countless facts (especially about yourself), a dynamic *process* in which you face a number of obstacles on the road:

Table 14-1 The Journey to CULTURALCOMPETENCE

Collisions	Head-ons—meeting dense cultural conflicts and barriers—can be fatal Rear-enders—come at you from behind to sabotage efforts Fender benders—slips and blunders Side swipes—minor, but hurtful frustrations
Conditions	Culture + Climate—Social/Institutional attitudes Weather (rain, snow, fog, sun)—Heritage—Race/Ethnicity/Religion/Socialization
Curves	The unknown—inability to anticipate the real responses, verbal vs. nonverbal
Destination	Physical, Mental, Spiritual—a realization of and respect for holistic HEALTH
Hills	The process of gaining CULTURALCOMPETENCY—content and experience—an up and down experience
Lights	Slow, and controls the progress

No Signs	Road twists and turns and no identifying markings
Open Highway	Cruise along—but not too fast
Other Drivers	Slow you down or speed you up on the road to CULTURALCARE
Pot Holes	Frequent blocks to smooth movement, often unseen, filled with water or covered with ice
Rush Hour	Institutional and provider clogs
Ruts	When cruising along, the unexpected hits and it is often difficult to break free
Speed Limits	Analogous to Institutional and Professional restraints—do not go too fast or too slow or you are in trouble and everyone is behind you
Tolls	Expensive—pay for books, travel, objects, admissions, tools
Unexpected Events	Negative—radar, accidents, ice—anger, "isms" Positive—enduring friendships with people you may have never met Knowledge far deeper than ever anticipated Wisdom Deep love of life and people

CULTURALCARE is the term I have coined to express all that is inherent in this text. Countless conflicts in the health care delivery arenas are predicated on cultural misunderstandings. Although many of these misunderstandings are related to universal situations, such as verbal and nonverbal language misunderstandings, the conventions of courtesy, sequencing of interactions, phasing of interactions, objectivity, and so forth, many cultural misunderstandings are unique to the delivery of health care. The necessity to provide CULTURALCARE—professional health care that is culturally sensitive, culturally appropriate, and culturally competent—is essential as we live in this millennium, and it demands that providers be able to assess and interpret a given patient's health/HEALTH beliefs and practices. CULTURALCARE alters the perspective of health care delivery as it enables the provider to understand, from a cultural perspective, the manifestations of the patient's HEALTH care beliefs and practices. Note, that the terms CULTURALCOMPETENCY and CULTURALCARE are written in small capitals to indicate that the view is holistic—three dimensional rather than two.

■ CULTURALCOMPETENCY

You'll know you are on the road to CULTURALCOMPETENCY when you understand that:

■ even when you are a part of a group, social or professional, you are a person who has your own HERITAGE—your own culture, ethnicity, and religion;

- you have been socialized, first by your parents then by schools/teachers and later by society at large, to be who you are;
- you have your own HEALTH and ILLNESS beliefs and practices;
- there are countless ways to protect and maintain your HEALTH other than those prescribed by the dominant culture;
- amulets are commonly used by people from many heritages;
- there are countless ways to restore your HEALTH other than those prescribed by the dominant culture's allopathic health care system;
- herbal remedies, teas, aromatherapy, and so on are used by people from countless traditional heritages;
- religion plays a profound role in the HEALTH and HEALING beliefs and practices of traditional people from all walks of life; and,
- shrines, either secular or religious, are inherent in the HEALING process of countless people.

I should like to reiterate that this book was written with the hope that by sharing the material I have learned and taught for nearly forty years, some small changes will be made in the thinking of all health care providers who read it. There is nothing new in these pages. Perhaps it is simply a recombination of material with which the reader is familiar, but I hope it serves its purpose: the sharing of beliefs and attitudes, and the stimulation of lots of consciousness raising concerning issues of vital concern to health care providers who must confront the needs of patients with diverse cultural backgrounds.

Explore 🌐 MediaLink

Go to the Student Resource Site at nursing.pearsonhighered.com for chapter-related review questions, case studies, and activities. Contents of the CULTURALCARE Guide and CULTURALCARE Museum can also be found on the Student Resource Site. Click on Chapter 14 to select the activities for this chapter.

■ References

Kassirer, J. P. (2005). *On the take*. Oxford: University Press.

Reid, T. R. (2010). *The healing of America: A global quest for better and cheaper, and fairer health care*. NY: Penguin.

Appendix A   Selected Key Terms Related to Cultural
             Diversity in Health and Illness   354

Appendix B   Calendar: Cultural and Religious Holidays
             That Change Dates   364

Appendix C   Suggested Course Outline   367

Appendix D   Suggested Course Activity—Urban Hiking   373

Appendix E   Heritage Assessment Tool   376

Appendix F   Quick Guide for CULTURALCARE   379

Appendix G   Data Resources   381

Appendix A

Selected Key Terms Related to Cultural Diversity in Health and Illness

The following terms have been defined to help you in the development of CULTURALCOMPETENCY. They are the "bricks" that comprise the steps that must be climbed in the process of developing CULTURALCOMPETENCY. They are the language of CULTURALCARE.

Aberglaubish or *aberglobin*—The traditional German term for the "evil eye."

Access—Gaining entry into a system; the term used in this text refers to access into the modern health care system. *Access* also means entry into a profession, education, employment, housing, and so forth.

Acculturation—The process of adapting to another culture; to acquire the majority group's culture.

Acupuncture—The traditional Chinese medical way of restoring the balance of *yin* and *yang* that is based on the therapeutic value of cold. Cold is used in a disease where there is an excess of *yang*.

Ageism—Being against people of a certain age.

Alcoholismo—Alcoholism.

Alien—Every person applying for entry to the United States; anyone who is not a U.S. citizen.

Allopathic Philosophy—Health beliefs and practices that are derived from current scientific models and involve the use of technology and other modalities of present-day health care, such as immunization, proper nutrition, and resuscitation.

Allopathy—The treatment of a disease by using remedies that cause the opposite effects of the disease.

Alternative health system—A system of health care a person may use that is not predicated within his or her traditional culture but is not allopathic.

Amulet—An object with magical powers, such as a charm, worn on a string or chain around the neck, wrist, or waist to protect the wearer from both physical and psychic illness, harm, and misfortune.

Anamnesis—The traditional Chinese medical way of diagnosing a health problem by asking questions.

Apparel—Traditional clothing worn by people for cultural or religious beliefs on a daily basis, such as head coverings.

Aromatherapy—Ancient science that uses essential plant oils to produce strong physical and emotional effects in the body.

Assimilation—To become absorbed into another culture and to adopt its characteristics. To develop a new cultural identity.

Ataque de nervios—An attack of nerves, or a nervous breakdown.

Average charge—Average amount of monetary charge in hospital bills for discharged patients.

Average length of stay—The typical number of days a patient stays in the hospital for a particular condition.

Ayurvedic—Four-thousand-year-old method of healing originating in India, the chief aim of which is longevity and quality of life. The most ancient existing medical system that uses diet, natural therapies, and herbs.

Balance (or equilibrium)—each aspect of the person—physical, mental, and spiritual—carries equal magnitude.

Bankes—Small, bell-shaped glass that is used to create a vacuum, placed on a person's chest, to loosen chest secretions.

Biofeedback—The use of an electronic machine to measure skin temperatures. The patient controls responses that are usually involuntary.

Biological variations—Biological differences that exist among races and ethnic groups in body structure, skin color, biochemical differences, susceptibility to disease, and nutritional differences.

Borders—Legal, geographic separations between nations.

Botanica—Traditional Hispanic pharmacy where amulets, herbal remedies, books, candles, and statues of saints may be purchased.

Bruja—A witch.

Caida de la mollera (fallen fontanel)—Traditional Hispanic belief that the fontanel falls if the baby's head is touched.

Calendar—Dates of religious holidays. Many of these dates of observance can change from year to year on the Julian calendar.

Care—Factors that assist, enable, support, or facilitate a person's needs to maintain, improve, or ease a health problem.

Celos—Jealousy.

Census—The U.S. Census Bureau counts every resident in the United States. The data collected by the decennial census determine the number of seats each state has in the U.S. House of Representatives and is also used to distribute billions in federal funds to local communities.

Charm—Objects that combine the functions of both amulets and talismans but consist only of written words or symbols.

Chinese doctor—Physician educated in China who uses traditional herbs and other therapeutic modalities in the delivery of health care.

Chiropractic—A form of health care that believes in the use of "energy" to treat diseases.

Complementary medicine—Treatment modalities used to complement allopathic regimens.

Citizen—a citizen of the United States is a native-born, foreign-born child of citizens, or a naturalized person who owes allegiance to the United States and who is entitled to its protection.

Conjure—To effect magic.

Coraje—Rage.

Costs—The monetary price of an item or the consequences of ignoring social factors.

CULTURALCARE—A concept that describes holistic HEALTH care that is culturally sensitive, culturally appropriate, and culturally competent. CULTURALCARE is critical to meeting the complex nursing care needs of a person, family, and community. It is the provision of health care across cultural boundaries and takes into account the context in which the patient lives as well as the situations in which the patient's health problems arise.

Culturally appropriate—Implies that the health care provider applies the underlying background knowledge that must be possessed to provide a given patient with the best possible HEALTH care.

CULTURALLYCOMPETENT—Implies that within the delivered care the health care provider understands and attends to the total context of the patient's situation. CULTURALCOMPETENCE is a complex combination of knowledge, attitudes, and skills.

Culturally sensitive—Implies that the health care providers possess some basic knowledge of and constructive attitudes toward the HEALTH traditions observed among the diverse cultural groups found in the setting in which they are practicing.

Culture—Nonphysical traits, such as values, beliefs, attitudes, and customs, that are shared by a group of people and passed from one generation to the next; a meta-communication system.

Culture shock—Disorder that occurs in response to transition from one cultural setting to another. Former behavior patterns are ineffective in such a setting, and basic cues for social behavior are absent.

Curandera(o)—Traditional Hispanic holistic healer.

Curing*—Two-dimensional phenomenon that results in ridding the body or mind (or both) of a given disease.

Decoction—A simmered tea made from the bark, root, seed, or berry of a plant.

Demographic disparity—A variation below the percentages of the profile of the total population with a specific entity, such as poverty, or professional, such as nursing. Comparison with the demographic profile of the total population.

Demographic parity—An equal distribution of a given entity, such as registered nurses, and the demographic profile of the total population.

Demographics—The population profile of the nation, state, county, or local city or town.

---

*These terms are defined with their traditional connotations, rather than with modern denotations (compiled over time by R. Spector).

Demography—The statistical study of populations, including statistical counts of people of various ages, sexes, and population densities for specific locations.

Determinism—Believing that life is under a person's control.

Diagnosis—The identifying of the nature or cause of something, especially a problem.

Disadvantaged background—Both educational and economic factors that act as barriers to an individual's participation in a health professions program.

Discrimination—Denying people equal opportunity by acting on a prejudice.

Divination—Traditional American Indian practice of calling on spirits or other forces to determine a diagnosis of a health problem.

Documentation—The papers necessary to prove one's citizenship or immigration status.

Duklij—A turquoise or green malachite amulet that may be used among American Indians to ward off evil spirits.

Dybbuk—Wandering, disembodied soul that enters another person's body and holds fast.

Emerging majority—People of color—Blacks; Asians/Pacific Islanders; American Indians, Eskimos, or Aleuts; and Hispanics—who are expected to constitute a majority of the American population by the year 2020.

Emic—Person's way of describing an action or event, an inside view.

Empacho—Traditional Hispanic belief that a ball of food is stuck in the stomach.

Envidia—Traditional Hispanic belief that the envy of others can be the cause of illness and bad luck.

Environmental control—Ability of a person from a given cultural group to actively control nature and to direct factors in the environment.

Epidemiology—The study of the distribution of disease.

Epilepsia—Epilepsy.

Ethnicity—Cultural group's sense of identification associated with the group's common social and cultural heritage.

Ethnocentrism—Tendency of members of one cultural group to view the members of other cultural groups in terms of the standards of behavior, attitudes, and values of their own group. The belief that one's own cultural, ethnic, professional, or social group is superior to that of others.

Ethnomedicine—Health beliefs and practices of indigenous cultural development. Not practiced in many of the tenets of modern medicine.

Etic—The interpretation of an event by someone who is not experiencing that event, an outside view.

Evil eye—Belief that someone can project harm by gazing or staring at another's property or person.

Excessism—Desiring to live with numerous possessions and material goods.

Exorcism—Ceremonious expulsion of an evil spirit from a person.

Faith—Strong beliefs in a religious or other spiritual philosophy.

Fatalism—Believing that life is not under a person's control.

Fatigue—Asthma-like symptoms.

Folklore—Body of preserved traditions, usually oral, consisting of beliefs, stories, and associated information of people.

Fundamentalism—Strict belief in the traditions of a heritage.

Garments—Sacred clothing that a person may wear.

Gender specific care—Care provided to another person by a person of the same gender—may be a religious mandate or personal preference.

Geophagy—Eating of nonfood substances, such as starch.

Glossoscopy—Traditional Chinese medical way of diagnosing a health problem by examining the tongue.

Green card—Documentation that a person is a legally admitted immigrant and has permanent resident status in the United States.

Gris-gris—Symbols of voodoo. They may take numerous forms and be used either to protect a person or to harm that person.

Halal—A designation for meat from animals that has been slaughtered in the ritual way by Islamic law so that it is suitable to be eaten by traditional Islamic people and follows Islamic dietary laws.

Haragei—Japanese art of using nonverbal communication.

HEALING*—Holistic, or three-dimensional, phenomenon that results in the restoration of balance, or harmony, to the body, mind, and spirit, or between the person and the environment.

HEALTH*—The balance of the person, both within one's being—physical, mental, and spiritual—and in the outside world—natural, communal, and metaphysical.

Herbrias—A person who sells herbs.

Heritage—The family culture, ethnicity, and/or religion that one is born into.

Heritage consistency—Observance of the beliefs and practices of one's traditional cultural belief system.

Heritage inconsistency—Observance of the beliefs and practices of one's acculturated belief system.

Hex—Evil spell, misfortune, or bad luck that one person can impose on another.

Histeria—Hysteria.

Homeopathic Philosophy—Health beliefs and practices derived from traditional cultural knowledge to maintain health, prevent changes in health status, and restore health.

Homeopathic medicine—In the practice of homeopathic medicine, the person, not the disease, is treated.

Homeopathy—System of medicine based on the belief that a disease can be cured by minute doses of a substance, which, if given to a healthy person in large doses, would produce the same symptoms that the person being treated is experiencing.

Hoodoo—A form of conjuring and a term that refers to the magical practices of voodoo outside New Orleans.

Hydrotherapy—The use of water in the maintenance of health and treatment of disease.

Hypnotherapy—The use of hypnosis to stimulate emotions and control involuntary responses, such as blood pressure.

Iatrogenic—The unexpected symptom or illness that can result from the treatment of another illness.

ILLNESS*—State of imbalance among the body, mind, and spirit. A sense of disharmony both within the person and with the environment.

Immigrant—Alien entering the United States for permanent (or temporary) residence.

Indigenous—People native to an area.

Kineahora—Word spoken by traditional Jewish people to prevent the "evil eye."

Kosher—A designation for food that has been prepared so that it is suitable to be eaten by traditional Jewish people and follows Jewish dietary laws.

Kusiut—A reference term for an American Indian medicine man. A "learned one."

Lay midwife—A person who practices lay midwifery.

Lay midwifery—Assisting childbirth for compensation.

Legal Permanent Resident (LPR)—Green card recipient. A person who has been granted lawful permanent residence in the United States.

Limpia—Traditional Hispanic practice of cleansing a person.

Locura—Craziness.

Macrobiotics—Diet and lifestyle from the Far East adapted for the United States by Michio Kushif. The principles of this vegetarian diet consist of balancing *yin* and *yang* energies of food.

Magico-religious folk medicine—Use of charms, holy words, and holy actions to prevent and cure illness.

Mal ojo (bad eye)—Traditional Hispanic belief that excessive admiration by one person can bring harm to another person.

Massage therapy—Use of manipulative techniques to relieve pain and return energy to the body.

Materialism—Taking great pleasure from having more than is necessary.

Medically underserved community—Urban or rural population group that lacks adequate health care services.

Melting pot—The social blending of cultures.

Mental—The aspect of the person that is related to thinking and cognition.

Meridians—Specific points of the body into which needles are inserted in the traditional Chinese medical practice of acupuncture.

Mesmerism—Healing by touch.

Metacommunication system—Large system of communication that includes both verbal language and nonverbal signs and symbols.

Milagros—Small figures of body parts or other objects that are offered to Saints for thanksgiving.

Minimalism—Knowing how to live with few possessions and material goods.

Miracle—Supernatural, unexplained event.

Modern—Present-day health and illness beliefs and practices of the providers within the American, or Western, health care delivery system.

Modernism—Adherence to modern ways and a belief that other values no longer exist.

Motion in the hand—An example of a traditional American Indian practice of moving the diagnostician's hands in a ritual of divination.

Moxibustion—Traditional Chinese medical way of restoring the balance of *yin* and *yang* that is based on the therapeutic value of heat. Heat is used in a disease where there is an excess of *yin*.

Multicultural nursing—Pluralistic approach to understanding relationships between two or more cultures to create a nursing practice framework for broadening nurses' understanding of health-related beliefs, practices, and issues that are part of the experiences of people from diverse cultural backgrounds.

Mysticism—Aspect of spiritual healing and beliefs.

Natural folk medicine—Use of the natural environment and use of herbs, plants, minerals, and animal substances to prevent and treat illness.

Naturalization—The process by which U.S. citizenship is conferred upon foreign citizens or nationals after fulfilling the requirements established by Congress.

Nonimmigrant—People who are allowed to enter the country temporarily under certain conditions, such as crewmen, students, and temporary workers.

Occult folk medicine—The use of charms, holy words, and holy actions to prevent and cure illness.

Orisha—Yoruba god or goddess.

Osphretics—Traditional Chinese medical way of diagnosing a health problem by listening and smelling.

Osteopathic medicine—School of medical practice that directs recuperative power of nature that is within the body to cure a disease.

Overheating therapy (hyperthermia)—Used since the time of the ancient Greeks. The natural immune system is stimulated with heat to kill pathogens.

Partera—A Mexican American or Mexican lay midwife.

Pasmo—Traditional Hispanic disease of paralysis of the face or limbs.

Physical—The aspect of a person one can see such as the face, eyes, ears, and so forth; and internal organs such as the heart, liver, spleen and so forth.

Pluralistic society—A society comprising people of numerous ethnocultural backgrounds.

Poultice—A hot, soft, moist mass of herbs, flour, mustard, and other substances spread on muslin and placed on a sore body part.

Powwow—A form of traditional HEALING practiced by German Americans.

Prejudice—Negative beliefs or preferences that are generalized about a group and that leads to "prejudgment."

Promesa—A deep and serious promise.

Racism—The belief that members of one race are superior to those of other races.

Rational folk medicine—Use of the natural environment and use of herbs, plants, minerals, and animal substances to prevent and treat illness.

Raza-Latina—A popular term used as a reference group name for people of Latin American descent.

Reflexology—Natural science that manipulates the reflex points in the hands and feet that correspond to every organ in the body in order to clear the energy pathways and the flow of energy through the body.

Refugee—A refugee is any person who is outside his or her country of nationality who is unable or unwilling to return to that country because of persecution or a well-founded fear of persecution.

Religion—Belief in a divine or superhuman power or powers to be obeyed and worshipped as the creator(s) and ruler(s) of the universe.

Remedies—Natural folk medicines that use the natural environment—herbs, plants, minerals, and animal substances to treat illnesses. Natural remedies have come to the United States from every corner of the world—the East and the West. They may be purchased in pharmacies, markets, and natural food stores.

Resident alien—A lawfully admitted alien.

Resiliency—The state of being strong and able to resist the consequences of an adverse event or emotional or physical danger.

Restoration—Process used by a person to return health.

Risk adjustment—Complex sets of data are put into terms whereby they are compared apples to apples.

Sacred objects—Objects, such as amulets and *milagros,* that have a spiritual purpose.

Sacred places—Places where people take petitions for favors or offer prayers of thanksgiving for the granting of a request.

Sacred practices—Religious practices, such as dietary taboos or lighting of candles, that a person is commanded to follow.

Santeria—A syncretic religion comprising both African and Catholic beliefs.

Santero(a)—Traditional priest and healer in the religion of *Santeria*.

Secular—Beliefs and practices that are not under the auspices of a religious body.

Self-denialism—Taking great pleasure from having less than is necessary.

Senoria—A woman who is knowledgeable about the causes and treatment of illness.

Sexism—Belief that members of one sex are superior to those of the other sex.

Shrine—A place—natural, secular, and/or affiliated with a religious tradition— where people make spiritual journeys or pilgrimages for the purposes of giving thanks or petitioning for favors. They are related to magico-religious folk medicine, and the use of charms, holy words, and holy actions, such as prayer, may be observed.

Singer—A type of traditional American Indian healer who is able to practice singing as a form of treating a health problem.

Skilly—An agent that is believed to cause disease by traditional Cherokee people.

Social organization—Patterns of cultural behavior related to life events, such as birth, death, childrearing, and health and illness, that are followed within a given social group.

Socialization—Process of being raised within a culture and acquiring the characteristics of the group.

Soul loss—Belief that a person's soul can leave the body, wander around, and then return.

Space—Area surrounding a person's body and the objects within that area.

Spell—A magical word or formula or a condition of evil or bad luck.

Sphygmopalpation—Traditional Chinese medical way of diagnosing a health problem by feeling pulses.

Spirit—The noncorporeal and nonmental dimension of a person that is the source of meaning and unity. The source of the experience of spirituality and every religion.

Spirit possession—Belief that a spirit can enter people, possess them, and control what they say and do.

Spiritual—Ideas, attitudes, concepts, beliefs, and behaviors that are the result of a person's experience of the spirit.

Spirituality—The experience of meaning and unity.

Stargazing—Example of a traditional American Indian practice of praying the star prayer to the star spirit as a method of divination.

Stereotype—Notion that all people from a given group are the same.

Superstition—Belief that performing an action, wearing a charm or an amulet, or eating something will have an influence on life events. These beliefs are upheld by magic and faith.

Susto (soul loss)—Traditional Hispanic belief that the soul is able to leave a person's body.

Szatan—The traditional Polish term for the "evil eye."

Taboo—A culture-bound ban that excludes certain behaviors from common use.

Talisman—Consecrated religious object that confers power of various kinds and protects people who wear, carry, or own them from harm and evil.

Tao—Way, path, or discourse. On the spiritual level, the way to ultimate reality.

Time—Duration, interval of time. Instances, or points in time.

Tirisia—Anxiety.

Title VI—Under the provisions of Title VI of the Civil Rights Act of 1964, people with Limited English Proficiency (LEP) who are cared for in such health care settings as extended care facilities, public assistance programs, nursing homes, and hospitals and are eligible for Medicaid, other health care, or human services cannot be denied assistance because of their race, color, or national origin.

Tradition—The handing down of statements, beliefs, legends, customs, and information, from generation to generation, especially by word of mouth or by practice.

Traditional—Ancient, ethnocultural-religious beliefs and practices that have been handed down through the generations.

Traditional epidemiology—Belief in agents other than those of a scientific nature, causing disease. These could be such agents as "envy," "jealousy," and "hate."

Traditionalism—Belief in the traditional HEALTH, ILLNESS, and HEALING methods of a given cultural cohort.

Tui Na—A complex Chinese system of massage, "pushing and pulling," using meridian stimulation used to treat orthopedic and neurological problems.

Undocumented alien—Person of foreign origin who has entered the country unlawfully by bypassing inspection or who has overstayed the original terms of admission.

Universalism—Open beliefs in many domains that may not be part of a given personal heritage.

Unlocking—Steps taken to help break down and understand the definitions of the terms *health/HEALTH* and *illness/ILLNESS* in a living context. It consists of persistent questioning: What is health? No matter what the response, the question "What does that mean?" is asked. Initially, this causes much confusion, but as each term is analyzed the process makes sense.

Voodoo—A religion that is a combination of Christianity and African Yoruba religious beliefs.

Vulnerability—The state of being weak or prone to an adverse event or emotional or physical danger.

Witched—Example of a traditional American Indian belief that a person is harmed by witches.

Xenophobia—Morbid fear of strangers.

Yang—Male, positive energy that produces light, warmth, and fullness.

Yin—Female, negative energy that produces darkness, cold, and emptiness.

Yoruba—The African tribe whose myths and rites are the basis of *Santeria*.

Appendix B

Calendar: Cultural and Religious Holidays That Change Dates

There are many Holy Days observed by people from many different cultural and religious heritages that do not fall on the same dates of the Julian calendar on an annual basis. This is because some religions, such as Judaism, follow the lunar calendar; and others, such as Islam, follow both the lunar and solar calendars. Given the increasing amount of cultural and religious diversity in this country, it is imperative that consideration be given to this fact. Religious leaders of a given faith community must be contacted regarding the Julian dates of a given holiday. Cultural and religious holidays have a significant impact on the lives of both patients and workers. Surgical procedures and extensive tests ought to be avoided on holidays and large professional meetings and other activities must not be scheduled at that time to cause conflict.

Heritage	Holiday	Approximate Date
Islam	Eid al-Fitr and Al Hisrah (New Year)	Varies
Chinese	Sending Off the Kitchen God Day	January
Islam	Laylat al-Qadr	January
Sikh	Guru Gobind Singh Ji's Birthday	January
Hindu	Makara Sakranti/Pongal	January
Chinese	New Year: Chinese, Korean, Tibetan, Vietnamese	February
Chinese	Lantern Festival	February
Baha'i	Intercalary Days	February or March
Hindu	Maha Shivaratri (Shiva's Night)	March
Christian	Shrove Monday	March
Christian	Shrove Tuesday	March
Christian	Ash Wednesday	March
Eastern Orthodox	Beginning of Lent, Eastern Orthodox Christian	March
Hindu	Holi	March
Iranian	Now Rouz	March
Chinese	Respect for Ancestors (Ch'ing-ming)	April
Islam	Muharram	April

Heritage	Holiday	Approximate Date
Vietnamese	Thanh Minh (Respect for Ancestors Day)	April
Hindu	Ramanavami	April
Cambodian	New Year	April
Hindu	Vaisakhi (Solar New Year)	April
Sikh	Baisakhi (New Year)	April
Jain	Mahavir Jayanti	April
Christian	Palm Sunday	April
Jewish	Passover begins at sundown	April
Jewish	Passover	April
Christian	Good Friday	April
Baha'i	Festival of Ridvan	April
Christian	Easter	April
Eastern Orthodox	Palm Sunday	April (a week after Christian Palm Sunday)
Christian	Easter Monday	April
Eastern Orthodox Christian	Good Friday	April (a week after Christian Good Friday)
Eastern Orthodox	Easter: Eastern Orthodox, also known as Pascha	April
Buddhist	Visakaha Day	May
Chinese	Dragon Boat Festival	June
Eastern Orthodox	Ascension Day	June
Jewish	Shavuoth begins at sundown	May or June
Christian	Pentecost	June
Islam	Maulid an-Nabi	June
Eastern Orthodox	Pentacost	June
Chinese	Seventh Night	August
Jewish	Tisha B' Av Fast Day	July or August
Hindu	Janmashtami	August
Korean	Chusok	September
Coptic Christian	Coptic New Year	September
Chinese	Midautumn Moon Festival—Chung-ch'iu	September
Jewish	Rosh Hashanah begins at sundown	September
Hindu	Durga Puja	October
Jewish	Yom Kippur begins at sundown	September or October
Jewish	Yom Kippur	October
Jewish	Sukkoth begins at sundown	October
Baha'i	Birthday of the Bab	October
Jewish	Shmini Atzeret begins at sundown	October
Jewish	Simchat Torah begins at sundown	October

(continued)

Heritage	Holiday	Approximate Date
Hindu	Diwali	October
Sikh	Nanak's Birthday	November
Baha'i	Birthday of Baha'u'llah	November
Islam	Ramadan	Varies

Source: Adapted from *Multicultural resource calendar.* (2011). Amherst, MA: Amherst Educational Publishing, 800-865-5549 or visit http://www.diversityresources.com/index.php. An annual calendar is available with the exact dates and explanations for the given holidays. There is an electronic version of this calendar that has numerous features including global religious, cultural, commemorative, and public holidays, pronunciations, food information, and resource information.

There are numerous observances that must also be considered. The following is a list of these observances:

■ African-American History Month (February)
■ Women's History Month (March)
■ Irish-American Heritage Month (March)
■ Asian/Pacific American Heritage Month (May)
■ Older Americans Month (May)
■ Anniversary of Americans With Disabilities Act (July 26)
■ Hispanic Heritage Month (Sept. 15-Oct. 15)
■ American Indian/Alaska Native Heritage Month (November)

These are available from the United States Census Bureau's Facts for Features series and can be accessed from http://www.census.gov/newsroom/releases/archives/facts_for_features_special_editions/cb11-ff13.html.

Appendix C

Suggested Course Outline

▇ Capstone[1]: Holistic Living

Culture is the soul of life. It is what gives us roots, gives our lives meaning, and binds us to each other.

—*Hillary Rodham Clinton, 12/5/98, Clinton Library, Little Rock, Arkansas*

The purposes of this course are to:

1. Examine spirituality, community, personal and family relationships, and education through the lenses of cross-cultural holistic HEALTH[2] and HEALING practices.
2. Bring the student into a direct relationship with health care consumers from various cultural backgrounds—American Indian and Alaska Native, Asian/ Pacific Islander, Black, Hispanic, and White populations.

Selected readings, films, and field visits will assist you to visualize the relationship of HEALTH to the holistic aspects of your life and that of the multicultural communities in which you will live and work. Through this study, the course will provide insight into the nature of health/HEALTH, the comparisons of health/HEALTH and healing/HEALING practices cross-culturally, and the consequences of health/HEALTH–related choices.

The course content includes discussion of the following topics:

- ▪ Cultural heritage and its contribution to health/HEALTH beliefs and practices
- ▪ Diversity, demographic and economic, existing in contemporary society

---

[1]Capstone courses are university courses, coordinated in the Theology Department of Boston College and open to senior students throughout the university. A Capstone Seminar is an intensely personal experience for seniors and is just as intensely a shared experience with their peers and professor. The seminar is kept to about 15 students to promote that sharing. The format of the seminar combines a deep exploration of the self with a disciplined academic exercise in substantive reading, writing, and discussion. Each seminar prompts the student to look both backward and forward. It asks, "What have you made of your Boston College education? What has it made of you?" It also inquires, "How will you carry out the lifelong commitments you have begun to envision?" These questions go to the heart of the seniors' concerns. Thus, Capstone Seminars provide a place where students can ponder ultimate questions within a community of discourse.

[2]*HEALTH* used in this manner connotes the balance of the person, both within one's being—physical, mental, and spiritual—and in the outside environment—natural, familial and communal, and metaphysical.

■ Health care providers' and patients' ways of understanding the maintenance, protection, and restoration of health/HEALTH and illness/ILLNESS and related problems

■ Cultural and institutional factors that affect the patients' access to and use of health care resources

Course Purpose and Process

Capstone courses are designed to provide you with the opportunity to reflect upon and integrate your education and life experiences in preparation for your future life. This course aims at studying spirituality, the duties of citizenship, vocation/career, education, and personal relationships through the lenses of HEALTH and holistic living.

Two of the most significant tasks of your adult life will be:

1. The development of CULTURALCOMPETENCY, given the dramatic demographic changes occurring in the United States and the globalization of the marketplace
2. Negotiating and advocating for comprehensive HEALTH care for
   a. Self and family
   b. Patients/clients from diverse cultural backgrounds

In fact, the development of an understanding of diversity within a HEALTH-centered focus leads to a broad understanding of and sensitivity to issues related to the larger issues of multiculturalism.

Ordinarily, a course dedicated to both HEALTH and holistic living would be structured to examine health practices and methods that may be employed to modify your health behaviors and choices. But, in this course, we will examine your HEALTH from a much deeper perspective and explore ways of expanding this concept to include social justice and work and the relationship that these concepts have to HEALTH. In each of the areas, we will use novels or films, guest speakers, and/ or field trips to broaden your perspectives of HEALTH, holistic living, and cultural diversity. You will see the relationships of HEALTH to the holistic aspects of your life and that of the communities in which you will live and work.

Course Objectives

On completion of this course, the student will:

1. Discuss the meanings of culture, ethnicity, religion, and socialization and their contribution to health/HEALTH beliefs and practices.
2. Discuss the diversity, demographic and economic, existing in contemporary society.
3. Discuss his or her ethnocultural heritage and socialization.
4. Analyze selected aspects of the modern health care delivery system.
5. Understand more fully the perception and meaning of health/HEALTH and illness among recipients of health care.
6. Deepen his or her understanding about self and reflect on what has been learned about personal HEALTH and cultural diversity.

7. Explore his or her existing knowledge about personal HEALTH care and holistic living.
8. Develop a long-term awareness about his or her role in citizenship, vocation/career, education, and personal relationships that is impacted on by both HEALTH and cultural diversity.
9. Develop an understanding and respect for the HEALTH traditions of people from many different cultural heritages.
10. Develop an understanding of the similarities and differences of culturally determined HEALTH traditions (beliefs and practices) and the relevance to overall cultural competency.

Texts

The following texts should be read in their entirety:

Spector, R. E. (2013). *Cultural diversity in health and illness* (8th ed.). Upper Saddle River, NJ: Prentice Hall Health.

Fadiman A. (1997). *The spirit catches you and you fall down.* New York: Farrar, Straus, Giroux.

Kassirer, J. P. (2005). *On the take.* New York: Oxford University Press.

Skloot, R. (2011). *The immortal life of Henrietta Lacks.* New York: Broadway Paperbacks.

Course Content

 I. Culture, Diversity, and Heritage Consistency
 II. Perceptions of Health/HEALTH and Illness/ILLNESS
 III. Ethnocultural Familial Beliefs—Roots
 IV. Allopathic versus Homeopathic Philosophies
 V. Modern Health Care Delivery
 VI. Health/HEALTH and Illness/ILLNESS in Selected Populations

Teaching and Learning Methods

reading assignments	web assignments	field trips
discussion	films	seminars
academic project/paper		

Course Assignments

1. Class attendance and participation is mandatory.			25%
2. Weekly reflection & Web assignment			25%
3. Class presentation (with text)	Day of class		25%
4. Final integrating essay	Last class		25%

Films

Required:

> *Talk to Her*, Pedro Almodovar
>
> *Sicko*, Michael Moore
>
> *Unnatural Causes,* Documentary Series, http://www.unnaturalcauses.org/about_the_series.php
>
> *Slavery by another name – The Public Broadcasting Series*
>
> View all programs at - http://video.pbs.org/program/slavery-another-name/

Class Schedule and Assignments

The first 4 weeks set the stage with primary reflections on yourself and your family over time—what it was like as a child, in high school, and later, through the lenses of health/HEALTH.

> Week 1—Introductions:
>> To each other, to Capstone, and to health/HEALTH and illness/ILLNESS and spirituality
>
> Week 2—Culture, Ethnicity, Religion, and Diversity
>> Readings: Spector, Preface, Unit I Introduction, Chapters 1, 2, and 3
>
> Week 3—Health and Illness
>> Readings: Spector, Chapter 4
>
> Week 4—Health and HEALTH of our parents and ancestors
>> Spector, Unit II Introduction, Chapter 5, 6, and 7

The second 4 weeks explore the dynamics of moving to the duties of citizenship, vocation/career, education, and personal relationships again through the lenses of health/HEALTH and illness/ILLNESS.

> Week 5—Traditional (Homeopathic) Medicine and Spiritual HEALTH Care and Discuss Ethnohealth Family Interviews
>> Reading: Review, Spector, Chapters 4 & 5
>
> Weeks 6 and 7—The Western (Modern) Health Care System
>> Reading: Spector, Chapter 8, and *On the Take*
>>
>> Film: *Sicko*
>
> *Unnatural Causes,* Documentary Series, http://www.unnaturalcauses.org/about_the_series.php
>
> Week 8—Midterm Discussion: The Spirit Catches You and You Fall Down and Film—*Talk to Her*

The remainder of this class explores the spiritual aspects of HEALTH by examining spirituality as it is found in the HEALTH traditions of selected ethnocultural populations. The comparison to your own experiences of spirituality, primarily in respect to the notion of Holistic Living, will become the central focus of reflection.

> Week 9—American Indian HEALTH Traditions
>> Reading: Spector, Unit III Introduction and Chapter 9; Suggested Film—*Dances with Wolves*

Week 10—Asian American HEALTH Traditions

Reading: Spector, Chapter 10; Suggested Film—*The Joy Luck Club*

Week 11—Black American HEALTH Traditions

Reading: Spector, Chapter 11; Suggested Film—*Slavery by another name – The Public Broadcasting Series*

View all programs at—http://video.pbs.org/program/slavery-another-name/

Reading: Skloot, R. (2011). *The immortal life of Henrietta Lacks.* New York: Broadway Paperbacks.

Week 12—Hispanic American HEALTH Traditions

Reading: Spector, Chapter 12; Suggested Film—*El Norte*

Week 13—White or European American HEALTH Traditions

Reading: Spector, Chapter 13; Suggested Film—*The Sorceress*

Week 14—Implications for Your Personal and Professional Future Life

Reading—Spector, Chapter 14

Week 15—HEALTH Traditions Cultural Banquet

EthnoHEALTH Family Interview

In preparation for the week 5 class, I am asking each of you to interview your *maternal* grandmother, your mother, or a *maternal* aunt. Please ask her for the following information:

1. Ethnic background

   Country of origin

   Religion

   Number of generations in U.S.

2. What does she do to *maintain* HEALTH? Also, if she can remember, what did her mother do?

3. What does she do to *protect* HEALTH? Also, if she can remember, what did her mother do?

4. What "home remedies" does she use to *restore* HEALTH? Also, if she can remember, what did her mother do?

5. How do her religious/spiritual beliefs define *birth*? What rituals accompany this event?

6. How do her religious/spiritual beliefs define *illness*? What rituals accompany this event?

7. How do her religious/spiritual beliefs define *healing*? What rituals accompany this event?

8. How do her religious/spiritual beliefs define *death*? What rituals accompany this event?

(Since I retired from the Boston College Connell School of Nursing in 2003, I have continued to teach this class at Boston College in the Theology Department to nursing, premed, and students from many other majors, including education, management, psychology, and political science. The course has been oversubscribed and well received by the students.)

Appendix D

Suggested Course Activity— Urban Hiking

We simply need that wild country available to us, even if we never do more than drive to its edge and look in. For it can be a means of reassuring ourselves of our sanity as creatures, a part of the geography of hope.

—*Wallace Stegner,*
plaque on Forest Service sign, Maroon Bells, Aspen, Colorado

Urban hiking—what is this? It is taking skills, knowledge, and curiosity applied to the great outdoors and applying it to peopled areas. It is an extraordinary way to tantalize your senses as you:

1. See—the infrastructure of a new or familiar place, the housing stock, the stores and small businesses, the markets, the transportation system, the pharmacies, houses of worship, and so forth.
2. Hear—listen to the symphony of voices, traffic, and music.
3. Taste—new foods by eating in neighborhood restaurants.
4. Smell—food as it is prepared on the streets, in homes, or in restaurants.
5. Feel—the textures of different fabrics and objects.

It is a way to witness and learn about cultural diversity and the New America and to erase fears of the unknown social and cultural phenomena that may impede your ability to embrace the demographic changes occurring in the United States today and to embrace the vitality and excitement of change, for, as Stegner looks to the "wild country," one can look to the streets of a city or town and successfully realize that "this is a means of reassuring ourselves of our sanity as creatures," a part of the geography of American LIFE!

Needed: a good street map, a good bus map, comfortable walking shoes, comfortable clothing, personal identification, and small amount of money for transportation, water, and food. There is no need to pack a lunch; restaurants are more than plentiful. And, of course, the greatest importance is a **good sense of humor and adventure.**

Indeed, the study of cultural diversity comes alive the moment you leave the confines of the classroom and go out into the community. This is the way to appreciate a given ethnoreligious community. It is extraordinary to go into a community and observe firsthand what daily life is like for a member of the community. The following outline can serve as an assessment guide to the target community and facilitate the understanding of CulturalCare.

Demographic data
Total population size of entire city or town
Breakdown by areas—residential concentrations
Specific focus on demographics of the target community
Breakdown by ages
Other breakdowns
Education
Occupations
Income
Nations of origin of residents of the location and the target neighborhood
Traditional health/HEALTH and illness/ILLNESS beliefs and practices
- Definition of *health/HEALTH*
- Definition of *illness/ILLNESS*
- Overall health status
Traditional causes of illness/ILLNESS, such as
- Poor eating habits
- Wrong food combinations
- Punishment from God
- The evil eye
- Hexes, spells, or envy
- Witchcraft
- Environmental changes
- Exposure to drafts
- Grief and loss
Traditional methods of maintaining health/HEALTH
Traditional methods of protecting health/HEALTH
Traditional methods of restoring health/HEALTH
Home remedies
Visits to physicians, nurse practitioners, traditional healers, or other health care resources
Health care resources, such as neighborhood health centers
Traditional pharmacies, such as a *botanica*
Childbearing beliefs and practices
Childrearing beliefs and practices
Rituals and beliefs surrounding death and dying

Go on a "hike" through the community. Identify the various services that are available. If possible, visit a community health care provider, visit a church or community center within the neighborhood, visit grocery stores and pharmacies and point out differences in foods and over-the-counter remedies, and eat a meal in a neighborhood restaurant.

I have shared this experience with many groups of students over the years, and the experience has been well received.

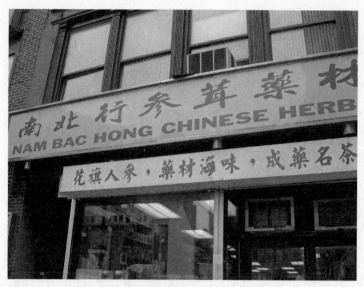

Figure D-1   Boston's Chinatown

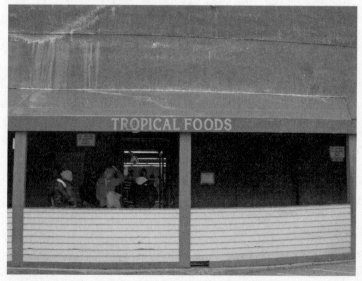

Figure D-2   Boston's Caribbean Neighborhood

Appendix E

Heritage Assessment Tool

This set of questions is to be used to describe a person's—or your own—ethnic, cultural, and religious background. In performing a *heritage assessment* it is helpful to determine how deeply a person identifies with his or her traditional heritage. This tool is very useful in setting the stage for assessing and understanding a person's traditional HEALTH and ILLNESS beliefs and practices and in helping determine the community resources that will be appropriate to target for support when necessary. The greater the number of positive responses, the greater the degree to which the person may identify with his or her traditional heritage. The one exception to positive answers is the question about whether a person's name was changed. The background rationale for the development of this tool is found in Chapter 1.

1. Where was your mother born? _____

2. Where was your father born? _____

3. Where were your grandparents born? _____

    A. Your mother's mother? _____

    B. Your mother's father? _____

    C. Your father's mother? _____

    D. Your father's father? _____

4. How many brothers _____ and sisters _____ do you have?

5. What setting did you grow up in? Urban _____ Rural _____

6. What country did your parents grow up in?

    Father _____

    Mother _____

7. How old were you when you came to the United States?

8. How old were your parents when they came to the United States?

    Mother _____

    Father _____

9. When you were growing up, who lived with you? _____

_____

10. Have you maintained contact with

    A. Aunts, uncles, cousins?   (1) Yes ____ (2) No ____
    B. Brothers and sisters?   (1) Yes ____ (2) No ____
    C. Parents?   (1) Yes ____ (2) No ____
    D. Your own children?   (1) Yes ____ (2) No ____

11. Did most of your aunts, uncles, and cousins live near your home?
    (1) Yes ____
    (2) No ____

12. Approximately how often did you visit family members who lived outside of your home?
    (1) Daily ____
    (2) Weekly ____
    (3) Monthly ____
    (4) Once a year or less ____
    (5) Never ____

13. Was your original family name changed?
    (1) Yes ____
    (2) No ____

14. What is your religious preference?
    (1) Catholic ____
    (2) Jewish ____
    (3) Protestant ____ Denomination _____
    (4) Other ____
    (5) None ____

15. Is your spouse the same religion as you?
    (1) Yes ____
    (2) No ____

16. Is your spouse the same ethnic background as you?
    (1) Yes ____
    (2) No ____

17. What kind of school did you go to?
    (1) Public ____
    (2) Private ____
    (3) Parochial ____

18. As an adult, do you live in a neighborhood where the neighbors are the same religion and ethnic background as you?
    (1) Yes ____
    (2) No ____

19. Do you belong to a religious institution?
    (1) Yes ____
    (2) No ____

20. Would you describe yourself as an active member?
    (1) Yes ____
    (2) No ____

21. How often do you attend your religious institution?
    (1) More than once a week ____
    (2) Weekly ____
    (3) Monthly ____
    (4) Special holidays only ____
    (5) Never ____

22. Do you practice your religion in your home?
    (1) Yes ____ (if yes, please specify by checking activities below)
    (2) No ____
    (3) Praying ____
    (4) Bible reading ____
    (5) Diet ____
    (6) Celebrating religious holidays ____
    (7) Other _____

23. Do you prepare foods special to your ethnic background?
    (1) Yes ____
    (2) No ____

24. Do you participate in ethnic activities?
    (1) Yes ____ (if yes, please specify by checking activities below)
    (2) No ____
    (3) Singing ____
    (4) Holiday celebrations ____
    (5) Dancing ____
    (6) Festivals ____
    (7) Costumes ____
    (8) Other ____

25. Are your friends from the same religious background as you?
    (1) Yes ____
    (2) No ____

26. Are your friends from the same ethnic background as you?
    (1) Yes ____
    (2) No ____

27. What is your native language other than English? ____

28. Do you speak this language?
    (1) Prefer ____
    (2) Occasionally ____
    (3) Rarely ____

29. Do you read your native language?
    (1) Yes ____
    (2) No ____

Appendix F

Quick Guide for CULTURALCARE

Preparing

- Understand your own cultural values, biases, and traditional health/ HEALTH beliefs and practices.
- Acquire basic knowledge of cultural values and health/HEALTH beliefs and practices for the populations you serve.
- Be respectful of, interested in, and understanding of other cultures' health/ HEALTH beliefs and practices without being judgmental. Understand that health/HEALTH beliefs and practices vary both within and between ethno-cultural and religious populations.

Enhancing Communication

- Determine the person's level of fluency in English and arrange for a competent interpreter, when needed.
- Ask how the person prefers to be addressed—that is, Mr./Mrs. or by first name. Do not refer to a person as "sweetie," "darling," "guy," "honey," or any other local popular terms.
- Allow the person to choose seating for comfortable personal space and eye contact. If the person prefers *not* to establish eye contact, do not become upset. In many cultures, it is considered polite to avoid eye contact.
- Avoid body language and gestures that may be offensive or misunderstood.
- Speak directly and quietly to the person, whether an interpreter is present or not.
- Choose a speech rate and style that promotes understanding and demonstrates respect for the person.
- Avoid slang, technical jargon, and complex sentences.
- Use open-ended questions or questions phrased in several ways to obtain information.
- Determine the person's reading ability before using written materials in the teaching process.
- Provide reading material that is easily read in the person's native language. Do not use cartoons and cartoon characters for illustrations.

Promoting Positive Change

■ Build on cultural HEALTH practices, reinforcing those that are positive and promoting change only in those that are potentially harmful.

■ Check for person understanding and acceptance of recommendations.

■ Remember: Not all seeds of knowledge fall into a fertile environment to produce change. Of those that do, some will take years to germinate.

Source: (Adapted for nursing) Schilling, B., & Brannon, E. (1986). *Cross-cultural counseling—A guide for nutrition and health counselors.* Alexandria, VA: U.S. Department of Agriculture, U.S. Department of Health and Human Services, Nutrition and Technical Services Division. Adapted with permission.

Appendix G

Data Resources

Countless invaluable resources are available in both the public and private sectors. These resources are available on the Internet and their addresses are included. It is important to note that the URLs change; however, the new addresses are usually linked to the old site. The spotlight here is on the agencies within the federal government that are useful for information regarding health and diversity.

1. The United States Census Bureau—provides information related to Census 2010, Statistical Abstract, Census Maps, and so forth; American Community Survey, and American FactFinder are sources for population, housing, economic, and geographic data from Census 2010, Census 2000, and the 1990 Decennial Census.

   The U.S. Census Bureau—http://www.census.gov/

   The American Community Survey—http://www.census.gov/acs/www/

   The New American Factfinder—http://factfinder2.census.gov/faces/nav/jsf/pages/searchresults.xhtml?refresh=t

2. United States Citizenship and Immigration Services—USCIS—provides immigration information, grants benefits, promotes awareness and understanding of *citizenship* and ensures the integrity of the immigration process.

   http://www.uscis.gov/portal/site/uscis

3. United States Department of Homeland Security—This agency has responsibility for information regarding immigration, commerce and trade, and emergency preparedness.

   http://www.dhs.gov/index.shtm

4. Office for Civil Rights—located within the U.S. Department of Health and Human Services, is responsible for enforcing the nondiscrimination requirements of **Title VI of the Civil Rights Act of 1964.**

   http://www.hhs.gov/ocr/

5. National Center for Health Statistics—*Healthy People 2020*—describes the ways that *Healthy People* 2020 is planning to improve the health of all Americans in the 10 years (2010–2020).

   http://www.healthypeople.gov/2020/default.aspx

6. National Center for Health Statistics—provides U.S. public health statistics including diseases, pregnancies, births, aging, and mortality.

   http://www.cdc.gov/nchs/

7. Health Resources and Services Administration—HRSA—is the primary federal agency for improving access to health care services for people who are uninsured, isolated, or medically vulnerable.

   http://www.hrsa.gov/index.html

8. The Office of Minority Health—OMH—advises the Secretary and the Office of Public Health Science on public health issues affecting American Indians and Alaska Natives, Black and African Americans, Asian Americans, and Hispanic Americans; and the elimination of racial and ethnic health disparities.

   http://minorityhealth.hhs.gov/

9. National Center for Complementary and Alternative Medicine—NCCAM—part of the U.S. National Institutes of Health that is undertaking research, training, and dissemination of data relevant to the public and professionals on the use and efficacy of complimentary and alternative medicine.

   http://nccam.nih.gov/

10. HealthFinder—Since 1997, HealthFinder has been recognized as a key resource for finding the best government and nonprofit health and human services information on the Internet. There are links to carefully selected information and Web sites from over 1,500 health-related organizations.

    http://www.healthfinder.gov

11. Center for Medicare & Medicaid Services—The mission of this agency is to ensure effective, up-to-date health care coverage and to promote quality care for beneficiaries.

    http://www.cms.hhs.gov

12. Centers for Disease Control—CDC—The mission of the CDC is saving lives, protecting people, and saving money through prevention. The CDC seeks to accomplish its mission by working with partners throughout the nation and the world to monitor health, detect and investigate health problems, conduct research to enhance prevention, and so forth.

    http://www.cdc.gov/

Bibliography

Abelson, R. (2007, June 14). In health care, cost isn't proof of high quality. *New York Times*, p. A-1.

Abraham, L. K. (1993). *Mama might be better off dead: The failure of health care in urban America*. Chicago, IL: University of Chicago Press.

Abrahams, P. (1954). *Tell freedom: Memories of Africa*. New York: Knopf.

Abramson, H. J. (1980). Religion. In S. Thernstrom (Ed.), *Harvard encyclopedia of American ethnic groups* (pp. 869–874). Cambridge, MA: Harvard University Press.

Achebe, C. (1959). *Things fall apart*. Greenwich, CT: Fawcett Crest.

Achebe, C. (1987). *Anthills of Savannah*. New York: Anchor Press/Doubleday.

Achterberg, J., Dossey, B., & Kolkmeier, L. (1994). *Rituals of healing: Using imagery for health and wellness*. New York: Bantam Books.

Aday, L. A. (1993). *At risk in America—The health and health care needs of vulnerable populations in the United States*. San Francisco, CA: Jossey-Bass.

Aiken, L. G. (1981). *Health policy and nursing practice*. New York: McGraw-Hill.

Aiken, R. (1980). *Mexican folk tales from the borderland*. Dallas, TX: Southern Methodist University Press.

Albrecht, G. L., & Higgens, P. C. (Eds.). (1979). *Health, illness, and medicine*. Chicago, IL: Rand McNally.

Alcott, W. A. (1839). *The house I live in; or the human body*. Boston, MA: George W. Light.

Alksen, L., Wellin, E., Suchman, E., et al. (n.d.). *A conceptual framework for the analysis of cultural variations in the behavior of the ill*. Unpublished report, New York City Department of Health, New York.

Allende, I. (1993). *The house of the spirits*. New York: Bantam Books.

Allison, D. (1992). *Bastard out of Carolina*. New York: Plume.

Allport, G. W. (1958). *The nature of prejudice (abridged)*. Garden City, NY: Doubleday

Alvarez, H. R. (1975). *Health without boundaries*. Mexico: United States-Mexico Border Public Health Association.

Alvarez, J. (1992). *How the Garcia girls lost their accents*. New York: Plume.

Ameer Ali, S. (1922, 1978). *The spirit of Islam*. Delhi, India: IDARAH-I-ADABIYAT-I-DELLI.

American Nurses' Association. (1979, June 9–10). *A strategy for change*. Papers presented at the conference of the Commission on Human Rights, Albuquerque, NM.

American Nurses' Association, Council on Cultural Diversity in Nursing Practice. (1993). *Proceedings of the invitational meeting, multicultural issues in the nursing workforce and workplace*. Washington, DC: Author.

American Psychiatric Association. (1994). *Diagnostic and statistical manual of mental disorders* (4th ed.). Washington, DC: Author.

Anderson, D. M. (1995). *Maasai people of cattle*. San Francisco, CA: Chronicle Books.

Anderson, E. T., & McFarlane, J. M. (1988). *Community as client*. Philadelphia, PA: J. B. Lippincott.

Anderson, J. Q. (1970). *Texas folk medicine*. Austin, TX: Encino Press.

Andrade, S. J. (1978). *Chicano mental health: The case of cristal*. Austin, TX: Hogg Foundation for Mental Health.

Andrews, E. D. (1953). *The people called Shakers*. New York: Dover.

Andrews, M. M., & Boyle, J. S. (1995). *Transcultural concepts in nursing care* (2nd ed.). Philadelphia, PA: J. B. Lippincott.

Angelou, M. (1970). *I know why the caged bird sings*. New York: Random House.

Annas, G. J. (1975). *The rights of hospital patients*. New York: Avon.

Appelfeld, A. (1990). *The healer*. New York: Grove Weidenfeld.

Apple, D. (Ed.). (1960). *Sociological studies of health and sickness: A source book for the health professions*. New York: McGraw-Hill, Blakiston Division.

Archer, S. E., & Fleshman, R. P. (1985). *Community health nursing* (3rd ed.). Monterey, CA: Wadsworth.

Armstrong, D., & Armstrong, E. M. (1991). *The great American medicine show.* New York: Prentice Hall.

Arnold, M. G., & Rosenbaum, G. (1973). *The crime of poverty.* Skokie, IL: National Textbook Co.

Ashely, J. (1976). *Hospitals, paternalism, and the role of the nurse.* New York: Teachers College Press.

Astin, J. A. (1998, May 20). Why patients use alternative medicine: Results of a national study. *Journal of the American Medical Association, 279*(19), 1548–1553.

Aurand, A. M., Jr. (n.d.). *The realness of witchcraft in America.* Lancaster, PA: Aurand Press.

Ausubel, N. (1964). *The book of Jewish knowledge.* New York: Crown.

Bahti, T. (1974). *Southwestern Indian ceremonials.* Las Vegas, NV: KC Publications.

Bahti, T. (1975). *Southwestern Indian tribes.* Las Vegas, NV: KC Publications.

Bakan, D. (1968). *Disease, pain, and sacrifice: Toward a psychology of suffering.* Chicago, IL: University of Chicago Press.

Baker, G. C. (1994). *Planning and organizing for multicultural instruction* (2nd ed.). Menlo Park, CA: Addison-Wesley.

Balch, J. F., & Balch, P. A. (1990). *Prescription for nutritional healing.* Garden City Park, NY: Avery.

Baldwin, R. (1986). *The healers.* Huntington, IN: Our Sunday Visitor.

Banks, J. A. (Ed.). (1973). *Teaching ethnic studies.* Washington, DC: National Council for Social Studies.

Bannerman, R. H., Burton, J., & Wen-Chieh, C. (1983). *Traditional medicine and health care coverage.* Geneva, Switzerland: World Health Organization.

Barden, T. E. (Ed.). (1991). *Virginia folk legends.* Charlottesville, VA: University Press of Virginia.

Barnes, J. S., & Bennett, C. E. (2002). *The Asian population: 2000.* Washington, DC: U.S. Department of Commerce.

Basque, E., & Young, P. (1984). *Personal Interviews.* Boston: Boston Indian Council.

Bass, P. H., & Pugh, K. (2001). *In our own image—Treasured African-American traditions, journeys, and icons.* Philadelphia, PA: Running Press.

Bauwens, E. F. (1979). *The anthropology of health.* St. Louis, MO: C. V. Mosby.

Bear, S., & Bear, W. (1996). *The medicine wheel.* New York: Fireside.

Beaudoin, T. (1998). *Virtual Faith: The irreverent spiritual quest of generation X.* San Francisco, CA: Jossey-Bass.

Becerra, R. M., & Shaw, D. (1984). *The elderly Hispanic: A research and reference guide.* Lanham, MD: University Press of America.

Becker, M. H. (1974). *The health belief model and personal health behavior.* Thorofare, NJ: Slack.

Beimler, R. R. (1991). *The days of the dead.* San Francisco, CA: Collins Publishers.

Belgium, D. (Ed.). (1967). *Religion and medicine.* Ames, IA: Iowa State University Press.

Ben-Amos, D., & Mintz, J. R. (1970). *In praise of the Baal Shem Tov.* New York: Shocken Books.

Benedict, R. (1946). *Patterns of culture.* New York: Penguin Books.

Benjamin, G. G. (1910, 1974). *The Germans in Texas.* Austin, TX: Jenkins.

Bennett, C. I. (1990). *Comprehensive multicultural education* (2nd ed.). Boston, MA: Allyn and Bacon.

Benson, H. (1996). *Timeless healing.* New York: Scribner.

Berg, D. J. (Ed.). (1986). *Homestead hints.* Berkeley, CA: Ten Speed Press.

Berg, P. S. (Ed.). (1977). *An entrance to the tree of life.* Jerusalem, Israel: Research Center for Kabbalah.

Berman, E. (1976). *The solid gold stethoscope.* New York: Macmillan Co.

Bermann, E. (1973). *Scapegoat.* Ann Arbor, MI: University of Michigan Press.

Bernardo, A. (n.d.). *Lourdes: Then and now.* Trans. Rand, P. T. Lourdes. France: Etablissements Estrade.

Bernardo, S. (1981). *The ethnic almanac.* Garden City, NY: Doubleday.

Bertrand, J., Floyd, R. L., & Weber, M. K. (2005). Guidelines for identifying and referring persons with fetal alcohol syndrome. *MMWR, 54,* 11.

Berwick, D. M., Godfrey, A. B., & Roessner, J. (1990). *Curing health care.* San Francisco, CA: Jossey-Bass.

Bienvenue, R. M., & Goldstein, J. E. (1979). *Ethnicity and ethnic relations in Canada* (2nd ed.). Toronto, ON: Butter worths.

Bilagody, H. (1969). An American Indian looks at health care. In R. Feldman & D.

Buch (Eds.), *The ninth annual training institute for psychiatrist-teachers of practicing physicians* (pp. 20–23). Boulder, CO: WICHE. No. 3A30

Birnbaum, P. (1988). *Encyclopedia of Jewish concepts.* New York: Hebrew.

Bishop, G. (1967). *Faith healing: God or fraud?* Los Angeles: Shervourne Press.

Blackmon, D. A. (2008). *Slavery by another name.* New York: Doubleday.

Blattner, B. (1981). *Holistic nursing.* Englewood Cliffs, NJ: Prentice Hall.

Bloch, B., & Hunter, M. L. (1981, January–February). Teaching physiological assessment of black persons. *Nurse Educator, 6*(1), 24–27.

Bohannan, P. (1992). *We, the alien.* Prospect Heights, IL: Waveland Press, Inc.

Boney, W. (1939). *The French Canadians today.* London: J. M. Dent and Sons.

Bonfanti, L. (1974). *Biographies and legends of the New England Indians,* Vol. 4. Wakefield, MA: Pride.

Bonfanti, L. (1980). *Strange beliefs, customs, and superstitions of New England.* Wakefield, MA: Pride.

Bottomore, T. B. (1968). *Classes in modern society.* New York: Vintage Books.

Bowen, E. S. (1964). *Return to laughter.* Garden City, NY: Doubleday

Bowker, J. (1991). *The meanings of death.* Cambridge, MA: Cambridge University Press.

Boyd, D. (1974). *Rolling thunder.* New York: Random House.

Boyle, J. S., & Andrews, M. M. (1995). *Transcultural concepts in nursing care* (2nd ed.). Philadelphia, PA: J. B. Lippincott.

Bracq, J. C. (1924). *The evolution of French Canada.* New York: Macmillan.

Bradley, C. J. (1980). "Characteristics of Women and Infants Attended by Lay Midwives in Texas, 1971: A Case Comparison Study." Master's thesis, University of Texas Health Science Center at Houston, School of Public Health, Houston, TX.

Branch, M. F., & Paxton, P. P. (1976). *Providing safe nursing care for ethnic people of color.* New York: Appleton-Century-Crofts.

Brand, J. (1978). *The life and death of Anna Mae Aquash.* Toronto, ON: James Lorimer.

Brandon, G. (1997). *Santeria: From Africa to the New World.* Bloomington, IN: University of Indiana Press.

Brink, J., & Keen, L. (1979). *Feverfew.* London: Century.

Brink, P. J. (Ed.). (1976). *Transcultural nursing: A book of readings.* Englewood Cliffs, NJ: Prentice Hall.

Brown, D. (1970). *Bury my heart at Wounded Knee.* New York: Holt, Rinehart & Winston.

Brown, D. (1980). *Creek Mary's blood.* New York: Holt, Rinehart & Winston.

Browne, G., Howard, J., & Pitts, M. (1985). *Culture and children.* Austin, TX: University of Texas Press.

Browne, K., & Freeling, P. (1967). *The doctor–patient relationship.* Edinburgh, MI: E & S Livingstone.

Brownlee, A. T. (1979). *Community, culture, and care: A cross cultural guide for healthworkers.* St. Louis, MO: C. V. Mosby.

Bruchac, J. (1985). *Iroquois stories heroes and heroines monsters and magic.* Freedom, CA: Crossing Press.

Bryant, C. A. (1985). *The cultural feast: An introduction to food and society.* St. Paul, MN: West.

Buchman, D. D. (1979). *Herbal medicine: The natural way to get well and stay well.* New York: Gramercy.

Budge, E. A. W. (1978). *Amulets and superstitions.* New York: Dover.

Bullough, B., & Bullough, V. L. (1972). *Poverty, ethnic identity, and health care.* New York: Appleton-Century-Crofts.

Bullough, V. L., & Bullough, B. (1982). *Health care for other Americans.* New York: Appleton-Century-Crofts.

Butler, H. (1967). *Doctor gringo.* New York: Rand McNally.

Buxton, J. (1973). *Religion and healing in Mandari.* Oxford: Clarendon Press.

Cafferty, P. S. J., Chiswick, B. R., Greeley, A. M., et al. (1983). *The dilemma, of American immigration: Beyond the golden door.* New Brunswick, NJ: Transaction Books.

Cahill, R. E. (1990a). *Olde New England's curious customs and cures.* Salem, MA: Old Saltbox Publishing House.

Cahill, R. E. (1990b). *Strange superstitions.* Salem, MA: Old Saltbox Publishing House.

Calhoun, M. (1976). *Medicine show.* New York: Harper and Row.

Califano, J. (1994). *Radical surgery.* New York: Random House.

Campos, E. (1955). *Medicina popular: Supersticione credios e meizinhas*

(2nd ed.). Ro de Janeiro: Livraria-Editora da Casa.

Candill, H. M. (1962). *Night comes to the Cumberlands.* Boston, MA: Little, Brown.

Carmack, R. M., Gasco, J., & Gossen, G. H. (1996). *The legacy of Mesoamerica.* Upper Saddle River, NJ: Prentice Hall.

Carnegie, M. E. (1987). *The path we tread: Blacks in nursing 1854–1984.* Philadelphia, PA: J. B. Lippincott.

Carson, V. B. (Ed.). (1989). *Spiritual dimensions of nursing practice.* Philadelphia, PA: W. B. Saunders.

Catlin, G. (1993). *North American Indian portfolios.* New York: Abbeville.

Chafets, Z. (1990). *Devil's night and other tales of Detroit.* New York: Vintage Books.

Chan, L. S., McCandless, R., Portnoy, B., et al. (1987). *Maternal and child health on the U.S.-Mexico border.* Austin, TX: The University of Texas.

Chan, P. K. (1988, August 3). *Herb specialist, interview by author.* New York City.

Chavira, L. (1975). *Curanderismo: An optional health-care system.* Edinburg, TX: Pan American University.

Chenault, L. R. (1938). *The Puerto Rican migrant in New York City.* New York: Columbia University Press.

Chiba, R. (1966). *The seven lucky gods of Japan.* Rutland, VT: Charles E. Tuttle Co.

Choron, J. (1964). *Death and modern man.* New York: Collier Books.

Chun, M. N. (1986). *Hawaiian medicine book.* Honolulu, Hawaii: Bess Press.

Chute, C. (1985). *The beans of Egypt, Maine.* New York: Ticknor & Fields.

Civil Rights Act of 1964, Pub. L No. 88-352, §601, 78 Stat. 252 (42 USC 2000d).

Clark, A. (1978). *Culture, childbearing health professionals.* Philadelphia, PA: F. A. Davis.

Clark, A. L. (1981). *Culture and child rearing.* Philadelphia, PA: F. A. Davis.

Clark, M. (1959). *Health in the Mexican-American culture: A community study.* Berkeley, CA: University of California Press.

Cobb, A. K. (1977). Pluralistic legitimation of an alternative therapy system: The case of chiropractic. *Medical Anthropology, 6*(4), 1–23.

Cohen, R. E. (1972, June). Principles of preventive mental health programs for ethnic minority populations: The acculturation of Puerto Ricans to the United States. *American Journal of Psychiatry, 128*(12), 79.

Comas-Diaz, L., & Griffith, E. E. H. (1988). *Clinical guidelines in cross-cultural mental health.* New York: Wiley.

Committee on Medical Care Teaching. (Eds.). (1958). *Readings in medical care.* Chapel Hill, NC: University of North Carolina Press.

Conde, M. I. (1992). *Tituba, black witch of Salem.* New York: Ballantine Books.

Conway, M. (1974). *Rise gonna rise.* New York: Anchor Books.

Conzen, K. N. (1980). Germans. In S. Thernstrom (Ed.), *Harvard encyclopedia of American ethnic groups* (pp. 405–425). Cambridge, MA: Harvard University Press.

Corish, J. L. (1923). *Health knowledge,* Vol. 1. New York: Domestic Health Society.

Cornacchia, H. J. (1976). *Consumer health.* St. Louis, MO: C. V. Mosby.

Corum, A. K. (1985). *Folk remedies from Hawai'i.* Honolulu, Hawaii: Bess Press.

Council of Churches. (1995). *Knowing my neighbor, religious beliefs and traditions at times of illness and death.* Springfield, MA: Visiting Nurse Hospice of Pioneer Valley.

Cowan, N. M., & Cowan, R. S. (1989). *Our parents' lives.* New York: Basic Books.

Cramer, M. E. (1923). *Divine science and healing.* Denver, CO: Colorado College of Divine Science.

Crichton, M. (1970). *Five patients.* New York: Alfred A. Knopf.

Crispino, J. A. (1980). *Assimilation of ethnic group: The Italian case.* Newark, NJ: New Jersey Center for Migration.

Cross, T. (1994). Understanding family resiliency from a relational worldview. In *Resiliency in families: Racial and ethnic minority families in America* (pp. 143–157). Madison, WI: University of Wisconsin-Madison.

Crow Dog, L., & Erdoes, R. (1996). *Crow Dog.* San Francisco, CA: Harper.

Culpeper, N. (1889). *Culpeper's complete herbal.* London: W. Foulsham.

culture. (n.d.). *The American Heritage New Dictionary of Cultural Literacy* (3rd ed.). Retrieved January 31, 2011, from Dictionary.com website: http://dictionary.reference.com/browse/culture

Currier, R. L. (1966, March). The hot-cold syndrome and symbolic balance in Mexican and Spanish-American folk medicine. *Ethnology, 5,* 251–263.

Curry, M. A., project director. (1987). *Access to prenatal care: Key to preventing low birth weight*. Kansas City, MO: American Nurses Association.

Curtis, E. (1993). *Native American wisdom*. Philadelphia, PA: Running Press.

Cutter, C. (1850). *First book on anatomy, physiology, and hygiene, for grammar schools and families*. Boston, MA: Benjamin B. Mussey.

Danforth, L. M. (1982). *The death rituals of rural Greece*. Princeton, NJ: Princeton University Press.

Davies, P. (Ed.) (1976). *The American Heritage Dictionary of the English Language* (Paperback ed.). New York: Dell.

Davis, F. (Ed.). (1966). *The nursing profession: Five sociological essays*. New York: Wiley.

Davis, F., & Furtado, C. (2002, July 22). INS to enforce change-of-address rule. *Boston Globe*, p. A2.

Davis, R. (1998). *American voudou: Journey into a hidden world*. Denton, TX: University of North Texas Press.

DeBella, S., Martin, L., & Siddall, S. (1986). *Nurses' role in health care planning*. Norwalk, CT: Appleton-Century-Crofts.

De Castro, J. (1967). *The black book of hunger*. Boston, MA: Beacon Press.

Delaney, J., Lupton, M. J., & Toth, E. (1988). *The curse: A cultural history of menstruation*. Chicago, IL: University of Chicago Press.

Deller, B., Hicks, D., & MacDonald, G., coordinators. (1979). *Stone boats and lone stars*. Hyde Park, Ontario: Middlesex County Board of Education.

Deloria, V., Jr. (1969). *Custer died for our sins: An Indian manifesto*. New York: Avon Books.

Deloria, V., Jr. (1974). *Behind the trail of broken treaties*. New York: Delacorte.

DeLys, C. (1948). *A treasury of American superstitions*. New York: Philosophical Library.

Densmore, F. (1974). *How Indians use wild plants for food, medicine, and crafts*. New York: Dover.

Deren, M. (1953). *Divine horseman: The living gods of Haiti*. New York: McPherson.

Dey, C. (1982). *The magic candle*. Bronx, NY: Original Publications.

Dickerson, J. (1998). *Dixie's dirty secret*. Armonk, NY: Sharpe.

Dickison, R. (Ed.). (1987). *Causes, cures, sense, and nonsense*. Sacramento, CA: Bishop Publishing Co.

Dinnerstein, L., & Reimers, D. M. (1988). *Ethnic Americans* (3rd ed.). New York: Harper & Row.

Dioszegi, V. (1996). *Folk beliefs and shamanistic practices in Siberia*. Budapest, Hungary: Akademiai Kiado.

Doane, N. L. (1985). *Indian doctor book*. Charlotte, NC: Aerial.

Doka, K. J., & Morgan, J. D. (Eds.). (1993). *Death and spirituality*. Amityville, NY: Baywood.

Dolan, J. (1973). *Nursing in society: A historical perspective*. Philadelphia, PA: W. B. Saunders.

Donegan, J. B. (1978). *Women and men midwives: Medicine, morality, and misogyny in early America*. Westport, CT: Greenwood Press.

Donin, H. H. (1972). *To be a Jew*. New York: Basic Books.

Dorris, M. (1989). *The broken cord*. New York: Harper & Row.

Dorsey, P. R., & Jackson, H. Q. (1976). Cultural health traditions: The Latino/ Mexican perspective. In M. F. Branch & P. P. Paxton (Eds.), *Providing safe nursing care for ethnic people of color* (p. 56). New York: Appleton-Century-Crofts.

Dorson, R. H. D. (Ed.). (1972). *Folklore and folklife*. Chicago, IL: University of Chicago Press.

Dossey, L. (1993). *Healing words*. San Francisco, CA: Harper.

Dresser, N. (1993). *Our own stories: Cross-cultural communication practice*. White Plains, NY: Longman.

Dresser, N. (1996). *Multicultural manners*. New York: John Wiley & Sons, Inc.

Dresser, N. (1999). *Multicultural celebrations*. New York: Three Rivers Press.

Dubos, R. (1961). *Mirage of health*. Garden City, NY: Anchor Books, Doubleday and Co.

Dubos, R. (1968). *Man, medicine and environment*. New York: Mentor.

Dubos, R. J. (1965). *Man adapting*. New Haven, CT: Yale University Press.

Dunstin, B. (1969). Pica during pregnancy. In *Current concepts in clinical nursing* (Chapter 26). St. Louis, MO: C. V. Mosby.

Dworaczyk, E. J. (1979). *The first Polish colonies of America in Texas*. San Antonio, TX: The Naylor Company.

Eck, D. (1994). *African religion in America: On common ground.* New York: Columbia University Press.

Eck, D. L. (1998). *World religions in Boston* (2nd ed.). Cambridge, MA: Harvard University Press.

Eck, D. L. (2001). *A new religious America: How a "Christian country" has become the world's most religious diverse nation.* San Francisco, CA: Harper.

Eddy, M. B. (1875). *Science and health with key to the scriptures.* Boston, MA: Christian Science Publishing.

Egan, M. (1991). *Milagros.* Santa Fe: Museum of New Mexico Press.

Ehrenreich, B., & Ehrenreich, J. (1971). *The American health empire: Power, profits, and politics.* New York: Random House, Vintage Books.

Ehrenreich, B., & English, D. (1973). *Witches, midwives, and nurses: A history of women healers* (2nd ed.). Old Westbury, NY: Feminist Press.

Ehrlich, P. R. (1979). *The golden door: International migration, Mexico and the United States.* New York: Wideview Books.

Eichler, L. (1923). *The customs of mankind.* Garden City, NY: Doubleday, Page.

Eisenberg, D. (1985). *Encounters with Qi.* New York: W. W. Norton.

Eisinger, P. K. (1998). *Toward an end to hunger in America.* Washington, DC: Brookings Institution.

Eliade, M., & Couliano, I. P. (1991). *The Eliade guide to world religions.* San Francisco, CA: Harper.

Elling, R. H. (1977). *Socio-cultural influences on health and health care.* New York: Springer.

Elworthy, R. T. (1958). *The evil eye: The origins and practices of superstition.* New York: Julian Press. (Originally published by John Murray, London, 1915.)

Epstein, C. (1974). *Effective interaction in contemporary nursing.* Englewood Cliffs, NJ: Prentice Hall.

Erickson, E. E. (1941). Tarboro Free Press. *SFQ, 5,* 123.

Ergil, K. V. (1996). China's traditional medicine. In M. S. Micozzi (Ed.), *Fundamentals of complementary and alternative medicine* (pp. 208–296). New York: Churchill Livingstone.

Estes, G., & Zitzow, D. (1980, November). *Heritage consistency as a consideration in counseling Native Americans.* Paper read at the National Indian Education Association Convention, Dallas, TX.

ethnicity. (n.d.). *The American Heritage New Dictionary of Cultural Literacy* (3rd ed.). Retrieved January 31, 2011, from Dictionary.com website: http://dictionary.reference.com/browse/ethnicity

Evans, E. F. (1881). *The divine law of cure.* Boston, MA: H. H. Carter.

Fadiman, A. (1997). *The spirit catches you and you fall down.* New York: Farrar, Straus and Giroux.

Farge, E. J. (1975). *La vida Chicana: Health care attitudes and behaviors of Houston Chicanos.* San Francisco, CA: R and E Research Associates.

Feagin, J. R. (1975). *Subordinating the poor: Welfare and American beliefs.* Englewood Cliffs, NJ: Prentice Hall.

Feagin, J. R., & Feagin, C. B. (1978). *Discrimination American style.* Englewood Cliffs, NJ: Prentice Hall.

Feldman, D. M. (1986). *Health and medicine in the Jewish tradition.* New York: Crossroads.

Fejos, P. (1959). Man, magic, and medicine. In L. Goldston (Ed.), *Medicine and anthropology* (p. 43). New York: International University Press.

Finney, J. C. (Ed.). (1969). *Culture change, mental health, and poverty.* New York: Simon and Schuster.

Fleming, A. S., chairman, U.S. Commission on Civil Rights. (1980). *The tarnished golden door: Civil rights issues on immigration.* Washington, DC: Government Printing Office.

Flores, G. (2006). Language Barriers to health care in the United States. *New England Journal of Medicine, 355*(3), 229–231.

Flores-Peña, Y. (1991). *Personal interview.* Los Angeles, CA.

Flores-Pena, Y., & Evanchuk, R. J. (1994). *Santeria garments and altars.* Jackson: University of Mississippi Press.

Fonseca, I. (1995). *Bury me standing: The gypsies and their journey.* New York: Vintage.

Fontaine, K. L. (2003). *Mental health nursing* (5th ed.). Upper Saddle River, NJ: Prentice Hall.

Forbes, T. R. (1966). *The midwife and the witch.* New Haven, CT: Yale University Press.

Ford, P. S. (1971). *The healing trinity: Prescriptions for body, mind, and spirit.* New York: Harper & Row.

Fortney, A. J. (1977, January 23). Has White man's lease expired? *Boston Sunday Globe*, pp. 8–30.

Fox, M. (2001). *One river, many wells*. New York: Tarcher/Putnam.

Foy, F. A. (Ed.). (1980). *Catholic Almanac*. Huntington, IN: Our Sunday Visitor.

Francis, P., Jr. (1994). *Beads of the world*. Atglen, PA: Schiffer.

Frankel, E., & Teutsch, B. P. (1992). *The encyclopedia of Jewish symbols*. Northvale, NJ: Jason Aronson, Inc.

Frazer, J. G. (1923). *Folklore in the Old Testament*. New York: Tudor Publishing.

Freedman, L. (1969). *Public housing: The politics of poverty*. New York: Holt, Rinehart & Winston.

Freeman, H., Levine, S., & Reeder, L. G. (Eds.). (1972). *Handbook of medical sociology* (2nd ed.). Englewood Cliffs, NJ: Prentice Hall.

Friedman, M., & Friedland, G. W. (1998). *Medicine's ten greatest discoveries*. New Haven, CT: Yale University Press.

Freidson, E. (1971). *Profession of medicine*. New York: Dodd, Mead.

Freire, P. (1970). *Pedagogy of the oppressed*. Trans. M. B. Ramos. New York: Seabury Press.

Frost, M. (n.d.). *The Shaker story*. Canterbury, NH: Canterbury Shakers.

Fuentes, C. (1985). *The old gringo*. New York: Farrar, Straus and Giroux.

Fugh-Berman, A. (1996). *Alternative medicine: What works*. Tucson, AZ: Odonian Press.

Fuller, J. G. (1974). *Arigo: Surgeon of the rusty knife*. New York: Pocket Books.

Galloway, M. R. U. (Ed.). (1990). *Aunt Mary, tell me a story*. Cherokee, NC: Cherokee Communications.

Gambino, R. (1974). *Blood of my blood: The dilemma of Italian-Americans*. Garden City, NY: Doubleday.

Gans, H. J. (1962). *The urban villagers*. New York: Free Press.

Garcia, C. (1992). *Dreaming in Cuban*. New York: Ballantine Books.

Gardner, D. (1992). *Niño Fidencio: A heart thrown open*. Santa Fe, NM: Museum of New Mexico Press.

Garner, J. (1976). *Healing yourself* (6th ed.). Vashon, WA: Crossing Press.

Gaver, J. R. (1972). *Sickle cell disease*. New York: Lancer Books.

Gaw, A. (Ed.). (1982). *Cross-cultural psychiatry*. Boston, MA: John Wright.

Geissler, E. M. (1994). *Pocket guide: Cultural assessment*. St. Louis, MO: C. V. Mosby.

Geissler, E. M. (1998). *Pocket guide cultural assessment* (2nd ed.). St. Louis, MO: C. V. Mosby.

Gelfond, D. E., & Kutzik, A. (Eds.). (1979). *Ethnicity and aging: Theory, research and policy*. New York: Springer.

Genovese, E. D. (1972). *Roll, Jordan, Roll*. New York: Vintage Books.

Gibbs, J. T., Huang, L. N., Nagata, D. K., et al. (1988). *Children of color*. San Francisco, CA: Jossey-Bass.

Gibbs, T. (1996). *A guide to ethnic health collections in the United States*. Westport, CT: Greenwood.

Gifford, E. S. (1957, August). Evil eye in medicine. *American Journal of Ophthalmology, 44*(2), 238.

Giger, J. N., & Davidhizar, R. E. (1995). *Transcultural nursing assessment and intervention* (2nd ed.). St. Louis, MO: C. V. Mosby.

Giordano, J., & Giordano, G. P. (1977). *The ethno-cultural factor in mental health*. New York: New York Institute of Pluralism and Group Identity.

Giordano, J., & McGoldrick, M. (1996). Italian families. In M. McGoldrick, J. Giordano, & J. K. Pearce (Eds.), *Ethnicity and family therapy* (2nd ed., pp. 567–582). New York: Guilford.

Glazer, N., & Moynihan, D. (Eds.). (1975). *Ethnicity: Theory and experience*. Cambridge, MA: Harvard University Press.

Goldberg, B. (1993). *Alternative medicine: The definitive guide*. Puyallup, WA: Future Medicine.

Gonzalez-Wippler, M. (1982). *The Santeria experience*. Bronx, NY: Original Publications.

Gonzalez-Wippler, M. (1985). *Tales of the Orishas*. New York: Original Publications.

Gonzalez-Wippler, M. (1987). *Santeria: African magic in Latin America*. Bronx, NY: Original Publications.

Gordon, A. F., & Kahan, L. (1976). *The tribal beads: A handbook of African trade beads*. New York: Tribal Arts Gallery.

Gordon, D. M. (1972). *Theories of poverty and underemployment*. Lexington, MA: D. C. Heath.

Gordon, F. (1966). *Role theory and illness*. New Haven, CT: College and University Press.

Goswami, S. D. (1983). *Prabhupada: He built a house in which the whole world can live*. Los Angeles: The Bhaktivedanta Book Trust.

Grant, G. (1994). *Obake: Ghost stories in Hawaii*. Honolulu, Hawaii: Mutual.

Graunke, K. (2003, January 8). *Personal Interview*. Boston, Massachusetts.

Gray, K. (1992). *Passport to understanding*. Denver, CO: Center for Teaching International Relations.

Greeley, A. M. (1975a). *The Irish Americans*. New York: Harper & Row.

Greeley, A. M. (1975b). *Why can't they be like us? America's white ethnic group*. New York: E. P. Dutton.

Green, V. (1980). Poles. In S. Thernstrom (Ed.), *Harvard encyclopedia of American ethnic groups* (pp. 787–803). Cambridge, MA: Harvard University Press.

Greenhaw, W. (2000). *My heart is in the earth*. Montgomery, AL: River City.

Grier, W. H., & Cobbs, P. M. (1968). *Black rage*. New York: Bantam Books.

Griffin, J. H. (1960). *Black like me*. New York: Signet.

Gruber, R. (1987). *Rescue: The exodus of the Ethiopian Jews*. New York: Atheneum.

Gutman, H. G. (1976). *The black family in slavery and freedom, 1750–1925*. New York: Pantheon Books.

Gutmanis, J. (1994). *Kahuna La'au Lapa'au*. Aiea, Hawaii: Island Heritage Press.

Hailey, A. (1984). *Strong medicine*. Garden City, NY: Doubleday.

Haley, A. (1976). *Roots*. New York: Doubleday.

Hallam, E. (1994). *Saints*. New York: Simon & Schuster.

Hammerschlag, C. A. (1988). *The dancing healers*. San Francisco, CA: Harper & Row.

Hand, W. D. (1973). *American folk medicine: A symposium*. Berkeley, CA: University of California Press.

Hand, W. D. (1980). *Magical medicine*. Berkeley, CA: University of California Press.

Harney, R. F., & Troper, H. (1975). *Immigrants: A portrait of urban experience 1890–1930*. Toronto, ON: Van Nostrand Reinhold.

Harrington, C., & Estes, C. L. (1994). *Health policy and nursing*. Boston, MA: Jones & Bartlett.

Harris, L. (1985). *Holy days: The world of a Hasidic family*. New York: Summit Books.

Harwood, A. (1971). The hot-cold theory of disease: Implications for treatment of Puerto Rican patients. *Journal of the American Medical Asssociation, 216,* 1154–1155.

Harwood, A. (Ed.). (1981). *Ethnicity and medical care*. Cambridge, MA: Harvard University Press.

Haskins, J. (1978). *Voodoo and hoodoo*. Bronx, NY: Original Publications.

Hauptman, L. M., & Wherry, J. D. (1990). *The Pequots in Southern New England: The fall and rise of an American Indian nation*. Norman, OK: University of Oklahoma Press.

Hawkins, J. B. W., & Higgins, L. P. (1983). *Nursing and the health care delivery system*. New York: Tiresias Press.

Hecker, M. (1979). *Ethnic American, 1970–1977*. Dobbs Ferry, NY: Oceana.

Henderson, G., & Primeaux, M. (Eds.). (1981). *Transcultural health care*. Menlo Park, CA: Addison-Wesley.

Hennessee, O. M. (1989). *Aloe: Myth-magic medicine*. Lawton, OK: Universal Graphics.

Hernandez, C. A., Haug, M. J., & Wagner, N. N. (1976). *Chicanos' social and psychological perspectives*. St. Louis, MO: C. V. Mosby.

Herzlich, C. (1973). *Health and illness: A social psychological analysis*. Trans. D. Graham. New York: Academic Press.

Hiatt, H. H. (1987). *America's health in the balance: Choice or chance?* New York: Harper & Row.

Hickel, W. J. (1972). *Who owns America?* New York: Paperback Library.

Hicks, R., & Hicks, K. (1999). *Boomers, Xers, and other strangers*. Wheaton, IL: Tyndale House.

Himmelstein, D. U., & Woolhandler, S. (1994). *The national health program book: A source guide for advocates*. Monroe, ME: Common Courage Press.

Hirsch, E. D. (1987). *Cultural literacy: What every American needs to know*. Boston, MA: Houghton Mifflin.

Hongo, F. M. (Gen. Ed.). (1985). *Japanese American journey: The story of a people*. San Mateo, CA: Japanese American Curriculum Project.

Honychurch, P. N. (1980). *Caribbean wild plants and their uses*. London: Macmillan.

Hopkins, E., Woods, L., & Kelley, R. (1995). *Working with groups on spiritual themes*. Duluth, MN: Whole Person Associates.

Howard, M. (1980). *Candle burning* (2nd ed.). Weingborough, Northamptonshire, England: Aquarian Press.

Howe, I. (1976). *World of our fathers.* New York: Harcourt Brace Jovanovich.

Hufford, D. J. (1984). *American healing systems: An introduction and exploration.* Conference booklet. Philadelphia, PA: University of Pennsylvania.

Hughes, H. S. (1953). *The United States and Italy.* Cambridge, MA: Harvard University Press.

Hughes, L., & Bontemps, A. (Eds.). (1958). *The Book of negro folklore.* New York: Dodd, Mead.

Hunter, J. D. (1991). *Culture wars: The struggle to define America.* New York: Basic Books.

Hunter, J. D. (1994). *Before the shooting begins: Searching for democracy in America's culture war.* New York: Free Press.

Hurmence, B. (Ed.). (1984). *My folks don't want me to talk about slavery.* Winston-Salem, NC: John F. Blair.

Hutchens, A. R. (1973). *Indian herbalogy of North America.* Windsor, Ontario: Meico.

Hutton, J. B. (1975). *The healing power.* London: Leslie Frewin.

Hyatt, H. M. (1935). *Folklore from Adams County Illinois.* New York.

Illich, I. (1975). *Medical nemesis: The expropriation of health.* London: Marion Bogars.

Illich, I., Zola, I. K., McKnight, J., et al. (1977). *Disabling professions.* Salem, NH: Boyars.

Informational brochure. (1953). *Shrine of Our Lady of La Leche.* St. Augustine, FL. (personal visit, 1999)

Informational brochure. (1999). *Shrine of the Blessed Virgin Mary.* Christ of the Hills Monastery, Blanco, TX. (personal visit, 1997)

Iorizzo, L. J. (1980). *Italian immigration and the impact of the Padrone System.* New York: Arno Press.

Jackson, J. S., Chatters, L. M., & Taylor, R. J. (1993). *Aging in black America.* Newbury Park, CA: Sage.

Jaco, E. G. (Ed.). (1958). *Patients, physicians, and illness: Sourcebook in behavioral science and medicine.* Glencoe, IL: Free Press.

Jacobs, H. A. (1988). *Incidents in the life of a slave girl.* London: Oxford University Press.

Jacobs, L. (Ed.). (1990). *The Jewish mystics.* London: Kyle Cathie.

Jacques, G. (1976). Cultural health traditions: A Black perspective. In M. Branch & P. P. Paxton (Eds.), *Providing safe nursing care for ethnic people of color* (p. 116). New York: Appleton-Century-Crofts.

Jangl, A. M., & Jangl, J. F. (1987). *Ancient legends of healing herbs.* Coeur d'Alene, ID: Prisma Press.

Jarvis, D. C. (1958). *Folk medicine: A Vermont doctor's guide to good health.* New York: Henry Holt.

Jennings, P., & Brewater, T. (1998). *The twentieth century.* New York: Doubleday.

Jilek, W. G. (1992). *Indian healing: Shamanic ceremonialism in the Pacific Northwest today.* Blaine, WA: Hancock House.

Johnson, C. J., & McGee, M. G. (Eds.). (1991). *How different religions view death and afterlife.* Philadelphia, PA: Charles Press.

Johnson, C. L. (1985). *Growing up and growing old in Italian-American families.* New Brunswick, NJ: Rutgers University Press.

Johnson, E. A. (1976). *To the first Americans: The sixth report on the Indian health program of the U.S. Public Health Service.* Washington, DC: DHEW Pub. No. (HSA) 77–1000, 1976.

The Joint Commission. (2010). *Advancing effective communication, cultural competence, and patient- and family-centered care: A roadmap for hospitals.* Oakbrook Terrace, IL: Author.

Jonas, S., & Kovner, A. R. (Eds.). (1998). *Health care delivery in the United States.* New York: Springer.

Jordan, B., & Heardon, S. (1979). *Barbara Jordan: A self portrait.* Garden City, NY: Doubleday.

Jung, C. G. (Ed.). (1964). *Man and his symbols.* Garden City, NY: Doubleday.

Kain, J. F. (Ed.). (1969). *Race and poverty: The economics of discrimination.* Englewood Cliffs, NJ: Prentice Hall.

Kanellos, N. (1997). *Hispanic firsts.* Detroit: Visible Ink.

Kaptchuk, T., & Croucher, M. (1987). *The healing arts.* New York: Summit Books.

Karolevitz, R. F. (1967). *Doctors of the old, west.* New York: Bonanza Books.

Kassirer, J. P. (2005). *On the take.* New York: Oxford University Press.

Katz, J. H. (1978). *White awareness.* Norman, OK: University of Oklahoma Press.

Kaufman, B. N., & Kaufman, S. L. (1982). *A land, beyond tears*. Garden City, NY: Doubleday.

Kavanagh, K. H., & Kennedy, P. H. (1992). *Promoting cultural diversity: Strategies for health care professionals*. Newbury Park, CA: Sage.

Kearney, M., & Medrano, M. (2001). *Medieval culture and the Mexican American borderlands*. College Station: Texas A & M University Press.

Keith, J. (1982a). *Old people as people: Social and cultural influences on aging and old age*. Boston, MA: Little, Brown.

Keith, J. (1982b). *Old people, new lives*. Chicago, IL: The University of Chicago Press.

Kekahbah, J., & Wood, R. (Eds.). (1980). *Life cycle of the American Indian family*. Norman, OK: AIANA Publishing Co.

Kell, K. T. (1965). Tobacco cures. *Journal of American Folklore Society, 78*, 106.

Kelly, I. (1965). *Folk practice in North Mexico: Birth customs, folk medicine, and spiritualism in the Laguna Zone*. Austin, TX: University of Texas Press.

Kelsey, M. T. (1973). *Healing and Christianity*. New York: Harper & Row.

Kennedy, E. M. (1972). *In critical condition: The crises in America's health care*. New York: Simon & Schuster.

Kennett, F. (1976). *Folk medicine, fact and fiction*. New York: Crescent Books.

Kiev, A. (1964). *Magic, faith and healing: Studies in primitive psychiatry today*. New York: Free Press.

Kiev, A. (1968). *Curanderismo: Mexican-American folk psychiatry*. New York: Free Press.

Killens, J. O. (1988). *The cotillion*. New York: Ballantine.

Kilner, W. J. (1965). *The human aura*. Secaucus, NJ: Citadel Press.

Kincaid, J. (1988). *A small place*. New York: Farrar, Straus and Giroux.

King, D. H. (1988). *Cherokee heritage*. Cherokee, NC: Cherokee Communications.

Kingston, M. H. (1989). *Tripmaster monkey: His fake book*. New York: Knopf.

Kinney, E. D. (2010). For profit enterprise in health care: Can it contribute to health reform? *American journal of law and medicine, 36*, 405–435.

Kirkland, J., Matthews, H. F. M., Sullivan, C. W., III, et al. (Eds.). (1992). *Herbal and magical medicine: Traditional healing today*. Durham, NC: Duke University Press.

Klein, A. M. (1991). *Sugarball, the American game, the Dominican dream*. New Haven, CT: Yale University Press.

Klein, J. W. (1980). *Jewish identity and self-esteem: Healing wounds through ethnotherapy*. New York: Institute on Pluralism and Group Identity.

Klein, M. (1998). *A time to be born: Customs and folklore of Jewish birth*. Philadelphia, PA: Jewish Publication Society.

Kluckhohn, C. (1944). *Navaho witchcraft*. Boston: Beacon Press.

Kluckhohn, C., & Leighton, D. (1962). *The Navaho* (rev. ed.). Garden City, NY: Doubleday and Co.

Kmit, A., Luciow, L. L., Luciow, J., et al. (1979). *Ukrainian Easter eggs and how we make them*. Minneapolis, MN: Ukrainian Gift Shop.

Knowles, J. (1970, January). It's time to operate. *Fortune, 79*.

Knox, M. E., & Adams, L. (1988). *Traditional health practices of the Oneida Indian*. Oshkosh, WI: University of Wisconsin, College of Nursing.

Knudtson, P., & Suzuki, D. (1992). *Wisdom of the elders*. Toronto, ON: Stoddart.

Knutson, A. L. (1965). *The individual, society, and health behavior*. New York: Russell Sage Foundation.

Komisar, L. (1974). *Down and out in the USA: A history of social welfare*. New York: New Viewpoints.

Kordel, L. (1974). *Natural folk remedies*. New York: Putnam's.

Kosa, J., & Zola, I. K. (1976). *Poverty and health: A sociological analysis* (2nd ed.). Cambridge, MA: Harvard University Press.

Koschi, B. (n.d.) *UCLA archive of California and western folklore*. unpublished, Cannon, UT, no. 3173

Kotelchuck, D. (Ed.). (1976). *Prognosis negative*. New York: Vintage Books.

Kotlowitz, A. (1991). *There are no children here: The story of two boys growing up in the other America*. New York: Doubleday.

Kotz, N. (1971). *Let them eat promises*. Garden City, NY: Doubleday.

Kovner, A. (Ed.). (1990). *Health care delivery in the United States* (4th ed.). New York: Springer.

Kramer, R. M. (1969). *Participation of the poor*. Englewood Cliffs, NJ: Prentice Hall.

Kraut, A. M. (1994). *Silent travelers: Germs, genes, and the immigrant menace*. New York: Basic Books.

Kraybeill, D. B. (1989). *The riddle of Amish culture*. Baltimore: Johns Hopkins.

Kreiger, D. (1979). *The therapeutic touch*. Englewood Cliffs, NJ: Prentice Hall.

Krippner, S., & Villaldo, A. (1976). *The realms of healing*. Millbrae, CA: Celestial Arts.

Kronenfeld, J. J. (1993). *Controversial issues in health care policy*. Newbury Park, CA: Sage.

Kunitz, S. J., & Levy, J. E. (1991). *Navajo aging: The transition from family to institutional support*. Tucson, AZ: University of Arizona Press.

LaFrombose, T., Coleman, L. K., & Gerton, J. (1993). Psychological impact of biculturalism: Evidence and theory. *Psychological Bulletin, 114*(3), 395.

Lake, M. G. (1991). *Native healer initiation into an art*. Wheaton, IL: Quest Books.

Landmann, R. S. (Ed.). (1981). *The problem of the undocumented worker*. Albuquerque, NM: Latin American Institute, University of New Mexico.

Lasker, R. D. (1997). *Medicine and public health*. New York: New York Academy of Medicine.

Lassiter, S. (1995). *Multicultural clients*. Westport, CT: Greenwood.

Last, J. M. (1987). *Public health and human ecology*. Norwalk, CT: Appleton.

Lau, T. (1979). *The handbook of Chinese horoscopes*. Philadelphia, PA: Harper & Row.

Lavelle, R. (Ed.). (1995). *America's new war on poverty: A reader for action*. San Francisco, CA: KQED Books.

Lawless, E. J. (1988). *God's peculiar people*. Lexington, MA: University of Kentucky Press.

Lee, J., & Bell, K. (2011). The impact of cancer on family relationships among chinese patients. *Journal of Transcultural Nursing, 22*(3), 225–234.

Lee, K. (1951). Greek supernatural. *Journal of American Folklore Society, 64*, 309.

Lee, P. R., & Estes, C. L. (Eds.). (1994). *The nation's health* (4th ed.). Boston, MA: Jones & Bartlett.

Leek, S. (1975). *Herbs: Medicine and mysticism*. Chicago, IL: Henry Regnery.

Lefcowitz, E. (1990). *The United States immigration history timeline*. New York: Terra Firma Press.

Leff, S., & Leff, V. (1957). *From witchcraft to world health*. New York: Macmillan.

Leininger, M. (1970). *Nursing and anthropology: Two worlds to blend*. New York: Wiley.

Leininger, M. (1978). *Transcultural nursing: Concepts, theories, and practices*. New York: Wiley.

Leong, L. (1974). *Acupuncture: A layman's view*. New York: Signet.

Leontis, A. (2009). *Culture and customs of Greece*. Westport, CT: Greenwood Press.

Lerner, M. (1994). *Choices in healing*. Cambridge, MA: MIT Press.

Leslau, C., & Leslau, W. (1985). *African proverbs*. White Plains, NY: Peter Pauper Press.

Lesnoff-Caravaglia, G. (Ed.). (1987). *Realistic expectations for long life*. New York: Human Sciences Press.

Letter from Poland—of faith healers and miracle workers. (1983, August 21). *Boston Globe*, p.15.

Levin, J. (2001). *God, faith, and health*. New York: John Wiley & Sons.

Lewis, O. (1959). *Five families: Mexican case studies in the culture of poverty*. New York: New American Library Basic Books.

Lewis, O. (1961). *The children of Sanchez: Autobiography of a Mexican family*. New York: Random House.

Lewis, O. (1966a). *A death in the Sanchez family*. New York: Random House.

Lewis, O. (1966b). *La vida: A Puerto Rican family in the culture of poverty—San Juan and New York*. New York: Random House.

Lewis, T. H. (1990). *The medicine men: Oglala Sioux ceremony and healing*. Lincoln: University of Nebraska Press.

Lich, G. E. (1981). *The German Texans*. San Antonio, TX: The Institute of Texan Cultures.

Lieban, R. W. (1967). *Cebuano sorcery*. Berkeley, CA: University of California Press.

Lin, K. M. (1982). Cultural aspects in mental health for Asian Americans. In A. Gaw (Ed.), *Cross-cultural psychiatry* (pp. 69–83). Boston: John Wright.

Linck, E. S., & Roach J. G. (1989). *Eats: A folkhistory of Texas foods*. Fort Worth: Texas Christian University Press.

Lipson, J. G., Dibble, S. L., & Minarik, P. A. (1996). *Culture and nursing care: A pocket guide*. San Francisco, CA: UCSF Nursing Press.

Litoff, J. B. (1978). *American midwives 1860 to the present*. Westport, CT: Greenwood Press.

LittleDog, P. (1994). *Border healing woman: The story of Jewel Babb* (2nd ed.). Austin, TX: University of Texas Press.

Littlejohn, Hawk. (1979). *Personal Interview.* Boston, MA.

Livingston, I. L. (Ed.). (1994). *Handbook of black American health.* Westport, CT: Greenwood Press.

Logan, P. (1981). *Irish country cures.* Dublin: Talbot Press.

Lorenz, A. J. (1957). Scurvy in the gold rush. *Journal History of Medicine, 12,* 503.

Louv, R. (1980). *Southwind: The Mexican migration.* San Diego, CA: San Diego Union.

Lovering, A. T. (1923). *The household physician,* Vols. 1 & 2. Boston, MA: Woodruff.

Lucero, G. (1975, March). *Health and illness in the Mexican community.* Lecture given at Boston College School of Nursing, Chestnut Hill, MA.

Lum, D. (1992). *Social work practice and people of color: A process-stage approach* (2nd ed.). Pacific Grove, CA: Brooks/ Cole.

Lynch, L. R. (Ed.). (1969). *The cross-cultural approach to health behavior.* Rutherford, NJ: Fairleigh Dickenson University Press.

Lyon, W. S. (1996). *Encyclopedia of native American healing.* New York: Norton.

Mackintosh, J. (1836). *Principles of pathology and practice of physics* (3rd ed.), Vol. 1. Philadelphia, PA: Key & Biddle.

MacNutt, F. (1974). *Healing.* Notre Dame, IN: Ave Maria Press.

MacNutt, F. (1977). *The power to heal.* Notre Dame, IN: Ave Maria Press.

Maduro, R. J. (1976, January). *Curanderismo: Latin American folk healing,* Conference, San Francisco, CA.

Magida, A. J. (Ed.). (1996). *How to be a perfect stranger, Vol. 1.* Woodstock, VT: Jewish Lights Publishing.

Malinowski, B. (1956). *Magic, science, and religion.* Garden City, NY: Doubleday.

Maloney, C. (Ed.). (1976). *The evil eye.* New York: Columbia University Press.

Malpezzi, F. M., & Clement, W. M. (1992). *Italian American folklore.* Little Rock, AR: August House Publishers.

Mandell, B. R. (Ed.). (1975). *Welfare in America: Controlling the "dangerous classes."* Englewood Cliffs, NJ: Prentice Hall.

Manderschied, R. W., & Sonnenschein, M. A. (Eds.). (1992). *Mental health, United States, 1992.* Washington, DC: Center for Mental Health Services and National Institute of Mental Health. Government Printing Office, DHHS Pub. No. (SMA) 92- 1942, 1992.

Mann, F. (1972). *Acupuncture: The Ancient Chinese art of healing and how it works scientifically.* New York: Vintage Books.

Marquez, G. G. (1998). *Love in the time of cholera.* New York: Alfred A. Knopf.

Marsella, A. B., & Pedersens, P. B. (Eds.). (1982). *Cross cultural counseling and psychotherapy.* New York: Pergamon.

Marsella, A. J., & White, G. M. (Eds.). (1982). *Cultural conceptions of mental health therapy.* London: D. Reidel.

Martin, J., & Todnem, A. (1984). *Cream and bread.* Hastings, MN: Redbird Productions.

Martin, J. A. (1995). Birth characteristics for Asian or Pacific Islander subgroups, 1992. Monthly vital statistics report, *National Center for Health Statistics, 43*(10), 1.

Martin, J. L. (1995). *They had stories, we had chores.* Hastings, MN: Caragana Press.

Martin, J. L., & Nelson, S. J. (1994). *They glorified Mary, we glorified rice.* Hastings, MN: Caragana Press.

Martin, L. C. (1984). *Wildflower folklore.* Charlotte, NC: East Woods Press.

Martinez, R. A. (Ed.). (1978). *Hispanic culture and health care.* St. Louis, MO: C. V. Mosby

Matlins, S. M., & Magida, A. J. (Eds.). (1997). *How to be a perfect stranger,* Vol. 2. Woodstock, VT: Jewish Lights Publishing.

Matsumoto, M. (1988). *The unspoken way.* Tokyo: Kodansha International.

Matthiessen, P. (1980). *In the spirit of Crazy Horse.* New York: Viking Press.

McBrid, I. R. (1975). *Practical folk medicine of Hawaii.* Hilo: Petroglyph Press.

McBride, J. (1996). *The color of water.* New York: Riverhead Books.

McCall, N. (1995). *Makes me wanna holler.* New York: Vintage Books.

McClain, M. (1988). *A feeling for life: Cultural identity, community, and the arts.* Chicago, IL: Urban Traditions.

McCubbin, H. I., Thompson, E. A., Thompson, A. I., et al. (1994a). *Resiliency in ethnic minority families. Vol. 1, Native and immigrant American families.* Madison, WI: University of Wisconsin.

McCubbin, H. I., Thompson, E. A., Thompson, A. I., et al. (1994b). *Sense of coherence and resiliency.* Madison, WI: University of Wisconsin.

McCubbin, H. I., Thompson, E. A., Thompson, A. I., et al. (1995). *Resiliency in ethnic minority families. Vol. 2,*

African-American families. Madison, WI: University of Wisconsin Center.

McGill, O. (1977). *The mysticism and magic of India.* South Brunswick, NJ, and New York: A. S. Baines.

McGoldrick, M., Giordano, J., & Pearce, J. K. (1996). *Ethnicity and family therapy* (2nd ed.). New York: Guilford Press.

McGregor, J. H. (1940). *The Wounded Knee massacre from the viewpoint of the Sioux.* Rapid City, SD: Fenwyn Press.

McLary, K. (1993). *Amish style.* Bloomington, IN: Indiana Press.

McLemore, S. D. (1980). *Racial and ethnic relations in America.* Boston, MA: Allyn & Bacon.

Means, R. (1995). *Where white men fear to tread.* New York: St. Martin's Press.

Mechanic, D. (1968). *Medical sociology: A selective view.* New York: Free Press.

Melton, J. G. (2000). *American religions.* Santa Barbara, CA: A B C Clio.

Melville, H. (1851). *Moby Dick* (1967 ed.). New York: Bantam Books.

Menchu, R. (1983). *I, Rigoberta Menchu.* Trans. A. Wright. London: Verso.

Merrill, F. E. (1962). *Society and culture.* Englewood Cliffs, NJ: Prentice Hall.

Metraux, A. (1972). *Voodoo in Haiti.* New York: Schocken Books.

Meyer, C. E. (1985). *American folk medicine.* Glenwood, IL: Meyerbooks.

Micozzi, M. S. (1996). *Fundamentals of complementary and alternative medicine.* New York: Churchill.

Milio, N. (1975). *The care of health in communities: Access for outcasts.* New York: Macmillan.

Millman, M. (1977). *The unkindest cut.* New York: William Morrow.

Mindel, C. H., & Habenstein, R. W. (Eds.). (1976). *Ethnic families in America.* New York: Elsevier.

Miner, H. (1939). *St. Denis, a French Canadian parish.* Chicago, IL: University of Chicago Press.

Moldenke, H. N., & Moldenke, A. L. (1952). *Plants of the Bible.* New York: Dover Publications.

Montagu, A. (1971). *Touching.* New York: Harper & Row.

Montgomery, R. (1973). *Born to heal.* New York: Coward, McCann, and Geoghegan.

Born to hel. (1980, February). *Monthly Missalette, 15*(13), 38.

Moody, R. A. (1976). *Life after life.* New York: Bantam.

Mooney, J. (1982). *Myths of the Cherokee and sacred formulas of the Cherokees.* Nashville, TN, Charles and Randy Elder— Booksellers, and Cherokee, NC: Museum of the Cherokee Indian.

Morgan, H. T. (1942 [1972]). *Chinese symbols and superstitions.* Detroit, MI: Gale Research. (Reprint, S. Pasadena, CA: Ione Perkins.)

Morgan, M. (1991). *Mutant message down-under.* Lees Summit, MO: MM CO.

Morgenstern, J. (1966). *Rites of birth, marriage, death, and kindred occasions among the Semites.* Chicago, IL: Quadrangle Books.

Morley, P., & Wallis, R. (Eds.). (1978). *Culture and curing.* Pittsburgh, PA: University of Pittsburgh Press.

Morrison, T. (1981). *Tar baby.* New York: Alfred A. Knopf.

Morrison, T. (1987). *Beloved.* New York: Knopf/Random House.

Morton, L. T., & Moore, R. J. (1998). *A chronology of medicine and related sciences.* Cambridge, MA: University Press.

Mumford, E. (1973, November–December). Puerto Rican perspectives on mental illness. *Mount Sinai Journal of Medicine, 40*(6), 771–773.

Murray, P. (1987). *Song in a weary throat: An American pilgrimage.* New York: Harper & Row.

Mushkin, S. V. (1974). *Consumer incentives for health care.* New York: Prodist.

Naegele, K. (1970). *Health and healing.* San Francisco, CA: Jossey-Bass.

Nahin, R. L., Barnes, P. M., Stussman, B. J., & Bloom, B. (2009). Costs of complementary and alternative medicine (CAM) and frequency of visits to CAM practitioners: United States, 2007. *National Health Statistics Reports,* 18. Hyattsville, MD: National Center for Health Statistics.

Nall, F. C., II, & Spielberg, J. (1967). Social and cultural factors in the responses of Mexican-Americans to medical treatment. *Journal of Health and Social Behavior, 8,* 302.

National Center for Health Statistics. (1998). *Health United States 1998 with socioeconomic status and health chartbook.* Hyattsville, MD: Author.

National Center for Health Statistics. (2006). *Health, United States, 2006 with chartbook on trends in the health of Americans.* Hyattsville, MD: Author.

National Center for Health Statistics. (2007). *Health, United States, 2007 with chartbook on trends in the health of Americans.* Hyattsville, MD: Author.

National Center for Health Statistics. (2011). *Health, United States, 2010 with special feature on death and dying.* Hyattsville, MD: Author.

Needleman, J. (2003). *The American soul.* New York: Tarcher/Putman.

Neihardt, J. G. (1991—original 1951). *When the tree flowered.* Lincoln: University of Nebraska Press.

Neihardt, J. G. (1998—original 1961). *Black Elk speaks.* Lincoln: University of Nebraska Press.

Neihardt, N. (1993). *The sacred hoop.* Tekamah, NE: Neihardt.

Nelli, H. S. (1980). Italians. In S. Thernstrom (Ed.), *Harvard encyclopedia of American ethnic groups* (pp. 545–560). Cambridge, MA: Harvard University Press.

Nelli, H. S. (1983). *From immigrants to ethnics: The Italian Americans.* Oxford: Oxford University Press.

Nelson, D. (1985). *Food combining simplified.* Santa Cruz, CA: The Plan.

Nemetz-Robinson, G. L. (1988). *Crosscultural understanding.* New York: Prentice Hall.

Nerburn, K., & Mengelkoch, L. (Eds.). (1991). *Native American wisdom.* San Rafael, CA: New World Library.

Neugrossschel, J. (1991). *Great tales of Jewish occult and fantasy.* New York: Wings Books.

Newman, K. D. (1975). *Ethnic American short stories.* New York: Pocket Books.

Nieves, E. (2007, June 9). Indian reservation reeling in weave of youth suicides and attempts. *New York Times,* p. A-9.

Nightingale, F. (1860, 1946). *Notes on nursing—What it is, what it is not.* New York: Appleton-Century. (A fascimile of the first edition published by D. Appleton and Co.)

Noble, M. (1997). *Sweet grass lives of contemporary Native women of the Northeast.* Mashpee, MA: C. J. Mills.

Norman, J. C. (Ed.). (1969). *Medicine in the ghetto.* New York: Appleton- Century-Crofts.

North, J. H., & Grodsky, S. J. (Comp.). (1979). *Immigration literature: Abstracts of demographic, economic, and policy studies.* Washington, DC: U.S. Department of Justice, Immigration & Naturalization Service.

Novak, M. (1972). *The rise of the unmeltable ethnics.* New York: Macmillan.

Novak, M. (1973). How American are you if your grandparents came from Serbia in 1888? In S. Te Selle (Ed.), *The rediscovery of ethnicity: Its implications for culture and politics in America.* New York: Harper & Row.

Null, G., & Stone, C. (1976). *The Italian-Americans.* Harrisburg, PA: Stackpole Books.

O'Berennan, J., & Smith, N. (1981). *The crystal icon.* Austin, TX: Galahad Press.

Oduyoye, M. (1996). *Words and meaning in Yoruba religion.* London: Karnak House.

Office of Minority Health. (2001). *National standards for culturally and linguistically appropriate services in health care.* Washington, DC: U.S. Department of Health and Human Services.

Opler, M. K. (Ed.). (1959). *Culture and mental health.* New York: Macmillan.

Orlando, L. (1993). *The multicultural game book.* New York: Scholastic Professional Books.

Orque, M. S., Block, B., & Monrray, L. S. A. (1983). *Ethnic nursing care: A Multicultural approach.* St. Louis, MO: C. V. Mosby.

Osofsky, G. (1963). *Harlem: The making of a ghetto.* New York: Harper & Row.

Overfield, T. (1985). *Biologic variation in health and illness.* Menlo Park, CA: Addison-Wesley.

Ozaniec, N. (1997). *Little book of Egyptian wisdom.* Rockport, MA: Element.

Padilla, E. (1958). *Up from Puerto Rico.* New York: Columbia University Press.

Paley, V. G. (1979). *White teacher.* Cambridge, MA: Harvard University Press.

Palos, S. (1971). *The Chinese art of healing.* New York: Herter and Herter.

Pappworth, M. H. (1967). *Human guinea pigs: Experimentation on man.* Boston, MA: Beacon Press.

Parsons, T. (1966). Illness and the role of the physician: A sociological perspective. In W. R. Scott & E. H. Volkart (Eds.), *Medical care: Readings in the sociology of medical institutions* (p. 275). New York: John Wiley & Sons.

Parsons, T., & Clark, K. B. (1965). *The Negro American.* Boston, MA: Beacon Press.

Paul, B. (Ed.). (1955). *Health, culture, and community: Case studies of public reactions to health programs.* New York: Russell Sage Foundation.

Payer, L. (1988). *Medicine and culture.* New York: Penguin Books.

Pearsall, M. (1963). *Medical behavior science: A selected bibliography of cultural anthropology, social psychology, and sociology in medicine.* Louisville, KY: University of Kentucky Press.

Peltier, L. (1999). *Prison writings: My life is my sun dance.* New York: St. Martin's Press.

Pelto, P. J., & Pelto, G. H. (1978). *Anthropological research: The structure of inquiry* (2nd ed.). Cambridge, MA: Cambridge University Press.

Pelton, R. W. (1973). *Voodoo charms and talismans.* New York: Popular Library.

Perera, V. (1995). *The cross and the pear tree.* Berkeley, CA: University of California Press.

Petry, A. (1985). *The street.* Boston: Beacon Press.

Philpott, L. L. (1979). "A Descriptive Study of Birth Practices and Midwifery in the Lower Ro Grande Valley of Texas." Ph.D. diss., University of Texas Health Science Center at Houston School of Public Health, Houston, TX.

Pierce, R. V. (1983). *The people's common sense medical advisor in plain English, or medicine simplified* (12th ed.). Buffalo, NY: World's Dispensary.

Piven, F. F., & Cloward, R. A. (1971). *Regulating the poor: The functions of public welfare.* New York: Vintage Books.

Plotkin, M. J. (1993). *Tales of a shaman's apprentice.* New York: Viking.

Popenoe, C. (1977). *Wellness.* Washington, DC: YES!

Powell, C. A. (1938). *Bound feet.* Boston, MA: Warren Press.

Power, S. (1994). *The grass dancer.* New York: Putnam.

Prabhupada, A. C. (1970). *Bhaktivedanta Swami. KRSNA: The supreme personality of godhead,* Vol. 1. Los Angeles: The Bhaktivedanta Book Trust.

Progoff, I. (1959). *Depth psychology and modern man.* New York: McGraw-Hill.

Prose, F. (1977). *Marie Laveau.* New York: Berkeley Pub. Corp.

Proulx, E. A. (1996). *Accordion crimes.* New York: Scribner.

Purnell, L. D., & Paulanka, B. J. (1988). *Transcultural health care.* Philadelphia, PA: F. A. Davis.

Putnam, R. D., & Campbell, D. E. (2010). *American grace: How religion divides and unites us.* New York: Simon and Schuster.

Ragucci, A. T. (1981). Italian Americans. In A. Harwood (Ed.), *Ethnicity and medical care* (pp. 545–560). Cambridge, MA: Harvard University Press.

Rand, C. (1958). *The Puerto Ricans.* New York: Oxford University Press.

Read, M. (1966). *Culture, health, and disease.* London: Javistock Publications.

Rector-Page, L. G. (1992). *Healthy healing: An alternative healing reference* (9th ed.). San Fransisco, CA: Healthy Healing Publications.

Redman, E. (1973). *The dance of legislation.* New York: Simon & Schuster.

Reichard, G. A. (1977). *Navajo medicine-man sandpaintings.* New York: Dover.

Reid, T. R. (2010). *The healing of America: A global quest for better and cheaper, and fairer health care.* New York: Penguin.

religion. (n.d.). *The American Heritage New Dictionary of Cultural Literacy* (3rd ed.). Retrieved January 31, 2011, from Dictionary.com website: http://dictionary.reference.com/browse/religion

Reneaux, J. J. (1992). *Cajun folktales.* Little Rock, AR: August House Publishers.

Rist, R. C. (1979). *Desegregated schools: Appraisals of an American experiment.* New York: Academic Press.

Riva, A. (1974). *The modern herbal spellbook.* N. Hollywood, CA: International Imports.

Riva, A. (1985). *Magic with incense and powders.* N. Hollywood, CA: International Imports.

Riva, A. (1990). *Devotions to the saints.* Los Angeles: International Imports.

Rivera, J. R. (1977). *Puerto Rican tales.* Mayaquez, Puerto Rico: Ediciones Libero.

Roby, P. (Ed.). (1974). *The poverty establishment.* Englewood Cliffs, NJ: Prentice Hall.

Rodriquez, C. E. (1991). *Puerto Ricans born in the U.S.A.* Boulder, CO: Westview Press.

Roemer, M. I. (1990). *An introduction to the U.S. health care system* (2nd ed.). New York: Springer.

Rogler, L. H. (1972). *Migrant in the city.* New York: Basic Books.

Rohde, E. S. (1922, 1971). *The old English herbs.* New York: Dover.

Romo, R. G. (1995, May 3). *Hispanic health traditions and issues.* Paper presented at the Minnesota Health Educators Conference, Minneapolis, MN.

Rose, P. I. (1981). *They and we: Racial and ethnic relations in the United States* (3rd ed.). New York: Random House.

Rosen, P. (1980). *The neglected dimension: Ethnicity in American life.* Notre Dame, London: University of Notre Dame Press.

Rosenbaum, B. Z. (1985). *How to avoid the evil eye.* New York: St. Martin's Press.

Rosenstock, I. M. (1966, July). Why people use health services. *Millbank Memorial Fund Quarterly, 44*(3), 94–127.

Ross, N. W. (1960). *The world of Zen.* New York: Vintage Books.

Rossbach, S. (1987). *Interior design with Feng Shui.* New York: Arkana.

Roter, D. L., & Hall, J. A. (1993). *Doctors talking with patients.* Westport, CT: Auburn House.

Roy, C. (1999). *Nurse's handbook of alternative and complementary therapies.* Springhouse, PAS: Springhouse.

Rubel, A. J. (1964, July). The epidemiology of a folk illness: Susto in Hispanic America. *Ethnology, 3*(3), 270–271.

Rude, D. (Ed.). (1972). *Alienation: Minority groups.* New York: Wiley.

Russell, A. J. (1937). *Health in his wings.* London: Metheun.

Ryan, W. (1971). *Blaming the victim.* New York: Vintage Books.

S., E. M. (1927). *The house of wonder: A romance of psychic healing.* London: Rider.

Saltus, R. (1999, February 18). Managed, yes, but couple wonders, is care? *Boston Globe,* p. A-1.

Santillo, H. (1983). *Herbal combinations from authoritative sources.* Provo, UT: NuLife.

Santino, J. (1994). *All around the tear.* Chicago, IL: University of Illinois Press.

Santoli, A. (1988). *New Americans.* New York: Ballantine.

Sargent, D. A. (1904). *Health, strength, and power.* New York: HM Caldwell.

Saunders, L. (1954). *Cultural difference and medical care: The case of the Spanish-speaking people of the Southwest.* New York: Russell Sage Foundation.

Saunders, L. (1958). Healing ways in the Spanish southwest. In E. G. Jaco (Ed.), *Patients, physicians, and illness* (p. 13). Glencoe, IL: Free Press.

Saunders, R. (1927). *Healing through the spirit agency.* London: Hutchinson.

Schilling, B., & Brannon, E. (1986). Health-related dietary practices. In *Cross-cultural counseling: A guide for nutrition and health counselors.* Alexandria, VA: U.S. Department of Health and Human Services.

Schneider, M. (1987). *Self healing: My life and vision.* New York: Routledge & Kegan Paul.

Scholem, G. G. (1941). *Major trends in Jewish mysticism.* New York: Schocken Books.

School, B. F. (1924). *Library of health complete guide to prevention and cure of disease.* Philadelphia, PA: Historical.

Schrefer, S. (Ed.). (1994). *Quick reference to cultural assessment.* St. Louis, MO: C. V. Mosby.

Scott, W. R., & Volkart, E. H. (1966). *Medical care.* New York: Wiley.

Senior, C. (1965). *The Puerto Ricans: Strangers then neighbors.* Chicago, IL: Quadrangle Books.

Serinus, J. (Ed.). (1986). *Psychoimmunity and the healing process.* Berkeley, CA: Celestial Arts.

Sexton, P. C. (1965). *Spanish Harlem.* New York: Harper & Row.

Shames, R., & Sterin, C. (1978). *Healing with mind power.* Emmaus, PA: Rodale Press.

Shaw, W. (1975). *Aspects of Malaysian magic.* Kuala Lumpur, Malaysia: Muzium Negara.

Sheinkin, D. (1986). *Path of the Kabbalah.* New York: Paragon House.

Shelton, F. (1965). *Pioneer comforts and kitchen remedies: Oldtime highland secrets from the Blue Ridge and Great Smoky Mountains.* High Point, NC: Hutcraft.

Shelton, F. (Ed.). (1969). *Pioneer superstitions.* High Point, NC: Hutcraft.

Shenkin, B. N. (1974). *Health care for migrant workers: Policies and, politics.* Cambridge, MA: Ballinger.

Shepard, R. F., & Levi, V. G. (1982). *Live and be well.* New York: Ballantine Books.

Shih-Chen, L. (1973). *Chinese medicinal herbs.* Trans. F. P. Smith & G. A. Stuart. San Francisco, CA: Georgetown Press.

Shor, I. (1986). *Culture wars: School and society in the conservative restoration 1969–1984.* Boston, MA: Routledge & Kegan Paul.

Shorter, E. (1987). *The health century.* New York: Doubleday.

Shostak, A. B., Van Til, J., & Van Til, S. B. (1973). *Privilege in America: An end to inequality?* Englewood Cliffs, NJ: Prentice Hall.

Sklott, R. (2011) *The immortal cells of Henrietta Lacks.* New York: Broadway Books.

Silver, G. (1976). *A spy in the house of medicine*. Germantown, MD: Aspen Systems Corp.

Silverman, D. (1989). *Legends of Safed*. Jerusalem, Israel: Gefen.

Silverstein, M. E., Chang, I.-L., & Macon, N. (Trans.). (1975). *Acupuncture and moxibustion*. New York: Schocken Books.

Simmen, E. (Ed.). (1972). *Pain and promise: The Chicano today*. New York: New American Library.

Simmons, A. G. (n.d.). *A witch's brew*. Coventry, CT: Caprilands Herb Farm.

Skelton, R. (1985). *Talismanic magic*. York Beach, ME: Samuel Weiser.

Slater, P. (1970). *The pursuit of loneliness*. Boston: Beacon Press.

Smedley, B. D., Stith, A. Y., & Nelson, A. R. (2004). *Unequal treatment: Confronting racial and ethnic health disparities in health care*. Institute of Medicine Report. Washington, DC: National Academy Press.

Smith, H. (1958). *The religions of man*. New York: Harper & Row.

Smith, H. (1991—original 1958). *The world's religions*. San Francisco, CA: Harper.

Smith, L. (1963). *Killers of the dream*. Garden City, NY: Doubleday.

Smith, P. (1962). *The origins of modern culture, 1543–1687*. New York: Collier Books.

Sowell, T. (1981). *Ethnic America*. New York: Basic Books.

Sowell, T. (1996). *Migrations and cultures*. New York: Basic Books.

Spann, M. B. (1992). *Literature-based multicultural activities*. New York: Scholastic Professional Books.

Spector, M. (1979). Poverty: The barrier to health care. In R. E. Spector (Ed.), *Cultural diversity in health and illness* (pp. 141–162). New York: Appleton, Century & Crofts.

Spector, R. (1992). Culture, ethnicity, and nursing. In P. Potter & A. Perry (Eds.), *Fundamentals of nursing* (3rd ed., pp. 351–369). St. Louis: Mosby-Year Book.

Spector, R. (1996). *Cultural diversity in health and illness* (4th ed.). Stamford, CT: Appleton & Lange.

Spector, R. E. (1983). "A Description of the Impact of Medicare on Health-Illness Beliefs and Practices of White Ethnic Senior Citizens in Central Texas." Ph.D. diss., University of Texas at Austin School of Nursing, Ann Arbor, MI: University Microfilms International.

Spector, R. E. (1998). *CulturalCare: Maternal infant issues*. Baltimore: Williams & Wilkins (video).

Spencer, R. T., Nichols, L. W., Lipkin, G. B., et al. (1993). *Clinical pharmacology and nursing management* (4th ed.). Philadelphia, PA: Lippincott.

Spicer, E. (Ed.). (1977). *Ethnic medicine in the Southwest*. New York: Russell Sage Foundation.

Spurlock, J. (1988). Black Americans. In L. Comas-Diaz & E. E. H. Griffith (Eds.), *Cross-cultural mental health* (p. 173). New York: John Wiley & Sons.

Stack, C. B. (1974). *All our kin*. New York: Harper & Row.

Starr, P. (1982). *The social transformation of American medicine*. New York: Basic Books.

Steele, J. D. (1884). *Hygienic physiology*. New York: A. S. Barnes.

Steinberg, M. (1947). *Basic Judaism*. New York: Harcourt, Brace and World.

Steinberg, S. (2001) *The ethnic myth: Race, ethnicity, and class in America*. Boston, MA: Beacon Press.

Steiner, S. (1969). *La Raza: The Mexican Americans*. New York: Harper & Row.

Steinsaltz, A. (1980). *The thirteen petalled rose*. New York: Basic Books.

Stephan, W. G., & Feagin, J. R. (1980). *School desegregation past, present, future*. New York: Plenum.

Stevens, A. (1974). *Vitamins and remedies*. High Point, NC: Hutcraft.

Stewart, J. (Ed.). (1973). *Bridges not walls*. Reading, MA: Addison-Wesley.

Still, C. E., Jr. (1991). *Frontier doctor medical pioneer*. Kirksville, MO: Thomas Jefferson University Press.

Stoll, R. I. (1990). *Concepts in nursing: A Christian perspective*. Madison, WI: Inter varsity Christian Fellowship.

Stone, E. (1962). *Medicine among the American Indians*. New York: Hafner.

Storlie, F. (1970). *Nursing and the social conscience*. New York: Appleton-Century-Crofts.

Storm, H. (1972). *Seven arrows*. New York: Ballantine Books.

Strauss, A., & Corbin, J. M. (1988). *Shaping a new health care system*. San Francisco, CA: Jossey-Bass.

Strickland, C. J., & Cooper, M. (2011). Getting into trouble: perspectives on stress and suicide prevention among Pacific Northwest Indian youth. *Journal of Transcultural Nursing, 22*(3), 240–247.

Styron, W. (1966). *The confessions of Nat Turner.* New York: Random House.

Suchman, E. A. (1965, Fall). Stages of illness and medical care. *Journal of Health and Human Behavior, 6*(3), 114.

Sykes, J., & Kelly, A. P. (1979, June). Black skin problems. *American Journal of Nursing,* 1092–1094.

Swazey, J. P., & Reeds, K. (1978). *Today's medicine, tomorrow's science.* Washington, DC: U.S. Government Department of Health, Education, and Welfare.

Sweet, M. (1976). *Common edible plants of the west.* Happy Camp, CA: Naturegraph.

Szasz, T. S. (1961). *The myth of mental illness.* New York: Dell.

Takaki, R. (1993). *A different mirror: A history of multicultural America.* Boston, MA: Little, Brown.

Tallant, R. (1946). *Voodoo in New Orleans.* New York: Collier Books.

Tan, A. (1989). *The Joy Luck Club.* New York: Ivy Books.

Tan, A. (2001). *The bonesetter's daughter.* New York: Putnam & Sons.

ten Boom, C. (1971). *The hiding place.* Washington Depot, CT: Chosen Books.

Te Selle, S. (Ed.). (1973). *The rediscovery of ethnicity: Its implications for culture and politics in America.* New York: Harper & Row.

Thernstrom, S. (Ed.). (1980). *Harvard encyclopedia of American ethnic groups.* Cambridge, MA: Harvard University Press.

Thomas, C. (1983). *They came to Pittsburgh.* Pittsburgh, PA: Post-Gazette.

Thomas, P. (1958). *Down these mean streets.* New York: Signet Books.

Thomas, P. (1972). *Savior, Savior, hold my hand.* Garden City, NY: Doubleday.

Thompson, K. (1964). Body, boots, britches. *Journal of American Folklore Society, 77,* 305.

Thurston, H. (1955). Ghosts & poltergeists. *Journal of American Folklore Society, 68,* 97.

Tierra, M. (1990). *The way of herbs.* New York: Pocket Books.

Titmuss, R. M. (1971). *The gift relationship.* New York: Vintage.

Tomasi, S. M. (Ed.). (1980). *National directory of research centers, repositories, and organizations of Italian culture in the United States.* Torino: Fondazione Giovanni Agnelli.

Tompkins, P., & Bird, C. (1973). *The secret life of plants.* New York: Avon.

Tooker, E. (Ed.). (1979). *Native American spirituality of the eastern woodlands.* New York: Paulist Press.

Torrens, P. R. (1988). Historical evolution and overview of health services in the United States. In S. J. Williams & P. R. Torrens (Eds.), *Introduction to health services* (3rd ed., pp. 3–31). New York: John Wiley & Sons.

Torres, E. (1982). *Green medicine: Traditional Mexican-American herbal remedies.* Kingsville, TX: Nieves Press.

Torres-Gill, F. M. (1982). *Politics of aging among elder Hispanics.* Washington, DC: University Press of America.

Touchstone, S. J. (1983). *Herbal and folk medicine of Louisiana and adjacent states.* Princeton, LA: Folk-Life Books.

Trachtenberg, J. (1939). *Jewish magic and superstition.* New York: Behrman House.

Trachtenberg, J. (1983). *The devil and the Jews.* Philadelphia, PA: The Jewish Publication Society of America. (Original publication, New Haven, CT: Yale University Press, 1945.)

Trattner, W. I. (1974). *From poor law to welfare state: A history of social welfare in America.* New York: Free Press.

Trotter, R., II, & Chavira, J. A. (1981). *Curanderismo: Mexican American folk healing.* Athens, GA: University of Georgia Press.

Tucker, G. H. (1977). *Virginia supernatural tales.* Norfolk, VA: Donning.

Tula, M. T. (1994). *Hear my testimony.* Boston, MA: South End Press.

Twining, M. A., & Baird, K. E. (Eds.). (1991). *Sea Island roots: African presence in the Carolinas and Georgia.* Trenton, NJ: Africa World Press.

Unger, S. (Ed.). (1977). *The destruction of American Indian families.* New York: Association on American Indian Affairs.

U.S. Census Bureau. (2001). *Statistical abstract of the United States: 2001.* Washington, DC: Author.

U. S. Commission on Civil Rights. (1970). *Mexican Americans and the administration of justice in the Southwest.* Washington, DC: Government Printing Office.

U.S. Commission on Civil Rights. (1976). *Fulfilling the letter and spirit of the law.* Washington, DC: Government Printing Office.

U.S. Department of Commerce, Bureau of the Census. (1980). *Ancestry of the population by State: 1980.* Washington, DC: Government Printing Office.

U. S. Department of Commerce, Bureau of the Census. (1982, September). *Population profile of the United States: 1981.* "Population Characteristics," ser. 20, no. 374.

U. S. Department of Health and Human Services. (1992). *Healthy people 2000 national health promotion and disease prevention objectives: Full report with commentary.* Boston, MA: Jones and Bartlett.

U. S. Department of Health and Human Services. (1993). *Health United States 1992 and healthy people 2000 review.* Washington, DC: United States Department of Health and Human Services, Public Health Service Centers for Disease Control and Prevention. DHHS Pub. No. (PHS) 93-1232, 1993.

U.S. Department of Health and Human Services. (1997a). *Comprehensive health care program for American Indians and Alaska Natives.* Rockville, MD: Public Health Service, Indian Health Service.

U. S. Department of Health and Human Services. (1997b). *Regional differences in Indian health.* Rockville, MD: Public Health Service, Indian Health Service.

U. S. Department of Health and Human Services. (1997c). *Trends in Indian Health.* Rockville, MD: Public Health Service, Indian Health Service.

U.S. Department of Health, Education, and Welfare. *Health in America: 1776–1976.* Washington, DC: DHEW Pub. No. (HRA) 76-616, 1976.

U.S. Department of Justice, Immigration and Naturalization Service. (1979). *Immigration literature: Abstracts of demographic economic and policy studies.* Washington, DC: Government Printing Office.

Valentine, C. A. (1968). *Culture and poverty.* Chicago, IL: University of Chicago Press.

Van-Ravenswaay, C. (1955). Pioneer medicine in Missouri. *South Medical Journal, 48,* 36.

VanWart, A. F. (1948). Native cures. *Canadian Medical Association Journal, 59*(342), 575.

Wade, M. (1946). *The French-Canadian outlook.* New York: Viking Press.

Wade, M. (1955). *The French-Canadians, 1876–1945.* New York: Macmillan.

Walker, A. (1994). *The temple of my familiar.* New York: Harcourt, Brace, Jovanovich.

Wall, S. (1994). *Shadowcatchers.* New York: HarperCollins.

Wall, S., & Arden, H. (1990). *Wisdomkeepers meetings with native American spiritual elders.* Hillsboro, OR: Beyond Words Publishing Co.

Wallace, G. (1979, November). Spiritual care—A reality in nursing education and practice. *The Nurses Lamp, 5*(2), 1–4.

Wallace, R. B. (Ed.). *Public health and preventive medicine* (14th ed.). Stamford, CT: Appleton & Lange.

Wallnöfer, H., & von Rottauscher, A. (1972). *Chinese folk medicine.* Trans. M. Palmedo. New York: New American Library.

Warner, D. (1979). *The health of Mexican Americans in South Texas.* Austin, TX: Lyndon Baines Johnson School of Public Affairs, University of Texas at Austin.

Warner, D., & Red, K. (1993). *Health care across the border.* Austin, TX: LBJ School.

Warren, N. (Ed.). (1980). *Studies in cross-cultural psychology.* New York: Academic Press.

Webb, J. Y. (1971). *Letter.* Dr. J. R. Krevans to Y. Webb, 15 February 1967. Reported in Superstitious influence—VooDoo in particular—Affecting health practices in a selected population in southern Louisiana (Paper). New Orleans, LA.

Weible, W. (1983). *Medjugore: The message.* Orleans, MA: Paraclete Press.

Wei-kang, F. (1975). *The story of Chinese acupuncture and moxibustion.* Peking: Foreign Languages Press.

Weil, A. (1983). *Health and healing.* Boston, MA: Houghton Mifflin.

Weinbach, S. (1991). *Rabbenu Yisrael Abuchatzira: The story of his life and wonders.* Brooklyn, NY: ASABA- FUJIE publication.

Weinberg, R. D. (1967). *Eligibility for entry to the United States of America.* Dobbs Ferry, NY: Oceana.

Weiss, G., & Weiss, S. (1985). *Growing and using the healing herbs.* New York: Wings Books.

Welch, S., Comer, J., & Steinman, M. (1973, September). Some social and attitudinal correlates of health care among Mexican Americans. *Journal of Health and Social Behavior, 14,* 205.

Wheelwright, E. G. (1974). *Medicinal plants and their history.* New York: Dover.

Wiebe, R., & Johnson, Y. (1998). *Stolen life—The journey of a Cree woman*. Athens, OH: Ohio University Press.

Wilen, J., & Wilen, L. (1984). *Chicken soup and other folk remedies*. New York: Fawcett Columbine.

Williams, R. A. (Ed.). (1975). *Textbook of black-related diseases*. New York: McGraw-Hill.

Williams, S. J., & Torrens, P. R. (1990). *Introduction to health services* (3rd ed.). New York: Wiley.

Wilson, F. A., & Neuhauser, D. (1982). *Health services in the United States* (2nd ed.). Cambridge, MA: Ballinger.

Wilson, S. G. (1992). *The drummer's path: Moving the spirit with ritual and traditional drumming*. Rochester, VT: Destiny Books.

Winkler, G. (1981). *Dybbuk*. New York: Judaica Press.

Wintrob, R. (1972). Hexes, roots, snake eggs? M.D. vs. occults. *Medical Opinion, 1*(7), 54–61.

Wolfson, E. (1993). *From the earth to the sky*. Boston, MA: Houghton Mifflin.

Wright, E. (1984). *The book of magical talismans*. Minneapolis, MN: Marlar Publishing, Co.

Wright, R. (1937). *Black boy*. New York: Harper & Brothers.

Wright, R. (1940). *Native son*. New York: Grosset & Dunlop.

Wright-Hybbard, E. (1977–1992). *A brief study course in homeopathy*. Philadelphia, PA: Formur.

Wyman, L. C. (1966). Navaho diagnosticians. In W. R. Scott & E. H. Volkhart (Eds.), *Medical care* (pp. 8–14). New York: John Wiley & Sons.

Yamamoto, J. (1982). Japanese Americans. In A. Gaw (Ed.), *Cross-cultural psychiatry* (p. 50). Boston, MA: John Wright.

Yambura, B. S. (1960). *A change and a parting*. Ames, IA: University of Iowa Press.

Yoder, D. (1972). Folk medicine. In R. H. Dorson (Ed.), *Folklore and folklife* (pp. 191–193). Chicago, CA: University of Chicago Press.

Young, J. H. (1967). *The medical messiahs*. Princeton, NJ: Princeton University Press.

Zambrana, R. E. (Ed.). (1982). *Work, family, and health: Latina women in transition*. New York: Fordham University.

Zborowski, M. (1969). *People in pain*. San Francisco, CA: Jossey-Bass.

Zeitlin, S. J., Kotkin, A. J., & Baker, H. C. (1977). *A celebration of American family folklore: Tales and traditions from the Smithsonian collection*. New York: Pantheon Books.

Zitner, A. (1999, March 14). Demographers caught looking on US trends. *Boston Sunday Globe*.
Web References.

Zola, I. K. (1972a). The concept of trouble and sources of medical assistance to whom one can turn with what. *Social Science and Medicine, 6*, 673–679.

Zola, I. K. (1972b, November). Medicine as an institution of social control. *Sociological Review, 20*(4), 487–504.

Zola, I. K. (1996, October). Culture and symptoms: An analysis of patients presenting complaints. *American Sociological Review, 31*, 615–630.

Zolla, E. (1969). *The writer and the shaman*. New York: Harcourt Brace Jovanovich.

Zook, J. (1899). *Oneida, The people of the stone*. The Church's Mission to the Oneidas. Oneida Indian Reservation, WI.

Zook, J. (1972a). *Exploring the secrets of treating deaf-mutes*. Peking: Foreign Languages Press.

Zook, J. (1972b). *Your new life in the United States*. Washington, DC: Center for Applied Linguistics.

Zook, J., & Zook, J. (1978). *Hexology*. Paradise, PA: Zook.

Zuckoff, M. (1995, April 18). More and more claiming American Indian heritage. *Boston Globe*, p. A8.

Index

A

Aberglaubisch, 96
Aberglobin, 96
Acculturation, 31
Acculturation themes, 30–32
Acupuncture, 247, 248
*Advancing Effective Communication,
    Cultural Competence, and Patient and
    Family Centered Care: A Roadmap for
    Hospitals* (Joint Commission), 12–13
African Americans, 265–90
    age, 47
    background, 266–70
    birth control, 284
    black genocide, 284
    black Muslims, 277–79
    Catholic saints or relics, 276
    civil rights movement, 269
    coronary heart disease, 281
    cultural phenomena, 277
    defined, 45
    folk medicine, 273–74
    hair care needs, 285
    health and illness, 270–71
    health care manpower, 286–87
    health care system, 282–84
    health maintenance and protection,
        271–72
    health restoration, 272–77
    HIV/AIDS, 281
    home remedies, 272–73
    homicide, 281
    mental illness, 281–82
    morbidity, 279–80
    mortality, 281
    physiological assessment, 284–85
    population, 44, 47
    public housing, 267
    research on culture, 288
    rooting, 272
    sickle-cell anemia, 280–81
    skin conditions, 285
    special considerations for health care
        providers, 284–86
    voodoo, 272–73, 274
Age, 46–47
Ageism, 37
Alaska natives. *See* American Indians
Albacar, 308
Alcohol abuse, 227, 228
Alcoholism, 225–26
Allopathic health care system, 352
Allopathic philosophy, 108
Alpha-thalassemia, 334
Alternative Medicine (NCCAM), 113
Alternative medicines, 108–16
American Association of Colleges of Nursing
    (AACN), 15
American Indian Movement (AIM), 213
American Indians, 207–37
    age, 47
    alcoholism, 225–26
    American Indian Movement (AIM), 213
    background, 211–13
    causes of death, 226
    cultural phenomena, 222
    cultural/communication problems,
        231–32
    current health care problems, 222–28
    death rituals, 151
    defined, 45
    divination, 216
    domestic violence, 227–28
    drums, 221
    fetal alcohol syndrome, 226
    health, 213
    health care manpower, 232–34
    health care provider services, 228
    health care providers, 232–33
    herbal remedies, 220–21
    Hopi Indians, 214, 220
    IHS, 228–31
    illness, 214
    listening, 217
    Lost Colonies, 212
    medicine man or woman, 215
    mental illness, 224–26
    Micmac Indians, 221
    morbidity/mortality, 223
    motion in the hand, 216
    Navajo people, 214–15
    Oneida Indians, 221
    population, 44, 47
    religions, 151
    research on culture, 234
    selected health care indicators, 224
    stargazing, 216
    traditional healer, 215–18
    traditional remedies, 220–22
    treaties of peace, 212
    urban problems, 228
    witchcraft, 217, 218
Amulets, 97–99, 246, 352
Anger syndrome, 260
Argo starch, 276
Aromatherapy, 109, 113, 352
Asafetida, 271–72
Asian Americans, 238–64
    acupuncture, 247
    age, 47

amulets, 246
Ayurvedic medicine, 253–57
background, 239–41
bleeding, 248
blood, 259
causes of death, 259
Chinese immigration, 240
Chinese medicine, 241, 243, 244, 253, 258
Chinese pediatrics, 253
cultural phenomena, 243
cupping, 248
current health problems, 257–61
female shamans, 253
health and illness, 241–46
health care manpower, 261
health care providers, as, 261–62
health maintenance and protection, 246
health status indicators, 258
herbal remedies, 248, 251–52
jade, 239, 246
language difficulties, 258
massage, 248
mental illness, 260
moxibustion, 248
other Chinese remedies, 252
population, 44, 47
pulses, 246
religions, 242
research on culture, 262
Taoism, 241–43
traditional healers, 253
yin and *yang*, 243–45, 247–48
Assemblies of God, 150
Assimilation, 31–32
Assumption of the sick role stage, 80
Ataque, 309
Ayurvedic medicine, 113, 253–57

B
Babalow, 311
Bad gris-gris, 275
Baha'i, 130, 150
Bangles, 97–99
Baptism, 140
Baptist, 140, 150, 162, 164
Barriers to health care, 197–99
Becker's health belief model, 71
Belt, 324
Beta-thalassemia. *See* Cooley's anemia
Biofeedback, 109
Biological variations, 38
Biotechnology Industry Organization, 191
Birth control, 284
Birth rituals/beliefs, 138–47, 172–73
Birthing Stones in Kukaniloko, 159
Black cat oil, 275
Black cohosh, 115
Black genocide, 284
Black magic, 274
Black Muslims, 277–79
Black population. *See* African Americans

Bleeding, 248
Blessing of the Throats on Saint Blaise, 106
Blood, 332
Body language, 40
Botanicas, 314, 315
Boufée delirante, 282
Brain Fog, 282
Brown v. Board of Education, 268, 269
Brujas, 297
Buddhism, 242
Buddhist Churches of America, 131, 150, 151
Byodo-In Temple, 239

C
Caida de la mollera, 296–97
Cajitas/Materias, 130
Cajones, 130
Cajun. *See* Pennsylvania Dutch
CAM, 108–16
CAM USE in America survey, 116
Camomile tea, 308
Cancer, 114
Capstone courses, 367–72
Castiga, 333
Catholicism, 152, 163, 164, 165, 166–67,
        168, 169, 170, 172
Census 2010, 45–48
Center for Medicare & Medicaid Services, 382
Centers for Disease Control (CDC), 382
Chachayotel, 100
Chan, P. K., 243, 244
Chinatown, 240
Chinese pediatrics, 253
Chiropractic, 111
Choking, 105–6
Cholera, 106–7
Christian, 172
Christian Science, 112, 132, 152
Church of Christ, 140, 150
Church of Jesus Christ of Latter-day Saints,
        132–33, 140, 151, 152
Circumcision, 139–40
Citizen, 48
Civil Rights Act of 1964, 11
Civil Rights Law, 349
Civil rights movement, 269
Colored candles, 275
Commingling variables, 34–36
Communication, 38
Complementary and alternative medicines,
        113–16
Confucianism, 242
Congenital abnormalities, 332
Contamination, 332
Cooley's anemia, 334
Course outline (Capstone courses), 367–72
Cruzan, Nancy, 201
Cultural assimilation, 32
Cultural care, 13–17, 201–3
Cultural competence, 6–7, 11, 345–52
    according to Joint Commission, 13

health, illness, and healing, 14
journey to, 351
Cultural competency, 351–52
Cultural conflict, 36
Cultural phenomena
African Americans, 277
American Indians, 222
Asian Americans, 243
biological variations, 38
communication, 38
environmental control, 38–39
Hispanic Americans, 313
social organization, 38
space, 37
time orientation, 37
White Americans, 326
CULTURALCARE, 346–47, 350
Culturally and Linguistically Appropriate
Services (CLAS), 8, 54
Culturally appropriate, 11
Culturally sensitive, 11
Culture, 21–23
Cupping, 248–51
Curandera. See Espiritista
Curanderismo, 114, 298, 299–303, 306–7
Curandero(a), 301
Curanderos, 297, 298, 299–303
Curses. *See Castiga*
Cyanosis, 284
Cycle of poverty, 58–59

D
Daruma, 345
Data resources, 381–82
De Padua, Saint Anthony, 276
Death mask, 153
Death rituals/beliefs, 141–53, 172–73
Decade of birth, 34
Deer antlers, 252
Deliverance (exorcism), 136
Department of Health and Human Services.
See United States Department of
Health and Human Services
Dependent-patient role stage, 80
Depression, 114
Diet regimen, 99–101
Dissonance, 14
Divination, 216
Doctor of osteopathy (D.O.), 111
Domestic violence, 227–28
Drums, 221
Duklij, 214
Dybbuk, 96

E
Eastern Orthodox, 140
Ecchymosis, 284
Echinacea, 115
Eclectic medicine, 111
Eddy, Mary Baker, 112
El Nino Fidencio, 130

Empacho, 296, 306
Envidia, 298
Environmental control, 38–39
Envy, 96
Episcopalian, 140, 164
Erythema, 284
Espiritista, 313, 314
Ethnicity, 23–24
Ethnocentrism, 23, 37
Ethnocultural life trajectories, 32–34
European freedom revolutions, 327
Evil eye, 95–96, 98
Exorcism, 136
Ex-votos, 299
Eye contact, 40

F
Facultades, 311, 312
Fadiman, Anne, 3, 4
Falling-Out, 282
Familial health traditions, 158–77
birth beliefs, 172–73
consciousness raising, 171–74
death beliefs, 161–62
family health histories, 160–71
similarities, 171–74
Family health histories, 160–77
Father John's Medicine, 159
Fatigue, 309
Favism, 333
Federal poverty programs, 55
Fetal alcohol syndrome, 226
Financial burden, 348
Flying devil oil, 275
Folk diseases, 309, 313
Folk medicine, 104–8, 273–74
Folklife centers, 176–77
Food customs, 40
Food stamps, 55
Friends (Quaker), 140

G
Garlic and onion, 99–100
Geophagy, 276
Germ theory, 328
German Americans, 326–30
amusement, 328
causes of illness, 328
current health problems, 328–30
germ theory, 328
health and illness, 328
home remedies, 329–30
German ethnic community, 327
Gestures, 40
Ghost sickness, 224
Ginkgo, 115
Ginseng, 100
Ginseng root, 239, 248
Glossary, 354–63
Glucose-6-phosphate dehydrogenase, 333
Good gris-gris, 274–75

Greek Orthodox, 172
Green card, 49
Greetings, 40
Gris-gris, 274–75

H
Hahnemann, Samuel C., 109, 110
Hair care needs, 285
Hate, 96
Hawaiians. *See* Pacific Islanders
Hawk Littlejohn, 218–19
Healing of America: A Global Quest for Better and Cheaper, and Fairer Health Care, The (Reid), 348
Healing traditions, 120–47
    ancient forms of healing, 123
    birth rituals, 138–47
    death rituals, 141–53
    healing, 121–22
    intersection of health, healing and religion, 153–54
    Religion. *See* Religion
    traditional healer *vs.* allopathic physician, 137
    types of healing, 136–37
Health, 63–74, 85–86
Health and illness
    affordable health care, 185
    barriers to health care, 197–99
    development of health care system, 187–91
    finding appropriate care at reasonable price, 192
    finding one's way among various types of health care, 192–94
    finding out what the physician is doing, 194
    finding out what went wrong, 194–95
    health care costs, 182–87
    health care provider's culture, 179–82
    healthcare delivery problems, 191–95
    historical overview, 187–91
    is health care in America better, 185–87
    male chauvinism, 195
    maze of health care, 196, 197
    medical *vs.* cultural care, 201–3
    medicalization of society, 199–204
    medicine as institution of social control, 199–204
    in modern health care, 178–205
    national health care expenditures, 182, 183
    pathway to health services, 195–97
    paying for health care, 184–85
    per capita health expenditures, 182, 186
    racism, 195
Health belief model, 70–72
Health care costs, 182–87
Health care events, 191
Health care provider's culture, 179–82
Health disparities, 70
Health equity, 70
Health maintenance and protection, 67–68

Health maintenance organizations (HMOs), 190
Health Professionals Education Assistance Act, 189
Health protection, 95–101
Health Resources and Services Administration (HRSA), 382
Health restoration, 102
Health traditions, 89–119, 347
    allopathic philosophy, 108
    CAM, 108–16
    death/HEALTHCARE choices, 102–4
    diet regimens, 99–101
    evil eye, 95–96, 98
    folk medicine, 104–8
    health and illness, 91–92
    health protection, 95–101
    health restoration, 102
    health traditions model, 92–95
    homeopathic philosophy/schools, 108–13
    intersection of health, healing and religion, 153–54
    natural remedies, 108
    objects that protect health, 97–101
    religion and health, 101–2
    spiritual practices, 101
    traditional health maintenance, 93–95
Health traditions model, 92–95
HealthFinder, 382
Health-illness Continuum, Natural History of, 80–81
Healthy People 2020, 69–70
Herb teas, 272
Herbal remedies, 220–21, 248, 251–52
Herbology, 248
Herbrias, 297
Heritage assessment tool, 376–78
Heritage consistency:
    culture, 21–23
    ethnicity, 23–24
    examples, 26–29
    factors to consider, 27
    matrix of, 29–30
    religion, 25–26
Heterosexism, 37
Hexes, 96
Hill-Burton Act, 189
Hinduism, 132–33, 150, 152, 242
Hispanic Americans, 291–32
    age, 47
    background, 292–94
    barriers to health care, 315–17
    botanicas, 314, 315
    causes of death, 316
    cultural phenomena, 313
    curanderismo, 298, 299–303, 306–7
    current health problems, 315–17
    defined, 46
    diet, 100
    folk diseases, 309, 313
    health and illness, 295–98
    health care providers, as, 317–18

health professions data, 318
health restoration, 305–8
health status indicators, 316
hot-cold balance, 309–10
Mexicans, 294–308
milagros, 299, 302, 306
moral illness, 307
origins, 292, 293
parteras, 303–5, 307
population, 44, 47
population distribution, 292
Puerto Ricans, 308–18
religious rituals, 298–99
research in culture, 319–20
santeria/santero, 311–13, 314
traditional healer, 307
Holidays, 40
Home remedies. *See also* Herbal remedies
African Americans, 272–77
German Americans, 329–30
Polish Americans, 336–38
Homeland Security, 381
Homeopathic medicine, 110
Homeopathic philosophy/schools, 108–13
Hopi Indians, 214, 220
herbal treatments by, 220–21
Hot-cold balance, 309–10
Huang-ti Nei Ching, 243
Humors, body, 295–96
Hwa-byung, 260
Hydrotherapy, 111–12
Hypnotherapy, 109
Hypnotism, 112

I
IHS, 228–31
Illness, 74–81, 86
Illness experience, 77–80
Illness trajectory, 82
Immigration, 48–54
Immigration and Nationality Act
(INA), 49
Immigration history, 53–54
Immigration reform, 52–54
Indian Health Service (IHS), 228–31
area offices, 231
Inner healing, 136
Institute of Medicine (IOM), 12
Institutional mandates, 12–13
Islam, 133, 140, 151, 152, 166
Italian Americans, 330–34
cancer surgery, 332
death, 333
emotions, 333, 334
family, 331
genetic diseases in, 333–34
health and illness, 332–33
health related problems, 333–34
history of migration, 331–32
Italian population, 332
language problems in, 334
traditional beliefs, 332

J
Jade, 239, 246
Jaundice, 284
Jay Treaty, 231
Jealousy, 96
Jehovah's Witness, 133–34, 152
Jerusalem amulet, 98
Jimsonweed, 216
Johnson, Robert Wood, 16
Joint Commission, 5, 8, 12–13, 16, 22–23
Judaism, 134, 140, 151, 152, 162, 163–64

K
Kaiser Family Fund, 15
Kassirer, J. P., 348
Kayn aynhoreh, 96
Keloids, 285
Kennet, F., 158
Kevorkian, Jack, 201
Key terms, 354–63
Kineahora, 96
Knowles, John, 179
Koro, 260
Kosher diet, 100
Kusiut, 215

L
Language, 349
Language access services (LAS), 10
Lao-Tzu, 241
Latino. *See* Hispanic Americans
Lazarus, Saint, 292
Legal Permanent Residents (LPR), 49–51, 239
Lifestyle, 33
Lightning sickness, 216
Lime calcium, 252
Limited English Proficiency (LEP), 10
language barriers faced by, 11
Linguistic competence, 11–12
Listening, 217
Little Rock Nine, 270
Littlejohn, Hawk, 218–19
Loco, 311, 312
Lourdes, 128
Lourdes of America, 128
Lu Chih Ch'un Ch'iu, 241
Lu Pu Wei, 241
Luke, Saint, 335
Lutheran, 140, 151, 169, 172

M
Macrobiotics, 109
Madonna Della Cava, 331–32
Magdalene, Saint Mary, 276
Magico-religious folk medicine, 108
Mal ojo, 297, 307, 309
Male chauvinism, 195
Malocchio, 333
Mano milagroso, 97
Mano negro, 97
Manzanilla, 308

Marital assimilation, 20
Massage, 248
Massage therapy, 109
Materia, 303
Medicaid, 55
Medical care contact stage, 80
Medical *vs.* cultural care, 201–3
Medicalization of society, 199–204
Medicare, 184, 188–90
Medicine man or woman, 215
Melasma, 285
Mennonite, 134–35
Menopausal symptoms, 114
Mental health, 86
Mental illness
    African Americans, 281–82
    American Indians, 224–26
    Asian Americans, 260
Meridians, 247–48
Mesmer, Friedrich Anton, 112
Mesmerism, 112
Mesoamerican, 293–94
Methamphetamine, 224
Methodist, 140
Mexican Americans, 294–308. *See also*
        Hispanic Americans
    employment, 295
    health and illness, traditional, 295–98
    health restoration, 305–8
    mental illness, 307
    Mexico border, 294
    moral illness, 307
    religious rituals, 298–99
Michael, Saint, 276
Micmac Indians, 221
Milagros, 299, 302, 306
Mind cure, 112
Mistletoe, 112
Moral illness, 307
Morita therapy, 260
Mormons, 132, 140, 151, 152
Motion in the hand, 216
Moxibustion, 248

N
National Breast and Cervical Cancer Early
        Detection Program (NBCCEDP), 15
National Center for Complementary and
        Alternative Medicine (NCCAM),
        113, 382
National Center for Health Statistics, 381
National Center for Health Statistics
        (NCHS), 16
National health care expenditures, 182, 183
National Shrine of Our Lady of the Snows, 129
National standards, 8–10
    for Culturally and Linguistically
        Appropriate Services (CLAS), 8
Native peoples. *See* American Indians
Natural folk medicine, 104
Natural remedies, 108

Naturalization, 49
Navajo people, 214–18, 228. *See also*
        American Indians
Nei Ching, 243, 245

O
Obama, Barack, 36
Office for Civil Rights, 381
Office of Minority Health (OMH), 16, 382
Olbas, 328
On the Take (Kassirer), 348
Oneida Indians, 221
Orange leaves, 308
Orishas, 311, 312
Orthodox Christian, 162–63
Osteopathic medicine, 110–11
Outreach workers, 349

P
Pacific Islanders. *See also* Asian Americans
    age, 47
    defined, 46
    population, 44, 47
Pallor, 284
Palmer, Daniel David, 111
*Parents v. Seattle Schools and Meredith v.
        Jefferson Schools,* 268
Parsons, Talcott, 76
Parteras, 303–5, 307
Pasmo, 309
Patient advocates, 349
Penicillin, 296
Pennsylvania Dutch, 325
Pentecostal, 140
Per capita health expenditures, 182, 186
Perceived susceptibility, 73
Peregrine, Saint, 333
Permanent resident alien, 48–49
Personal space, 37
Phylacto, 159
Physical healing, 136
Pigmentary disorders, 285
Polish Americans, 334–39
    folk medicine, 339
    health and illness, 336–38
    health care problems, 338–39
    home remedies, 336–38
    Polish immigration, 335
    Swamp Root, 336, 338
    in Texas, 335
Polonia, 334
Population, 46–49
Poultices, 272
Poverty, 54–59
Pregnant woman, 332–33
Presidente, 311
Priessnitz, Vincent, 111
Primary structural assimilation, 32
Promesas. See Ex-votos
Proposition 187, 52
Protestantism, 152, 170–71

Pseudofolliculitis, 285
Puerto Ricans, 308–18. *See also* Hispanic
        Americans
    caliente (hot), 309–10
    current health problems, 315–17
    folk disease and treatment, 309–13
    folk practitioner, 313–14
    fresco (cool), 309–10
    frio (cold), 309–10
    mainland health systems, 313–15
    Pasmo, 309
Pulses, 246
Pysanka, 323

Q
Qi gong, 114
Quaker, 140
Quick guide for cultural care, 379–80
Quicksilver, 252

R
Racism, 37, 195
Reauthorization of the Elementary and
        Secondary Education Act, 36
Recovery or rehabilitation stage, 80
Reflexology, 109
Refugee, 48
Reid, T. R., 348
Reiki, 114
Religion, 352
    Asian religions, 242
    birth rituals/beliefs, 140, 172–73
    death rituals/beliefs, 150–52, 172–73
    family health histories, 158–77
    healing and, 124–36
    health protection, 101
    heritage consistency, 24–26
    holidays, 364–66
    intersection of health, healing and religion,
        153–54
    Mexican Americans, 298–99
    religious identification, 27
    responses to health events, 130–35
    saints, 125
    shrines/spiritual journeys, 125–36
Religious holidays that change dates, 364–66
Resources. *See* Data resources
Retalbo, 298, 301
Rheumatoid arthritis, 114
Rhinoceros horns, 252
Roman Catholicism, 131–32, 140, 151
Rooting, 272
Roots (Haley), 276
Rosenstock, Irwin M., 64
Russian Orthodox, 140

S
Saints, 125
SALUD, 86
Santeria/santero, 115, 311–13, 314
Sassafras tea, 272

Science and Health with Key to the Scriptures
        (Eddy), 112
Seahorses, 252
Secondary structural assimilation, 32
Section 8 low-income housing assistance, 55
Seminal events, 33
Senoria, 313, 314
Sexism, 37
Sexual abuse, 227
Shamanism, 242
Shen Nung, 244
Shinto, 173
Shrine of Our Lady of La Leche, 126–27
Shrine of our Lady of Montserrat, 128
Shrine of our Lady of San Juan, 127–28
Shrine of our Lord of Esquipulas, 128–29
Shrine of St. Peregrine for Cancer Sufferers,
        128–29
Shrines, 125–36, 352
Sick role, 76–77
Sickle-cell anemia, 280–81
SICKO (Moore), 348
Skin conditions, 285
Smiling, 40
Snake flesh, 252
Social class, 35
Social organization, 38
Social values, 33
Socialization, 31
Soul loss, 96
SPA, 112
Space, 37
Spearmint tea, 308
Spells, 96
Spirit Catches You and You Fall Down, The
        (Fadiman), 4
Spirit channeler. *See Materia*
Spirit possession, 96
Spiritual care, 121
Spiritual healing, 136
Spiritual health, 86
Spiritual journeys, 125–36
Spirituality, 101
St. Blaise, 124
St. John's wort, 115
Stargazing, 216, 217
Still, A. T., 110
Structural assimilation, 32
Substance Abuse and Mental Health Services
        Administration (SAMHSA), 226
Suchman, Edward A., 78
Susto, 297, 306, 309
Swamp Root, 336, 338
Sweet basil, 308
Symptom experience stage, 78
Szatan, 96

T
Taboo times, 39
Taijin kyofusho, 260
Talismans, 99

Tan, Amy, 238
TANF. *See* Temporary Assistance for Needy
    Families (TANF)
Tao, 241
Te de narranjo, 308
Temporary Assistance for Needy Families
    (TANF), 55
Terminology (glossary), 354–63
Thai Spirit Shrine, 345
Thalassemia syndromes, 334
Therapeutic Touch, The (Krieger), 121
Time orientation, 37
Tomb of Menachem Mendel Schneerson,
    126
Traditional (ethnocultural) care, 113–16
Traditional healer, 137, 215–18, 307
Transcultural Nursing Society, 16
Ts'ang, 244, 245
Tui Na, 248
Turtle shells, 252

U
Unitarian, 140
Unitarian/Universalist Church, 135
United Methodists, 1551
United States Census Bureau, 381
United States Citizenship and Immigration
    Services, 381
United States Department of Health and
    Human Services, 286
University of Michigan Health System, 17
Urban hiking, 373–75
Urea, 252

V
Virgin de San Juan del Valle shrine in San
    Juan, Texas, 298
Virgin of Guadalupe, 101
Voodoo, 115, 272, 274–76

Voodoo candles, 275
Voudou. *See* Voodoo

W
Wages, 35
War on Poverty, 189
We Believe in Niño Fedencio (film), 298
Weasel medicine, 220
White Americans, 323–44
    age, 47
    background, 324–26
    causes of death, 342
    cultural phenomena, 326
    defined, 45
    German Americans, 326–30
    health status, 339–42
    home remedies, 329–30, 336–38
    Italian Americans, 330–34
    Polish Americans, 334–39
    population, 44, 47, 324, 325
    research in culture, 343
White magic, 274
White non-Hispanic population, 324–25, 339
Witchcraft, 217, 218, 297
Witches. *See Brujas*
Women, Infants, and Children (WIC), 55
Workplace ethos, 33

X
Xenophobe, 23
Xenophobia, 23, 37

Y
Yerb Buena, 308
Yerberia, 298
Yin and *yang,* 101, 243–45, 247–48

Z
Zar, 282